Case Studies in Cardiology

Case Studies in Cardiology

Editor: August Hunter

AMERICAN
MEDICAL PUBLISHERS
www.americanmedicalpublishers.com

AMERICAN
MEDICAL PUBLISHERS
www.americanmedicalpublishers.com

Cataloging-in-Publication Data

Case studies in cardiology / edited by August Hunter.
p. cm.
Includes bibliographical references and index.
ISBN 979-8-88740-593-3
1. Cardiology. 2. Heart--Diseases. 3. Heart--Diseases--Treatment.
4. Clinical medicine. I. Hunter, August.
RC667 .C55 2023
616.1--dc23

American Medical Publishers,
41 Flatbush Avenue,
1st Floor, New York,
NY 11217, USA

ISBN 979-8-88740-593-3 (Hardback)

Contents

Preface

Cardiology refers to the branch of medicine that focuses on the diagnosis and treatment of conditions that affect blood vessels and the heart. It encompasses the study of a wide range of cardiovascular system disorders. Some of the major cardiovascular system disorders include acute coronary syndrome, myocardial infarction, atherosclerosis, restenosis, angina pectoris, coronary heart disease, cardiac arrest, disorders of the pericardium, disorders of the heart valves, congenital heart defects, and diseases of the blood vessels. Cardiology has several subspecialties including echocardiography, nuclear cardiology, cardiac electrophysiology, and interventional cardiology. Treatment of cardiovascular diseases makes use of a number of devices and instruments such as defibrillators and balloons, stethoscopes, pacemakers, and artificial hearts. This book provides comprehensive case studies related to various areas of cardiology including studies on valvular heart disease, congenital heart disease, hypertension, cardiomyopathy, arrhythmia, vascular disease, cardiac sarcoidosis, cardio-obstetrics, cardio-oncology, and congestive heart failure. The extensive content of this book provides the readers with a thorough understanding of the subject.

The researches compiled throughout the book are authentic and of high quality, combining several disciplines and from very diverse regions from around the world. Drawing on the contributions of many researchers from diverse countries, the book's objective is to provide the readers with the latest achievements in the area of research. This book will surely be a source of knowledge to all interested and researching the field.

In the end, I would like to express my deep sense of gratitude to all the authors for meeting the set deadlines in completing and submitting their research chapters. I would also like to thank the publisher for the support offered to us throughout the course of the book. Finally, I extend my sincere thanks to my family for being a constant source of inspiration and encouragement.

Editor

1

A Rare Case of Chylothorax after Heart Transplantation

Amit Alam,[1] Linle Hou,[2] Dreamy James,[3] Kanika Mody,[4] Deepa Iyer,[2] Aziz Ghaly,[5] and Jesus Almendral[3]

[1]Division of Cardiology, Baylor University Medical Center, Dallas, TX, USA
[2]Division of Cardiology, Rutgers-Robert Wood Johnson University Hospital, New Brunswick, NJ, USA
[3]Division of Cardiology, Jersey Shore University Medical Center, Neptune, NJ, USA
[4]Division of Cardiology, Hackensack University Medical Center, Hackensack, NJ, USA
[5]Department of Cardiothoracic Surgery, Rutgers-Robert Wood Johnson University Hospital, New Brunswick, NJ, USA

Correspondence should be addressed to Jesus Almendral; jalmendral1592@gmail.com

Academic Editor: Ertugrul Ercan

Chylothorax is an exceedingly rare but serious complication of orthotopic heart transplantation (OHT). Prompt diagnosis and appropriate management are essential for a good outcome. Management is similar to that of nontransplant patients, but special attention must be given to patients' nutritional and immunological status. Relevant literature on this topic is limited. We describe our experience in the management of chylothorax after OHT and provide a summary of reported cases of this complication after isolated heart and combined heart/lung transplant.

1. Introduction

Chylothorax is an uncommon but serious complication following cardiothoracic surgery. It presents with unilateral or bilateral pleural effusion, dyspnea, and increased pleural drain output and is sometimes associated with life-threatening tamponade. Chylothorax complicating OHT is exceedingly rare and has only been described in medical literature in case reports and small case series [1–5]. Chyle leakage is a challenge in these immunosuppressed patients given the concern for infection and the requirements of rigorous dietary modification. Prompt diagnosis and timely treatment are of paramount importance.

2. Case

A 61-year-old female with end-stage ischemic cardiomyopathy on home milrinone listed as status 1B was admitted for heart transplantation. She had coronary bypass surgery 6 years prior and had a left-sided defibrillator implanted 4 years previously. The operation was uneventful, and the defibrillator lead and generator were explanted at the time of transplant. She was extubated on postoperative day (POD) 2 and was placed on standard immunosuppression medications and infection prophylaxis as per our center's protocol. On POD 5, the patient was noted to have excessive milky output from the left pleural drain that was placed intraoperatively. Fluid analysis showed lymphocytic predominance with pleural fluid triglyceride of 470 mg/dl and plasma triglyceride of 85 mg/dl confirming chylous drainage. Fluid staining was negative for bacteria, mycobacteria, and fungi. Management with low-fat diet and subcutaneous octreotide 100 mcg every 8 hours was initiated, and subsequently, *nil per os* (NPO) with total parenteral nutrition (TPN) was attempted to reduce chyle production. However, the patient continued to have persistently high output after 7 days (550 to 1,520 ml/day). Invasive intervention was discussed with the patient but she refused. The high output persisted despite conservative management until the patient finally agreed to an intervention. As she was deemed to be a high surgical risk due to posttransplant immunosuppression, she underwent interventional radiology-guided lymphangiography on POD 21 which demonstrated thoracic duct laceration at the level of the left clavicle that was successfully embolized. The pleural drain output decreased substantially and the chest tube was subsequently removed. The patient was discharged home on POD 25 with no recurrence.

3. Discussion

First described by Olof Rudbeck and Jean Pecquet in the 17th century, the lymphatic system consists of the lymph glands, lymphatic vessels, cisterna chyli, and thoracic duct [6]. In the abdomen, the 4 main lymphatic trunks coalesce along the vertebral column at the level of L2 to form the cisterna chyli. From there, the lymph is transported to the chest via the thoracic duct which extends from L2 to the base of the neck. The duct is 2-5 mm in diameter and varies in length from 38 to 45 cm. It collects lymph from most of the body aside from the right side of the head and neck, right upper thorax, and right upper extremity which are drained by the right lymphatic duct. From its origin at the superior pole of the cisterna chyli, the thoracic duct traverses the aortic opening of the diaphragm between the aorta and azygous vein and ascends the posterior mediastinum to the right of the midline. At the T5 level, it gradually inclines to the left and ascends behind the aortic arch. In the neck, the thoracic duct forms an arch which rises 3-4 cm above the left clavicle and descends anterior to the first part of the left subclavian artery. It ends by the opening at the junction of the left subclavian and internal jugular veins [7].

The thoracic duct transports chyle and lymph from the gastrointestinal tract, abdominal wall, and lower extremities to the systemic venous system. Chyle contains large amounts of chylomicrons, triglycerides, fat-soluble vitamins, and cholesterol. Lymph, a constituent of chyle, contains significant amounts of immunoglobulins, lymphocytes, enzymes, and digestive products [8]. Chylothorax refers to injury to the thoracic duct as it transverses the thoracic cavity and the resulting leakage of chyle into the pleural space. The thoracic duct transports approximately 2.5 l of chyle a day, and any resulting injury could lead to the rapid accumulation of a large amount of fluid [9].

Postoperative chylothorax is a rare but serious complication with a reported incidence of 0.42% after general thoracic surgery [10]. It has been described following a broad range of surgical procedures with the highest rates (0.2-10.5%) reported following esophagectomy [11]. However, posttransplant chylothorax is exceedingly rare. An extensive literature search on MEDLINE and PubMed yielded only 7 reports of chylothorax after isolated heart or combined heart/lung transplant [1–5]. A summary of these reports, including the present case, is provided in Table 1. Four cases occurred after heart transplant and four after combined heart/lung transplantation. Patients were predominantly male (88%) with a mean age of 44 years (19-62 years old) presenting at a median of 9 days after surgery, mostly with a unilateral effusion. Three patients had prior cardiac surgery—one had an aneurysmectomy and endocardial resection, one had a left ventricular assist device implanted and replaced after 4 months, and one had prior coronary bypass surgery. Only one patient had acute rejection, and none developed an infection. Two cases required surgical reexploration via thoracotomy with suture ligation of the thoracic duct at the level of the carina in one case and ligation at the supradiaphragmatic level in the other. One had thoracic duct embolization (present case) while the rest resolved with conservative therapy. No patient had recurrence of chylothorax one year after treatment.

Chylous pleural effusion usually develops 1-2 weeks postoperatively and typically presents with dyspnea, chest discomfort, cough, or increased drainage if a chest tube is in place [8]. The effusion could be right-sided (52.7%), left-sided (25.7%), or bilateral (21.6%) depending on the location of the leak. Thoracic duct injury above the fifth thoracic vertebra causes a left-sided effusion while damage below this level leads to an effusion on the right side [12, 13].

Iatrogenic thoracic duct injury during thoracic surgery is the most common cause of traumatic chylothorax [8]. Significant embryological variation in thoracic duct anatomy is present in 35% of the population and is a key factor in inadvertent duct injuries [6, 13]. In addition, thoracic aortic reoperations and descending aortic repairs have been reported as risk factors for postoperative chylothorax likely due to the presence of adhesions and altered location of the thoracic duct after reoperation [14].

Chylothorax has also been reported with central venous cannulation of the neck vessels as well as with duct blockage from catheter-related venous thrombosis [13]. Lymphangiography, if performed, helps elucidate the site and mechanism of thoracic duct trauma. In our case, lymphangiography showed ethiodized oil extravasation at the level of the left clavicle. A central venogram performed at the same time showed occlusion of the left subclavian vein at the level of the thoracic outlet with nonvisualization of the ostium of the thoracic duct. As the patient did not have central venous catheterization in her left neck, we postulate that the thoracic duct injury and resulting subclavian vein thrombosis likely arose from the extraction of the defibrillator lead in her left upper chest at the time of heart transplant.

Diagnosing chylothorax can be sometimes elusive and a strong clinical suspicion is important. The classic milky fluid color present in our case is seen in less than half of patients. In a study by Maldonado et al., chylous effusion was described as milky in only 44% of patients, with the rest documented as serous (26%), serosanguinous (26%), or bloody (3%). In addition, although majority of the effusions are exudative, up to 14% may be transudative, most commonly in patients with cirrhosis [12]. Diagnosis typically requires fluid analysis of pleural fluid with a triglyceride level of >110 mg/dl having a 99% chance of being chylous while fluid with a triglyceride level of <50 mg/dl has a likelihood of only 5% [15]. For fluid with triglyceride levels of <110 mg/dl but >50 mg/dl, lipoprotein electrophoresis demonstrating chylomicrons is required to confirm or exclude the diagnosis, although this test may not be widely available [8].

It is important to recognize chylothorax after transplant as prompt diagnosis and a multidisciplinary approach are necessary for a favorable outcome. Untreated postoperative chylothorax is associated with mortality rates of 50-82% [11]. Prolonged chyle loss could lead to dehydration and malnutrition, as well as hyponatremia, acidosis, and hypocalcemia [8]. Patients are also at increased risk of infections due

TABLE 1

Reference	Age (yrs)	Gender	Transplanted organ	Days after transplant	Laterality	Prior cardiac surgery	Treatment	Outcome
Bowerman et al. [1]	62	Male	Heart	7	Left	Aneurysmectomy Endocardial resection	Chest tube NPO/feeding tube MCT	No recurrence Low lymphocyte count 300/mm^3
Twomey [2]	32	Male	Heart	18	Right	None	Chest tube NPO/TPN	No recurrence Acute rejection
Shitrit et al. [3]	53	Male	Heart/lung	120	Bilateral	None	Chest tube Oral low-fat diet	No recurrence No infection/rejection
Ziedalski et al. [4]	50	Male	Heart/lung	35	Bilateral	None	Chest tube Oral MCT IV octreotide Oral aminocaproic acid	No recurrence No infection/rejection
	27	Male	Heart/lung	7	Left	None	Chest tube NPO Left thoracotomy Duct ligation at the level of carina	No recurrence No infection/rejection
	19	Male	Heart/lung	10	Right	None	Chest tube NPO/TPN VATS pleurodesis Right thoracotomy Supradiaphragmatic duct ligation	No recurrence No infection/rejection
Berdy et al. [5]	47	Male	Heart	8	Mediastinal	Left ventricular assist device implant; device exchange after 4 mos	Mediastinal tube Oral low-fat diet	No recurrence No infection/rejection
Present report	61	Female	Heart	5	Left	Coronary artery bypass grafting	Chest tube Oral low-fat diet SC octreotide NPO/TPN Thoracic duct embolization	No recurrence No infection/rejection

to the loss of lymphocytes and immunoglobulins with resulting depression of both cellular and humoral immunity. Development of chylothorax is associated with a higher 30-day risk of sepsis, pneumonia, reintubation, reoperation, and death [16]. This is particularly problematic in posttransplant patients who are already immunosuppressed. Furthermore, prolonged lymphocyte losses could lead to a decrease in total lymphocytic count. This could lead to profound immune suppression particularly if lymphocyte-depleting antirejection medication is utilized posttransplant. In addition, cyclosporine, a common immunosuppression agent, is secreted in chyle [17]. In patients with prolonged and uncontrolled chyle loss, close drug level monitoring with appropriate dose adjustment is warranted.

Various treatment modalities for chylothorax, ranging from conservative to invasive interventions, have been described. Low-output chylothoraces (<1 l chyle/day) usually respond to conservative measures while high-output effusions (>1 l/day), commonly seen in postsurgical patients, typically need more invasive intervention [10]. With appropriate and timely intervention, mortality rates have decreased to 10-16% [11]. Management largely depends on experience from case reports and single-center case series as no comparative clinical trials of specific therapies are available.

The initial treatment of chylothorax involves thoracic cavity decompression via a chest tube (if one is not already in place) to relieve dyspnea and to quantitate daily chyle output to monitor response to treatment. Conservative management with dietary modification using low-fat diet and medium-chain fatty acids (MCFA) is usually attempted first. The MCFA diet is utilized because these fatty acids are absorbed directly into the portal venous system and bypass the lymphatic system including the thoracic duct. If this fails, temporary NPO with total parenteral nutrition to reduce chyle formation has been successful in some cases [8, 13].

Adjunctive therapy with somatostatin or its analogue octreotide, which was used in our case, is often utilized in addition to dietary modification. Somatostatin acts directly on vascular somatostatin receptors in order to minimize lymphatic fluid excretion. It also reduces lymphatic flow by increasing the splanchnic arteriolar resistance and decreasing gastrointestinal blood flow [6]. However, the dose, route of administration (subcutaneous, intravenous, or continuous infusion), or duration of treatment has not been established in prospective studies [18].

Conservative measures are aimed at reducing the formation and flow of chyle through the thoracic duct to allow the leak to close and eventually heal. It has a reported success rate of 16-75% [18]. However, surgical intervention should be strongly considered if the chyle output remains >1,000 ml/day (or > 10 ml/kg/day) for >5 days, chyle flow persists for >2 weeks, or if clinical signs of malnutrition or metabolic derangements occur [8, 10, 13, 16].

Operative treatment options include thoracic duct ligation and thoracic duct embolization or disruption. Thoracic duct ligation is traditionally performed via a thoracotomy. In a unilateral effusion, thoracotomy is made on the side of the effusion as the leak is likely located on that side. For bilateral chylothoraces, it is usually best to approach the right side. Given the morbidity and pain associated with thoracotomy, use of video-assisted thoracic surgery (VATS) has become an attractive alternative [19]. Regardless of the approach (thoracotomy or VATS), identification of the site of leakage is usually attempted preoperatively via lymphangiography or by enteral administration of cream or oil [9, 11]. Clips are then applied proximal and distal to the site of injury. If the leak cannot be easily identified, mass ligation of lymphatic tissue in the supradiaphragmatic region between the descending thoracic aorta and azygos vein should be performed [6]. In addition, fibrin glue is sometimes applied to the area [11]. With thoracic duct ligation, success rates of over 90% have been reported [6, 10].

For patients at high risk of reoperation, such as in our case, thoracic duct embolization or disruption is a viable alternative with a success rate of 46-74% [20]. It is a technically challenging procedure requiring lymphangiography via a pedal or intranodal approach to visualize the location of the leak. Cannulation of the thoracic duct can be difficult and is successful in about two-thirds of cases. In patients that can be cannulated, embolization with endovascular coils and/or liquid embolic agents resolves the chyle leak in 90% [21]. In cases where lymphatic catheterization is unsuccessful, duct disruption can be attempted using a 21- or 22-gauge needle to create holes in the thoracic duct to slow down lymphatic flow allowing for healing of the leak. Success rates with needle disruption range from 44 to 72%. Complication rates of 0% to 10.5% have been reported for thoracic duct embolization or disruption including embolization of the pulmonary artery and injection site infections after lymphangiography. Chronic diarrhea and leg and abdominal swelling have been reported as delayed complications [20].

For patients with refractory chylothorax, a pleuroperitoneal shunt may be effective with a success rate of approximately 80% [9]. It involves the creation of a subcutaneous or external connection between the pleura and peritoneum connected to a pump activated by light pressure [13]. The shunt can be removed once the chyle leak resolves.

In summary, we report a rare case of chylothorax following heart transplantation. Unexplained pleural effusion, either unilateral or bilateral, should raise suspicion even in the absence of the classic milky appearance of the pleural fluid. Elevated pleural fluid triglyceride level is a typical finding. Conservative management with chest tube placement and diet modification should first be attempted in conjunction with octreotide. Patients should be closely monitored for malnutrition, dehydration, and infections with adjustments made to immunosuppressive therapy accordingly. Lymphangiography may help identify the site and mechanism of thoracic duct injury. When conservative management fails, an invasive procedure to ligate the thoracic duct via thoracotomy, VATS, or IR-guided embolization should be considered early.

Abbreviations

MCFA: Medium-chain fatty acids
NPO: Nil per os
OHT: Orthotopic heart transplant
POD: Postoperative day
TPN: Total parenteral nutrition
VATS: Video-assisted thoracoscopic surgery.

References

[1] R. E. Bowerman, D. A. Solomon, D. Bognolo, and L. R. Brauner, "Chylothorax: report of a case complicating orthotopic heart transplantation," *The Journal of Heart and Lung Transplantation*, vol. 12, no. 4, pp. 665–668, 1993.

[2] C. R. Twomey, "Chylothorax in the adult heart transplant patient (a case report)," *American Journal of Critical Care*, vol. 3, no. 4, pp. 316–319, 1994.

[3] D. Shitrit, G. Izbicki, D. Starobin, D. Aravot, and M. R. Kramer, "Late-onset chylothorax after heart-lung transplantation," *The Annals of Thoracic Surgery*, vol. 75, no. 1, pp. 285-286, 2003.

[4] T. M. Ziedalski, T. A. Raffin, D. Y. Sze et al., "Chylothorax after heart/lung transplantation," *The Journal of Heart and Lung Transplantation*, vol. 23, no. 5, pp. 627–631, 2004.

[5] A. E. Berdy, N. J. Patel, C. A. German, A. Dutta, and B. A. Pisani, "Chylothorax as a post-operative complication of orthotopic heart transplantation," *Journal of Cardiac Failure*, vol. 24, no. 8, article S84, 2018.

[6] T. G. Pillay and B. Singh, "A review of traumatic chylothorax," *Injury*, vol. 47, no. 3, pp. 545–550, 2016.

[7] H. Hematti and R. J. Mehran, "Anatomy of the thoracic duct," *Thoracic Surgery Clinics*, vol. 21, no. 2, pp. 229–238, 2011.

[8] S. K. Nair, M. Petko, and M. P. Hayward, "Aetiology and management of chylothorax in adults," *European Journal of Cardio-Thoracic Surgery*, vol. 32, no. 2, pp. 362–369, 2007.

[9] I. E. Platis and C. E. Nwogu, "Chylothorax," *Thoracic Surgery Clinics*, vol. 16, no. 3, pp. 209–214, 2006.

[10] R. J. Cerfolio, M. S. Allen, C. Deschamps, V. F. Trastek, and P. C. Pairolero, "Postoperative chylothorax," *The Journal of Thoracic and Cardiovascular Surgery*, vol. 112, no. 5, pp. 1361–1366, 1996.

[11] S. A. Wemyss-Holden, B. Launois, and G. J. Maddern, "Management of thoracic duct injuries after oesophagectomy," *The British Journal of Surgery*, vol. 88, no. 11, pp. 1442–1448, 2001.

[12] F. Maldonado, F. J. Hawkins, C. E. Daniels, C. H. Doerr, P. A. Decker, and J. H. Ryu, "Pleural fluid characteristics of chylothorax," *Mayo Clinic Proceedings*, vol. 84, no. 2, pp. 129–133, 2009.

[13] E. E. McGrath, Z. Blades, and P. B. Anderson, "Chylothorax: aetiology, diagnosis and therapeutic options," *Respiratory Medicine*, vol. 104, no. 1, pp. 1–8, 2010.

[14] A. H. Allaham, A. L. Estrera, C. C. Miller III, P. Achouh, and H. J. Safi, "Chylothorax complicating repairs of the descending and thoracoabdominal aorta," *Chest*, vol. 130, no. 4, pp. 1138–1142, 2006.

[15] B. A. Staats, R. D. Ellefson, L. L. Budahn, D. E. Dines, U. B. Prakash, and K. Offord, "The lipoprotein profile of chylous and nonchylous pleural effusions," *Mayo Clinic Proceedings*, vol. 55, no. 11, pp. 700–704, 1980.

[16] R. D. Shah, J. D. Luketich, M. J. Schuchert et al., "Postesophagectomy chylothorax: incidence, risk factors and outcomes," *The Annals of Thoracic Surgery*, vol. 93, no. 3, pp. 897–904, 2012.

[17] R. Repp, H. H. Scheld, J. Bauer, H. Becker, J. Kreuder, and H. Netz, "Cyclosporine losses by a chylothorax," *The Journal of Heart and Lung Transplantation*, vol. 11, no. 2, Part 1, pp. 397-398, 1992.

[18] H. H. Schild, C. P. Strassburg, A. Welz, and J. Kalff, "Treatment options in patients with chylothorax," *Deutsches Ärzteblatt International*, vol. 110, no. 48, pp. 819–826, 2013.

[19] P. Misthos, M. A. Kanakis, and A. G. Lioulias, "Chylothorax complicating thoracic surgery: conservative or early surgical management?," *Updates in Surgery*, vol. 64, no. 1, pp. 5–11, 2012.

[20] M. Toliyat, K. Singh, R. C. Sibley, M. Chamarthy, S. P. Kalva, and A. K. Pillai, "Interventional radiology in the management of thoracic duct injuries: anatomy, techniques and results," *Clinical Imaging*, vol. 42, pp. 183–192, 2017.

[21] M. Itkin, J. C. Kucharczuk, A. Kwak, S. O. Trerotola, and L. R. Kaiser, "Nonoperative thoracic duct embolization for traumatic thoracic duct leak: experience in 109 patients," *The Journal of Thoracic and Cardiovascular Surgery*, vol. 139, no. 3, pp. 584–590, 2010.

2

A Case Series of Diverse Cardiac Abnormalities in Collegiate Athlete with COVID-19: Role for Multimodality Imaging

Vanessa-Rose G. Turpin,[1] Kyle Goerl,[2] Chen Hoe Chow,[3] and Carl J. Ade[1,4,5]

[1]*Department of Kinesiology, College of Health and Human Sciences, Kansas State University, USA*
[2]*Lafene Health Center, Kansas State University, USA*
[3]*Cotton O'Neil Heart Center, Stormont Vail Health, USA*
[4]*Physician Assistant Studies, College of Health and Human Sciences, Kansas State University, USA*
[5]*Johnson Cancer Center, Kansas State University, USA*

Correspondence should be addressed to Carl J. Ade; cade@ksu.edu

Academic Editor: Yigit Canga

Introduction. Since the COVID-19 pandemic there is concern for subclinical cardiac pathology in the absence of clinical symptoms in collegiate athletes, we present 4 cases of abnormal left ventricular global longitudinal strain (LVGLS), a "red-flag" for potential COVID-19 myocardial disease, following diagnosis with diverse abnormalities reported via multimodality imaging weeks into recovery. *Methods.* Cardiac imaging studies consisting of transthoracic echocardiography (TTE) and cardiovascular magnetic resonance imaging (CMR) were performed 10 days post-COVID-19 diagnosis and several weeks into recovery. *Results.* Initial TTE revealed abnormal left ventricular global longitudinal strain (LVGLS), an identified "red-flag" for potential COVID-19 myocardial disease. Further CMR imaging revealed potential recent/prior myocarditis in 1 athlete. Follow-up TTE several weeks later revealed a return to normal LVGLS. Conversely, 2 cases with normal CMR imaging had a LVGLS that remained abnormal >30 days into recovery. *Conclusions.* These individual cases highlight the substantial differences in echocardiographic and CMR abnormalities between athletes with confirmed COVID-19.

1. Introduction

With increased concerns for coronavirus disease-19-(COVID-19-) induced cardiac injury in athletes, numerous recommended screening procedures have been proposed; however, the differential pattern of cardiac abnormalities in individual athletes remains unknown [1]. Moreover, recent work suggests in the acute stage a presence of myocardial and pericardial inflammation in some athletes, but it is unknown if this persists into weeks of recovery. We describe a series of 4 competitive athletes with COVID-19 cardiac abnormalities. All patients provided written and verbal consent for this study which was approved by the Institutional Review Board of Kansas State University and conformed to the standards set forth by the Declaration of Helsinki.

2. Case 1

An 18-year-old male collegiate athlete presented with fever, cough, and sinus congestion but denied chest pain and shortness of breath. The test for COVID-19 returned positive. Ten days into recovery, he had normal sinus rhythm, was normotensive, and had a normal 12-lead ECG. High-sensitivity troponin T (hsTnT) was normal (<0.010). Transthoracic echocardiography (TTE) showed mild left ventricular (LV) hypertrophy and cavity dimensions, suggestive of athletic remodeling. Mild dilations of right atria (RA) and left atria (LA) were noted with mild tricuspid valve regurgitation. LV ejection fraction (LVEF) was normal, but global longitudinal strain (GLS) was abnormal (-16%) with normal diastolic function (Figure 1). Cardiovascular magnetic resonance

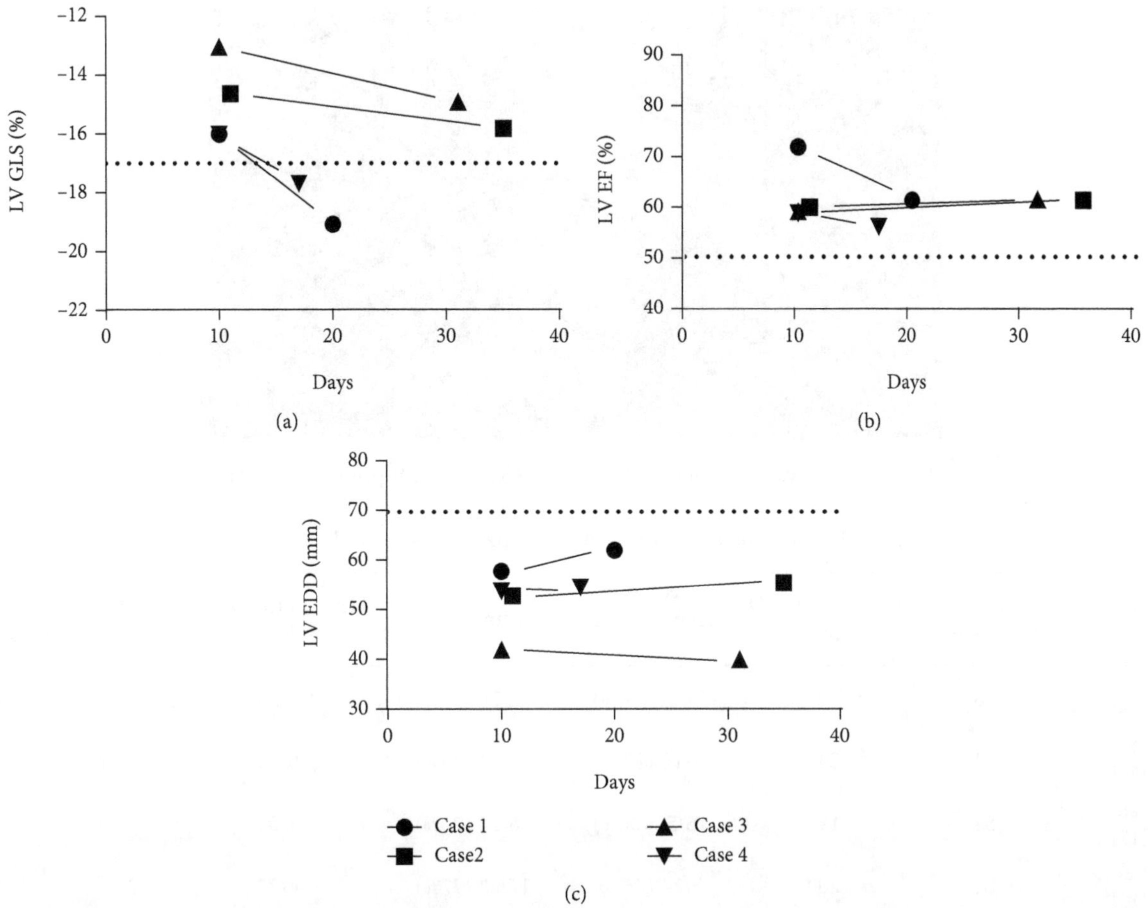

FIGURE 1: Transthoracic echocardiography findings following COVID-19 diagnosis. (a) LV GLS at ~10 days postinfection is abnormal in all cases [1]. (b) LVEF was normal in all cases. (c) LV dilation (LVEDD) [1] did not occur following infection.

imaging (CMR) was performed 20 days into recovery, showing mild dilation of the LV and RV along with mitral and tricuspid valve regurgitation but no signs of myocarditis (no edema, T1 alterations, or Late Gadolinium Enhancement (LGE)). A repeat TTE 31 days into recovery showed improved GLS (-19.1%) and normal LVEF.

3. Case 2

A 19-year-old male collegiate athlete tested positive for COVID-19, and 11 days into his recovery, there were no indications of arrhythmias or murmurs with normal hsTnT (<0.010). Contemporaneous TTE revealed a normal camber dimensions, LVEF, and diastolic function, but abnormal GLS (-14.6%) with mitral and tricuspid valve regurgitation was observed. CMR performed 19 days into recovery revealed no signs of myocarditis (no edema, T1 alterations, or Late Gadolinium Enhancement (LGE)). A repeat TTE 35 days into recovery showed a still abnormal but improved GLS of -15.8%, with normal LVEF%.

4. Case 3

A 20-year-old male collegiate athlete presented with symptoms of a headache, nausea, difficulty breathing, sore throat, and fatigue after testing positive for COVID-19 but denied any symptoms of chest pain or shortness of breath (SOB), and hsTnT was normal (<0.010). TTE was performed 10 days following diagnosis, and athlete reported continuing symptoms of a headache, stuffy nose, and fatigue. He was hypertensive (130/58 mmHg) but had a normal 12-lead ECG and LVEF. TTE showed mild dilation of the RV and RA and abnormal LV GLS of -13%. CMR was performed 22 days into recovery showing no signs of myocarditis (no edema, T1 alterations, or Late Gadolinium Enhancement (LGE)) and normal myocardial perfusion. Follow-up TTE, 31 days into recovery, revealed an abnormal but improved GLS (-14.9%).

5. Case 4

An 18-year-old male collegiate diagnosed with COVID-19 reported a mild cough during infection but denied chest pain, SOB, or fever. Ten days into recovery, he had a normal ECG and hsTnT (<0.010). TTE revealed an abnormal LVGLS of -16%, but normal LVEF and diastolic function. CMR performed 15 days into recovery showed an area of midmyocardial LGE, indicating potential recent/prior myocarditis, with normal LV wall motion and LVEF (Figure 2).

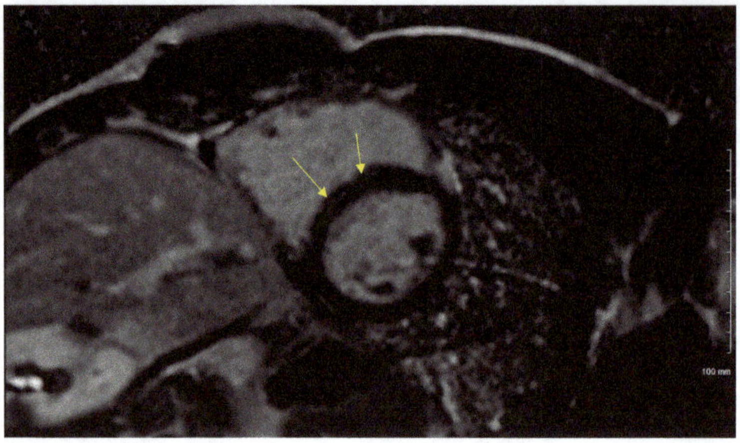

Figure 2: Typical CMR in case 4 of LGE-indicated recent/prior myocarditis.

Table 1: Recent reports on cardiac abnormalities in athletes with COVID-19.

First author (year)	No. of participants	Average age ± SD (years)	No. of asymptomatic (%)	No. of symptomatic (%)	Elevated troponin I or T levels	LGE presence	No. of myocarditis
Rajpal et al. (2020) [16]	26	19.5 ± 1.5	14/26 (54%)	12/26 (46%)	0/26	12/26	4
Vago et al. (2020) [25]	12	23	2/12 (17%)	10/12 (83%)	0/12	0/12	0
Brito et al. (2020) [17]	54	19	16/54 (30%)	38/54 (70%)	1/54	1/54	0
Clark et al. (2020) [15]	22	20	5/22 (23%)	17/22 (77%)	0/22	2/22	1

Each study analyzed serum troponin I or T levels and utilized CMR to evaluate LGE and other cardiac parameters. Only Clark et al. [15] performed transthoracic echocardiography in addition to hsTnT and CMR.

TTE was performed 2 days later and showed an improved and normal LVGLS of -17.7%.

6. Discussion

Early reports have indicated that SARS-CoV-2 infection elicits cardiac injury in up to 2 out of 5 hospitalized COVID-19 patients [2–9], with elevated cardiac troponin I, a marker of acute myocardial injury, within 24 hrs of hospital admissions associated with death (hazard ratio 3.23 and 95% CI 2.59-4.02) [2]. Moreover, data from China has revealed that mortality rate was higher among patients with vs. without cardiac injury, even after adjusting for age and prior comorbidities, with COVID-19-related cardiac injury associated a 5-fold increase in required ventilation [4, 6, 9–12]. Recent data from Puntmann et al. has also suggested that in middle-aged adults recently recovered from COVID-19, of which 33% required hospitalization, a majority of patients had cardiovascular involvement, as detected by CMR, with 60% exhibiting ongoing myocardial inflammation [13].

Unfortunately, to date, most of our knowledge on COVD-19-induced cardiovascular complications is limited to hospitalized patients, with a paucity of information on the use of imaging modalities for diagnosis and follow-up of myocardial involvement in younger nonhospitalized individuals. Recently, Joy et al. evaluated cardiac function in health-care workers (mean age 37 years) 6 months following COVID-19, of which 85% were mildly symptomatic and 15% asymptomatic at the time of diagnosis [14]. Their measurements of cardiac involvement via CMR scanning revealed no difference in cardiac structure, function, or tissue characterization between recovered COVID-19 individuals and matched controls. While CMR imaging provides valuable insight into cardiovascular involvement with COVID-19, it is not readily available in all clinical settings, with TTE more commonly used as the method for early cardiac screening following infection.

Assessment of COVID-19-induced cardiac abnormalities, against the background of athletic remodeling, presents a particularly unique challenge in identifying individuals at risk for pathologic outcomes following infection. In addition, most athletic departments do not have the capabilities or capacity for onsite cardiac evaluation following COVID-19. When follow-up evaluation for cardiac involvement is required, this challenge is further exacerbated when different imaging modalities are utilized. Thus, there is a critical need to improve our understanding on the differential pattern of cardiac abnormalities that may exist in this unique population. Here, we present 4 cases of abnormal LVGLS, an identified "red-flag" for potential COVID-19 myocardial disease [1]. CMR revealed potential recent/prior myocarditis in 1 case, but a return to normal LVGLS. Two cases had normal

CMR outcomes but LVGLS remained abnormal >30 days into recovery. This highlights the substantial variability in echocardiographic and CMR abnormalities between athletes with confirmed COVID-19. Recommendations for screening of athletes with COVID-19 include the use of hsTnT and echocardiographic assessment of chamber size, wall motion, and systolic and diastolic function, with subsequent CMR recommended when indicated [1]. We demonstrate variability in multimodality imaging in the characterization of potential COVID-19 cardiac injury in collegiate athletes, which highlights the challenges of managing COVID-19 and determining the appropriate workup in this population. At the individual patient level, an abnormal LVGLS and the temporal characteristics into recovery do not appear to be predictive of CMR-indicated myocarditis.

To date, there are a limited number of studies investigating the potential cardiac consequences of COVID-19 in the athletic populations, with fewer extending into recovery (Table 1). In a study of 22 COVID-19-positive athletes, all had normal troponin and LVGLS [15], with one exhibiting meeting CMR criteria for suggested myocarditis. In agreement, a recent study by Rajpal et al. looked at 26 COVID-19-positive student athletes and reported that no athlete had markers of elevated troponin, but 46% showed the presence of CMR-indicated LGE, further highlighting how variable CMR data is between studies and the potential for myocarditis in the absence of elevated biomarkers [16]. Others have reported ~40% of COVID-19 athletes exhibit late pericardial enhancement and with more than one-half of athletes showing subclinical myocardial and pericardial disease [17]. Additional work in professional athletes with COVID-19 revealed acute cardiac injury in 2.5% with CMR-confirmed inflammatory heart disease in 18.5%, myocarditis in 11.1%, and pericarditis in 7.4% [18].

To date, both direct and indirect effects of the SARS-CoV-2 virus on cardiovascular outcomes have been postulated but remain incompletely understood [19–22], thus limiting clinical decision-making regarding patient triage and treatment. Recent work by Greulich and Klingel suggests a very heterogenous presentation of myocardial inflammation in patients with a history of COVID-19 following endomyocardial biopsy, further highlighting the unknown pathogenesis of COVID-19-related cardiac inflammation [23]. Moreover, while CMR and other imaging modalities, like that used in the present study and previous work provide valuable prognostic insight, they often provide different pathological information relative to endomyocardial biopsy further complicating our understanding of the underlying mechanisms mediating COVID-19 myocardial injury [24]. Thus, this previous work, coupled with the divergent response reported in the present cases, highlights the challenges associated with the clinical evaluation of cardiac abnormalities in athletes following COVID-19 diagnosis.

The diverse temporal responses of our cases highlight our limited understanding of the time course of LV function changes as they relate to CMR parameters. Taken altogether, the consequences of COVID-19 infection still remain unclear and future research looking into the long-term effects of this disease is warranted, with clear indication that no screening modality provides a complete picture of potential cardiac abnormalities.

Authors' Contributions

All authors have read and approved the manuscript.

References

[1] D. Phelan, J. H. Kim, M. D. Elliott et al., "Screening of potential cardiac involvement in competitive athletes recovering from COVID-19: an expert consensus statement," *JACC: Cardiovascular Imaging*, vol. 13, no. 12, pp. 2635–2652, 2020.

[2] A. Lala, K. W. Johnson, J. Januzzi et al., "Prevalence and impact of myocardial injury in patients hospitalized with COVID-19 infection," 2020, https://www.medrxiv.org/content/10.1101/2020.04.20.20072702v2.

[3] L. Chen, X. Li, M. Chen, Y. Feng, and C. Xiong, "The ACE2 expression in human heart indicates new potential mechanism of heart injury among patients infected with SARS-CoV-2," *Cardiovascular Research*, vol. 116, no. 6, pp. 1097–1100, 2020.

[4] T. Guo, Y. Fan, M. Chen et al., "Cardiovascular implications of fatal outcomes of patients with coronavirus disease 2019 (COVID-19)," *JAMA cardiology*, vol. 5, no. 7, pp. 811–818, 2020.

[5] C. Huang, Y. Wang, X. Li et al., "Clinical features of patients infected with 2019 novel coronavirus in Wuhan, China," *Lancet*, vol. 395, no. 10223, pp. 497–506, 2020.

[6] S. Shi, M. Qin, B. Shen et al., "Association of cardiac injury with mortality in hospitalized patients with COVID-19 in Wuhan, China," *JAMA cardiology*, vol. 5, no. 7, pp. 802–810, 2020.

[7] D. Wang, B. Hu, C. Hu et al., "Clinical characteristics of 138 hospitalized patients with 2019 novel coronavirus-infected pneumonia in Wuhan, China," *JAMA*, vol. 323, no. 11, pp. 1061–1069, 2020.

[8] X. Yang, Y. Yu, J. Xu et al., "Clinical course and outcomes of critically ill patients with SARS-CoV-2 pneumonia in Wuhan, China: a single-centered, retrospective, observational study," *The Lancet Respiratory Medicine*, vol. 8, no. 5, pp. 475–481, 2020.

[9] F. Zhou, T. Yu, R. du et al., "Clinical course and risk factors for mortality of adult inpatients with COVID-19 in Wuhan, China: a retrospective cohort study," *Lancet*, vol. 395, no. 10229, pp. 1054–1062, 2020.

[10] N. Tang, D. Li, X. Wang, and Z. Sun, "Abnormal coagulation parameters are associated with poor prognosis in patients with novel coronavirus pneumonia," *Journal of Thrombosis and Haemostasis*, vol. 18, no. 4, pp. 844–847, 2020.

[11] A. K. Gupta, H. Jneid, D. Addison et al., "Current perspectives on coronavirus 2019 (COVID-19) and cardiovascular disease: a white paper by the *JAHA* editors," *Journal of the American Heart Association*, vol. 9, no. 12, article e017013, 2020.

[12] G. Lippi, C. J. Lavie, and F. Sanchis-Gomar, "Cardiac troponin I in patients with coronavirus disease 2019 (COVID-19): evidence from a meta-analysis," *Progress in Cardiovascular Diseases*, vol. 63, no. 3, pp. 390-391, 2020.

[13] V. O. Puntmann, M. L. Carerj, I. Wieters et al., "Outcomes of cardiovascular magnetic resonance imaging in patients recently recovered from coronavirus disease 2019 (COVID-19)," *JAMA Cardiology*, vol. 5, no. 11, pp. 1265 1273, 2020.

[14] G. Joy, J. Artico, H. Kurdi et al., "Prospective case-control study of cardiovascular abnormalities 6 months following mild COVID-19 in healthcare workers," *JACC: Cardiovascular Imaging*, vol. 14, no. 11, pp. 2155–2166, 2021.

[15] D. E. Clark, A. Parikh, J. M. Dendy et al., "COVID-19 myocardial pathology evaluation in athletes with cardiac magnetic resonance (COMPETE CMR)," *Circulation*, vol. 143, no. 6, pp. 609–612, 2021.

[16] S. Rajpal, M. S. Tong, J. Borchers et al., "Cardiovascular magnetic resonance findings in competitive athletes recovering from COVID-19 infection," *JAMA Cardiology*, vol. 6, no. 1, pp. 116–118, 2021.

[17] D. Brito, S. Meester, N. Yanamala et al., "High prevalence of pericardial involvement in college student athletes recovering from COVID-19," *JACC: Cardiovascular Imaging*, vol. 14, no. 3, pp. 541–555, 2021.

[18] M. W. Martinez, A. M. Tucker, O. J. Bloom et al., "Prevalence of inflammatory heart disease among professional athletes with prior COVID-19 infection who received systematic return-to-play cardiac screening," *JAMA cardiology*, vol. 6, no. 7, pp. 745–752, 2021.

[19] A. B. Patel and A. Verma, "COVID-19 and angiotensin-converting enzyme inhibitors and angiotensin receptor blockers," *JAMA*, vol. 23, no. 18, pp. 1769-1770, 2020.

[20] E. Driggin, M. V. Madhavan, B. Bikdeli et al., "Cardiovascular considerations for patients, health care workers, and health systems during the Coronavirus Disease 2019 (COVID-19) pandemic," *Journal of the American College of Cardiology*, vol. 75, no. 18, pp. 2352–2371, 2020.

[21] M. Vaduganathan, O. Vardeny, T. Michel, J. J. V. McMurray, M. A. Pfeffer, and S. D. Solomon, "Renin-angiotensin-aldosterone system inhibitors in patients with Covid-19," *The New England Journal of Medicine*, vol. 382, no. 17, pp. 1653–1659, 2020.

[22] D. Atri, H. K. Siddiqi, J. P. Lang, V. Nauffal, D. A. Morrow, and E. A. Bohula, "COVID-19 for the cardiologist: a current review of the virology, clinical epidemiology, cardiac and other clinical manifestations and potential therapeutic strategies," *JACC; Basic to Translational science*, vol. 5, no. 5, pp. 518–536, 2020.

[23] S. Greulich and K. Klingel, "COVID-19 and myocarditis: findings from cardiac magnetic resonance imaging and endomyocardial biopsies," *Hämostaseologie*, vol. 41, no. 5, pp. 366–370, 2021.

[24] P. Lurz, I. Eitel, J. Adam et al., "Diagnostic performance of CMR imaging compared with EMB in patients with suspected myocarditis," *JACC: Cardiovascular Imaging*, vol. 5, no. 5, pp. 513–524, 2012.

[25] H. Vago, L. Szabo, Z. Dohy, and B. Merkely, "Cardiac magnetic resonance findings in patients recovered from COVID-19: initial experiences in elite athletes," *JACC: Cardiovascular Imaging*, vol. 14, no. 6, pp. 1279–1281, 2021.

3

Squamous Cell Carcinoma of the Tongue with Metastasis to Myocardium

Ali Shafiq,[1] **Fatima Samad**,[1] **Eric Roberts**,[1] **Jonathan Levin**,[2] **Ubaid Nawaz**,[3] **and A. Jamil Tajik**[1]

[1]*Aurora Cardiovascular Services, Aurora Sinai/Aurora St. Luke's Medical Centers, Milwaukee, WI, USA*
[2]*BayCare Clinic Radiology, BayCare Health System, Green Bay, WI, USA*
[3]*Department of Hematology and Oncology, Vince Lombardi Cancer Clinic, Aurora BayCare Medical Center, Green Bay, WI, USA*

Correspondence should be addressed to A. Jamil Tajik; publishing14@aurora.org

Academic Editor: Assad Movahed

This is a case of a 43-year-old man who in 2014 was diagnosed with oral squamous cell carcinoma involving the tongue. He underwent extensive surgery that involved right tongue cancer resection and reconstruction with a free flap graft from his right forearm. He then was started on chemotherapy and radiation. Surveillance computed tomography in December 2016 showed a cardiac lesion in the left ventricular apex, which was confirmed by further echocardiography and cardiac magnetic resonance imaging. A biopsy of the mass revealed metastatic squamous cell carcinoma. He was deemed to not be a surgical candidate and continued on palliative chemotherapy. The patient had a very poor prognosis and eventually succumbed to the disease, highlighting the importance of surveillance imaging in such cases. A high index of suspicion on the part of the physician is needed to help in the early identification of these patients.

1. Introduction

Oral cancer is the 6th most common cancer in the world, with 9 out of every 10 oral cancers being oral squamous cell carcinomas (OSCCs). The tongue is involved in more than 50% of OSCCs [1, 2]. Although OSCCs may frequently metastasize to regional areas, distant metastasis—especially secondary involvement of the myocardium—is extremely rare. Most of these cases are generally diagnosed only at autopsy given that many patients are asymptomatic at the time of initial diagnosis. The risk factors most commonly associated with OSCCs are alcohol use, tobacco use, betel quid (combination of the betel leaf, areca nut, and lime), and female sex [2]. This is the main reason that OSCCs are prevalent in countries where there is frequent use of betel quid, such as on the Indian subcontinent. However, there has been a dramatic increase in the rate of OSCCs in the US over the last 30 years [3]. The most commonly cited reason for this rise is an increase in infection with high-risk human papilloma virus (HPV) [4]. We present a rare case of a young male diagnosed with OSCC, which, despite aggressive surgery and chemotherapy, eventually metastasized to his heart.

2. Case Presentation

A 43-year-old man with a history of leukoplakia underwent biopsy of his oral mucosa in 2010; it revealed moderate to severe dysplasia. He remained asymptomatic until 2014 when he felt a mass in his tongue. A computed tomography (CT) scan of the head and neck showed a density in the right tongue with no cervical lymphadenopathy. Biopsy of the tongue revealed moderately differentiated squamous cell carcinoma (SCC). A staging positron emission tomography (PET) scan demonstrated evidence of ipsilateral cervical lymph node involvement. He underwent tracheostomy, right neck dissection, right tongue cancer resection, and reconstruction with a free flap graft from his right forearm. Pathology revealed a 3 cm, invasive, well-differentiated SCC of the keratinizing subtype. The patient received 2 months of chemotherapy with

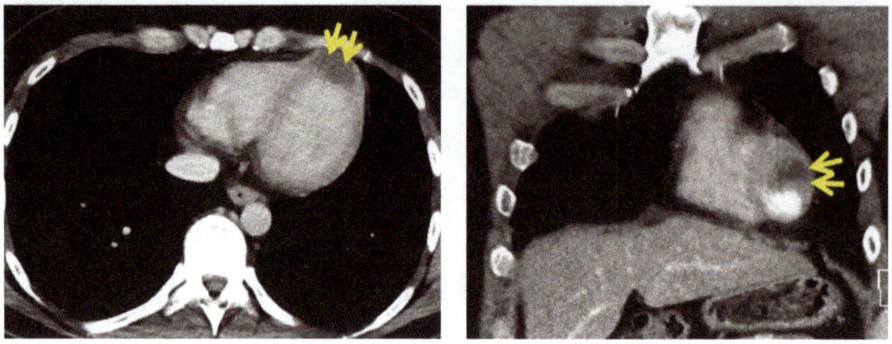

(a) (b)

Figure 1: (a, b) Chest computed tomography with contrast shows a mass in the apex of the left ventricle (arrows).

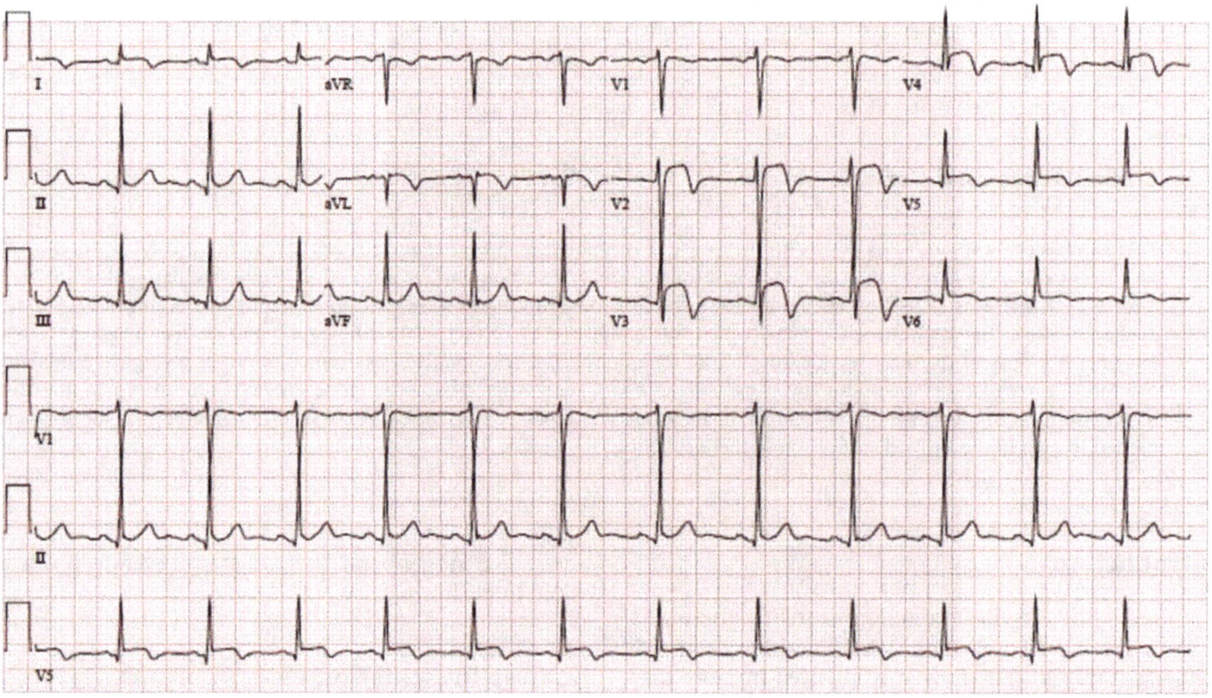

Figure 2: Electrocardiogram shows ST elevations in the anterior and lateral leads.

cisplatin and radiation. A PET scan was done in May 2015 that showed complete remission.

A surveillance CT scan done 1 year later, in May 2016, showed left lung lesions suspicious for metastatic disease, and bronchoscopy confirmed SCC of these lung lesions. He then underwent chemotherapy with 2 cycles of paclitaxel, carboplatin, and radiation. A repeat PET scan in September 2016 showed complete response, and the patient decided to proceed with observation. Another surveillance CT scan in December 2016 showed a cardiac lesion in the left ventricular (LV) apex (Figure 1). The patient was referred to our specialized cardiomyopathy clinic. In the clinic, the patient's physical examination was unremarkable but his electrocardiogram (ECG) showed ST elevations in the anterior and lateral leads suggestive of myocardial injury (Figure 2). He underwent a comprehensive transthoracic echocardiogram, which showed a 4.6×2.8 cm mass infiltrating the apical anteroseptal and anterolateral wall segments (Figure 3). The mass had an abnormal texture with less echodensity than the adjacent LV myocardium and was highly suspicious for metastatic disease. The patient underwent a cardiac magnetic resonance imaging (MRI) scan, which demonstrated a 3.3×4.2 cm infiltrating lesion within the apex of the LV without early or delayed enhancement (Figure 4(a)). The patient was referred for a right ventricular echocardiogram-guided myocardial biopsy. The

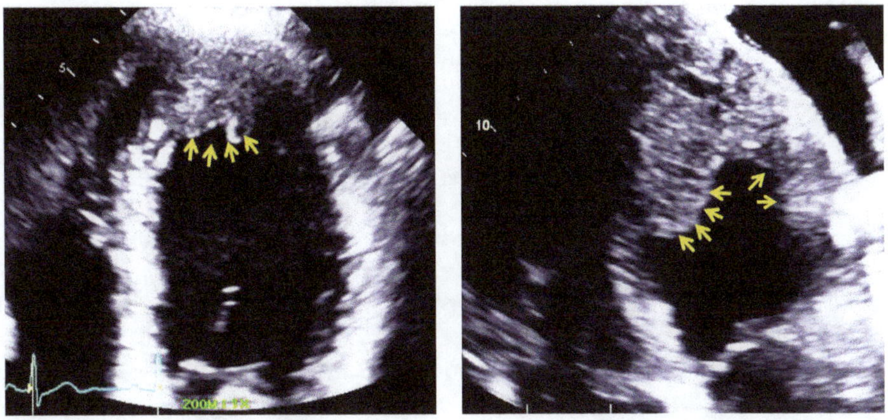

(a) (b)

FIGURE 3: (a) Transthoracic echocardiogram shows a 4.6 × 2.8 cm mass (arrows) infiltrating the apical, antero-septal-lateral wall segments. (b) Transthoracic echocardiogram shows interval progression of the mass (arrows).

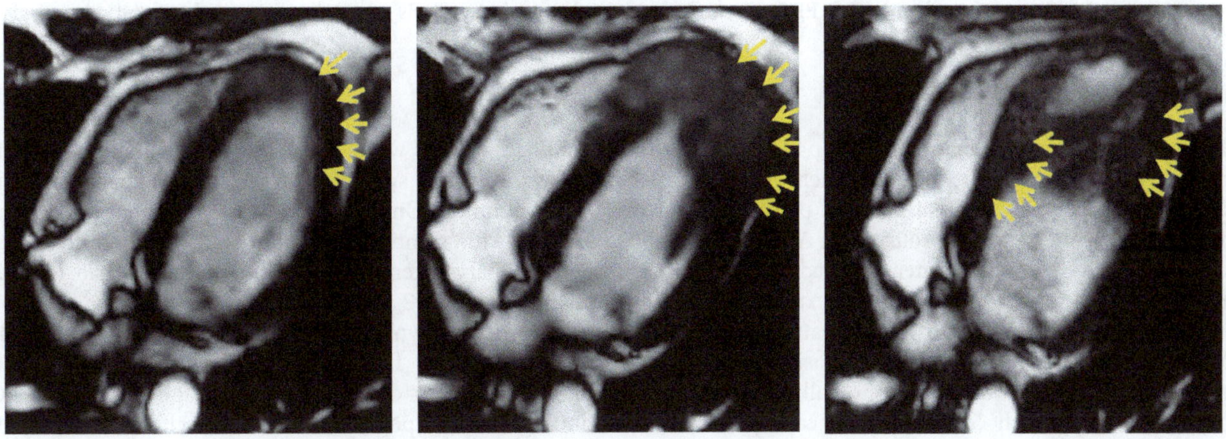

(a) (b) (c)

FIGURE 4: (a) Cardiac magnetic resonance imaging (MRI) demonstrates a 3.3 × 4.2 cm infiltrating lesion (arrows) within the apex of the left ventricle without early or delayed enhancement. (b) Cardiac MRI shows interval progression of the mass (arrows). (c) Cardiac MRI shows the infiltrative tumor mass involving the left ventricular myocardium with features suggesting central necrosis (arrows).

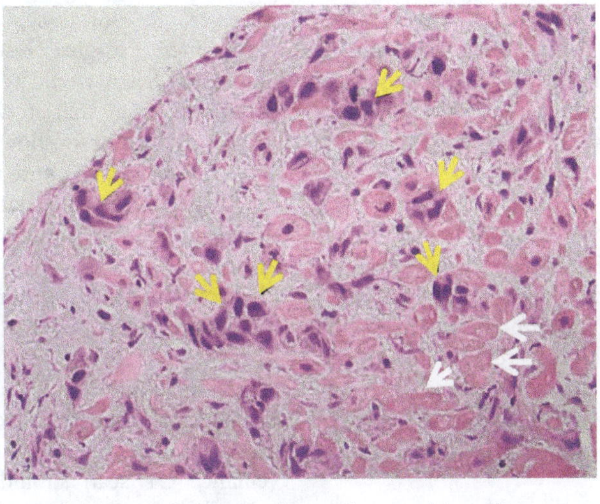

FIGURE 5: Pathology slide of right ventricular myocardial tissue shows pleomorphic malignant tumor cells (yellow arrows) and cardiac myocytes (white arrows).

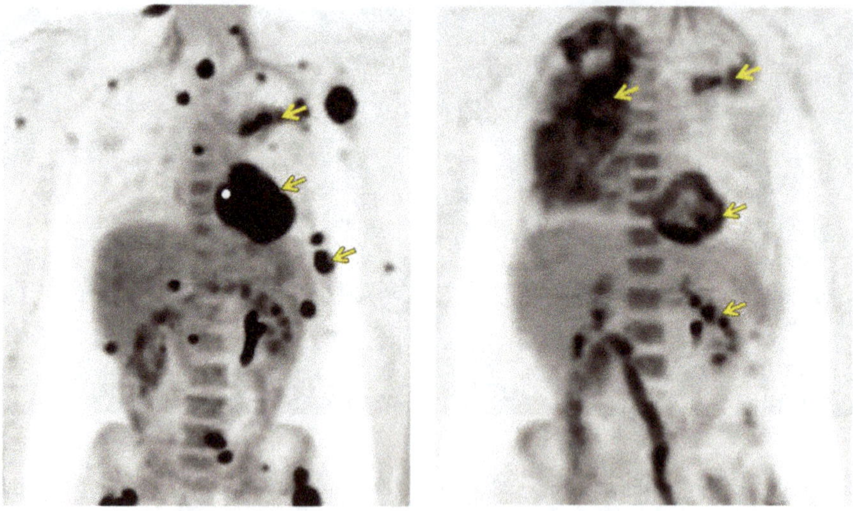

(a) (b)

Figure 6: (a) Fluorodeoxyglucose positron emission tomography/computed tomography (FDG PET/CT) shows development of widespread hypermetabolic metastases (arrows). (b) FDG PET/CT shows more widespread metastasis involving the right lung and adrenal glands (arrows).

pathology immunohistochemical stains (p40 and CK5/6) were consistent with myocardial involvement by metastatic SCC (Figure 5). The patient was started on palliative immunotherapy treatment with pembrolizumab. A follow-up cardiac MRI done 2 months later showed a substantial increase in the size of the mass as well as extension into the right ventricular apex (Figure 4(b)). A repeat PET scan done in March 2017 showed widespread metastasis (Figure 6(a)). The patient's treatment was switched to palliative combination chemotherapy with 5 fluorouracil, carboplatin, and cetuximab, to which he had a very good partial response. A repeat cardiac MRI done in July 2017 showed some improvement in the overall size of the cardiac mass. However, a cardiac MRI done in December 2017 showed interval progression of the infiltrative tumor mass involving the LV myocardium, with features suggesting central necrosis (Figure 4(c)). A follow-up PET scan showed multiple new metastatic lesions (Figure 6(b)). The patient was admitted to the hospital in February 2018 with worsening dyspnea and acute hypoxic respiratory failure. An echocardiogram showed interval progression of metastasis to the left and right ventricular cavities (Figure 4(c)).

3. Discussion

After the initial diagnosis of the OSCC, these patients usually have routine surveillance for the identification of any metastasis, but it is extremely rare to have secondary involvement of the myocardium. Through literature review, we found only 10 other patients (Table 1) who were found with an antemortem diagnosis of OSCC metastasis to the heart. We therefore present this unique case to raise awareness of this complication.

Among the previously reported cases, most patients were male and the patient age ranged from 36 to 73 years. Dyspnea, with or without congestive heart failure, appeared to be a frequent symptom at the time of diagnosis of the cardiac tumor. Only 1 patient [6] presented with typical angina, with symptoms attributed to the compression of her coronary arteries as a result of the anterior position of the tumor. In 2 patients, there were either no symptoms or nonspecific symptoms such as fever [11] and cardiac metastases were found incidentally on surveillance CT scans (similar to our patient). Although no specific ECG findings were reported, ST segment changes were noted in several of the patients (Table 1). Echocardiography was the cornerstone diagnostic modality to show the cardiac mass, and pericardial effusion appeared to be present in many of these patients [7, 8, 10, 11]. Cardiac MRI was used to define the extent of the cardiac mass in a few of the reported cases, as well as in our patient (Table 1). Surgical resection was attempted in a few of these patients; however, in our case, owing to extensive myocardial involvement, surgical resection was considered high risk and it was felt it would result in incomplete resection. Furthermore, given that it was not producing any degree of midventricular or outflow obstruction, palliative treatment was chosen and instituted.

Owing to the rare nature of cardiac involvement from primary OSCCs, routine cardiac imaging is usually not undertaken, often delaying this diagnosis. Surveillance CT scans often are done in patients with a primary malignancy and may help to unmask such rare cardiac involvement. Because of the variability in symptom presentation, a high index of suspicion on the part of the physician is needed to help in the early identification of these patients. Echocardiography supplemented with surveillance CT scan should be able to detect early lesions and allow better management strategy, including surgical excision.

Table 1: Comparison of characteristics between cases reported with oral squamous cell carcinoma with metastasis to the heart.

Variables	Martell et al. [5]	Werbel et al. [6]	Rivkin et al. [7]	Schwender et al. [8]	Onwuchekwa and Banchs [9] (patient 1)	Onwuchekwa and Banchs [9] (patient 2)	Hans et al. [10]	Nagata et al. [11] (patient 1)	Nagata et al. [11] (patient 2)	Shimoyama et al. [12]	Shafiq et al. (current study)
Age (y)	60	61	57	73	45	36	54	59	69	71	43
Sex	Male	Female	Male	Female	Female	Female	Male	Male	Male	Male	Male
Primary cancer	SCC of retromolar trigone	SCC of base of tongue	SCC of base of tongue	Buccal SCC	SCC of tongue	SCC of tongue	SCC of base of tongue	SCC of tongue	SCC of left palate	SCC of tongue	SCC of tongue
At time of diagnosis of cardiac mass											
Symptoms	Dyspnea and edema	Angina	Lower extremity edema	Weakness and dyspnea	Syncope	Palpitations and dyspnea	Dyspnea and hemoptysis	Fever	None	Ulceration of oral cavity	Incidental
ECG findings	Atrial fibrillation	ST depressions with T wave inversions	Atrial fibrillation and ST elevations V2-V6	Atrial fibrillation	Normal sinus rhythm	ST elevations anterolateral leads	Right bundle branch block	Normal	Right bundle branch block and Q wave	ST elevations I, aVL, and V5-V6 and ST depressions II, III, and Avf	ST elevation anterior and lateral leads
Echocardiographic findings	Large mass in RV	Anterior mediastinal mass compressing RV outflow tract plus mass in right atrium	Pericardial effusion and RV mass	Pericardial effusion and echodense adherent lesions of anterior pericardium	Large mass at base of RV	Large mass infiltrating anteroseptal LV	Pericardial effusion and hyperechogenic mass involving RV	Pericardial effusion and mass in left atrium	Pericardial effusion and right atrial mass	Multiple echodense masses in LV	Mass in LV apex
Cardiac MRI	Yes	No	Yes	No	No	No	No	No	Yes	No	Yes
Pathology of cardiac mass	Metastatic, poorly differentiated SCC	Grade I SCC	Moderately differentiated SCC	Metastatic SCC	Biopsy not done	Biopsy not done	Biopsy not done	SCC	N/A	SCC	SCC
Treatment	Palliative radiation and chemotherapy	Surgical resection attempted but unsuccessful	Palliative chemotherapy	Developed septic shock and died	Palliative radiation of brain metastasis	Palliative treatment	Palliative treatment	Surgical resection of mass but died 3 weeks after surgery	Refused treatment and died 3 weeks later	Palliative radiation and chemotherapy	Palliative chemotherapy

ECG: electrocardiogram; LV: left ventricular; MRI: magnetic resonance imaging; RV: right ventricular; SCC: squamous cell carcinoma.

Acknowledgments

The authors are grateful to Jennifer Pfaff and Susan Nord of Aurora Cardiovascular Services for editorial preparation of the manuscript and Brian Miller and Brian Schurrer of Aurora Research Institute for assistance with the figures.

References

[1] J. P. Shah and Z. Gil, "Current concepts in management of oral cancer - surgery," *Oral Oncology*, vol. 45, no. 4-5, pp. 394–401, 2009.

[2] E. Attar, S. Dey, A. Hablas et al., "Head and neck cancer in a developing country: a population-based perspective across 8 years," *Oral Oncology*, vol. 46, no. 8, pp. 591–596, 2010.

[3] N. Howlader, A. M. Noone, M. Krapcho, J. Garshell, D. Miller, S. F. Altekruse, C. L. Kosary, M. Yu, J. Ruhl, Z. Tatalovich, A. Mariotto, D. R. Lewis, H. S. Chen, E. J. Feuer, and K. A. Cronin, Eds., *SEER Cancer Statistics Review, 1975-2012*, National Cancer Institute, Bethesda, MD, USA, 2015, https://seer.cancer.gov/archive/csr/1975_2012/, based on November 2014 SEER data submission, posted to the SEER web site, April 2015.

[4] E. Benson, R. Li, D. Eisele, and C. Fakhry, "The clinical impact of HPV tumor status upon head and neck squamous cell carcinomas," *Oral Oncology*, vol. 50, no. 6, pp. 565–574, 2014.

[5] K. Martell, R. Simpson, and D. Skarsgard, "Solitary myocardial metastasis from locoregionally controlled squamous cell carcinoma of the oral cavity," *Cureus*, vol. 8, no. 6, article e650, 2016.

[6] G. B. Werbel, J. H. Skom, D. Mehlman, and L. L. Michaelis, "Metastatic squamous cell carcinoma to the heart. Unusual cause of angina decubitus and cardiac murmur," *Chest*, vol. 88, no. 3, pp. 468-469, 1985.

[7] A. Rivkin, J. G. Meara, K. K. Li, C. Potter, and R. Wenokur, "Squamous cell metastasis from the tongue to the myocardium presenting as pericardial effusion," *Otolaryngology–Head and Neck Surgery*, vol. 120, no. 4, pp. 593–595, 1999.

[8] F. T. Schwender, I. Wollner, L. P. Kunju, R. E. Nakhleh, and K. M. Chan, "Squamous cell carcinoma of the buccal mucosa with metastases to the pericardial cavity, lung and thyroid," *Oral Oncology*, vol. 38, no. 1, pp. 114–116, 2002.

[9] J. Onwuchekwa and J. Banchs, "Early cardiac metastasis from squamous cell carcinoma of the tongue in 2 patients," *Texas Heart Institute Journal*, vol. 39, no. 4, pp. 565–567, 2012.

[10] S. Hans, D. Chauvet, B. Sadoughi, and D. F. Brasnu, "Cardiac metastasis after squamous cell carcinoma of the base of tongue," *American Journal of Otolaryngology*, vol. 30, no. 3, pp. 206–208, 2009.

[11] S. Nagata, K. Ota, M. Nagata, and M. Shinohara, "Cardiac metastasis of head and neck squamous cell carcinoma," *International Journal of Oral and Maxillofacial Surgery*, vol. 41, no. 12, pp. 1458–1462, 2012.

[12] M. Shimoyama, F. Kitamura-Sasaka, and C. Shigemasa, "Metastatic cardiac squamous cell carcinoma arising in the left ventricle," *Heart*, vol. 85, no. 5, p. 507, 2001.

4

A Band that Causes Leaky Valves: Severe Mitral Regurgitation due to Left Atrial Fibrous Band

Christopher Nnaoma,[1] Gurdarshan Sandhu,[1] Christoph Sossou,[1] Ilan Vavilin,[2] Jose Bustillo,[1] and Anshu Garg[1]

[1]Newark Beth Israel Medical Center, Newark, NJ, USA
[2]St. George's University, Grenada

Correspondence should be addressed to Christopher Nnaoma; bobbyxcarry@gmail.com

Academic Editor: Ertugrul Ercan

Left atrial fibrous band is a rare clinical and echocardiographic finding characterized by the presence of a fibrous band attached to the mitral valve. Diagnosis is accomplished with transesophageal echocardiography (TEE), live 3D imaging, or cardiac MRI. Most patients are asymptomatic and incidental findings. However, in rare cases, an atrial fibrous band can produce symptoms such as dyspnea on exertion, fatigue, and lightheadedness secondary to mitral regurgitation (MR) which can lead to heart failure if unattended to. More serious complications such as cardioembolic phenomenon can occur. We herein report a case of a 55-year-old male with hypertension who presented with dyspnea on exertion and chest pain. Transthoracic echocardiography (TTE) showed mitral valve prolapse with moderate to severe mitral regurgitation. TEE showed an atrial fibrous band. Given the patient's poor exercise tolerance, he was taken to surgery for a mitral annuloplasty.

1. Introduction

The first case of left atrial fibrous band was reported in 1897 by Rollestone [1]. Left atrial fibrous bands are rare. Autopsy data suggest the prevalence of left atrial bands to be approximately 2% [2]. Its association with MR is exceedingly unique [2]. The clinical importance of these bands in the left atrium is still not clearly defined and should not be confused with the left ventricular false tendon [3]. A better understanding of the natural history and clinical implications of this condition may better help us to diagnose and manage these patients. We present a case of severe symptomatic mitral regurgitation caused by a left atrial fibrous band. The patient had surgical resection of the band and symptoms improved significantly post procedure.

2. Methods

In addition to the presented case report, we reviewed the literature to compare the clinical presentation and management of patients with a left atrial fibrous band. The review considered papers and publications written in the English language only. Keywords used for electronic search were left atrial fibrous band and mitral regurgitation. Definitions used for case inclusion were (a) diagnosis of left atrial band either by TTE, TEE, cardiac MRI, live 3D imaging, (b) abnormalities produced by left atrial bands, and (c) age greater than 18 years. Autopsy-reported cases were not included and no studies were excluded based on the date of publication.

3. Case Presentation

A 55-year-old male with a past medical history of hypertension reports exertional dyspnea for 8 months and nonexertional chest pain for 5 days. Physical exam revealed an afebrile patient; BP of 133/82 mmHg; heart auscultation revealed a new 3/6 systolic murmur, maximal at the apex radiating to the axilla; no leg swelling; and no jugular vein distention. The lungs were clear to auscultation. Pertinent

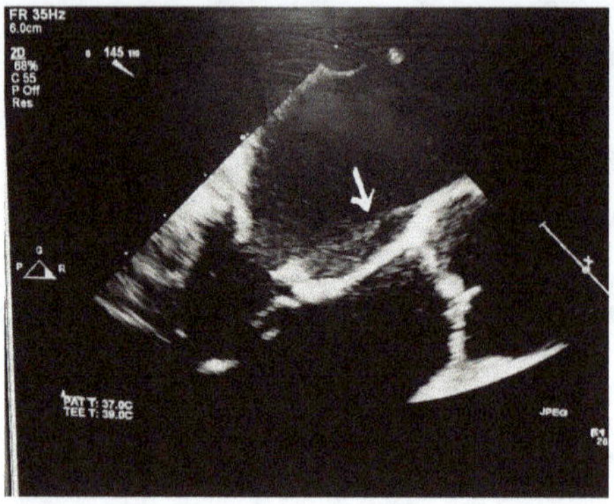

FIGURE 1: Preop ECHO showing mild focal bileaflet (anterior > posterior) leaflet prolapse with moderate to severe MR. EF was 45%.

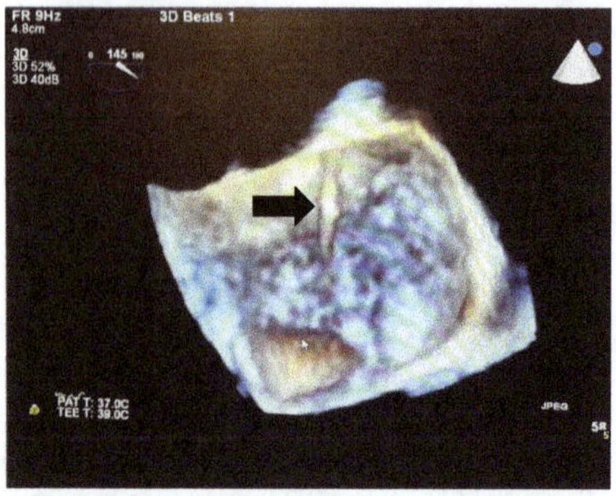

FIGURE 2: 3D live imaging of the left atrial fibrous band.

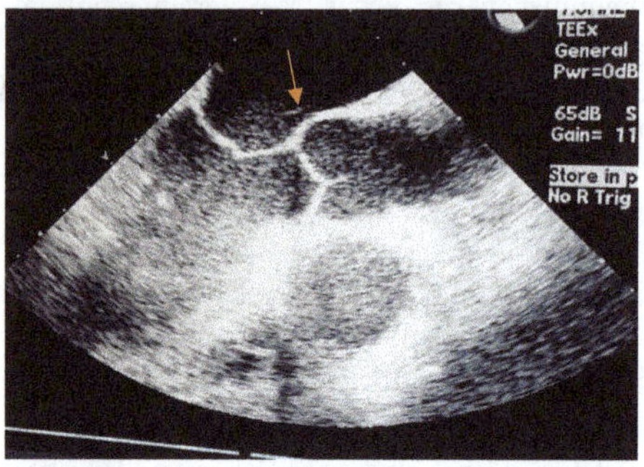

FIGURE 3: Intraoperative image of a thickened fibrous band from the atrial septum down to the edge of the A2 segment.

labs were a negative Troponin and BNP. CT angiography and cardiac catheterization were negative. Increased MR with exercise was noted. TTE revealed a moderate to severe posteriorly directed MR which was said to be functional in origin (Carpentier classification III). Ejection fraction (EF) was 45%. TEE showed a structure attached to the atrial surface of the anterior (A2, A3 component) leaflet of the mitral valve (Figure 1), most consistent with a left atrial fibrous band. The distal portion of the band was attached to the interatrial septum in close relation to the aortic valve. The band appeared to restrict the motion of the A2, A3 component with consequent MR, giving it a tented appearance, while 3D live imaging allowed for complete visualization of the band attaching to the mitral valve (Figure 2).

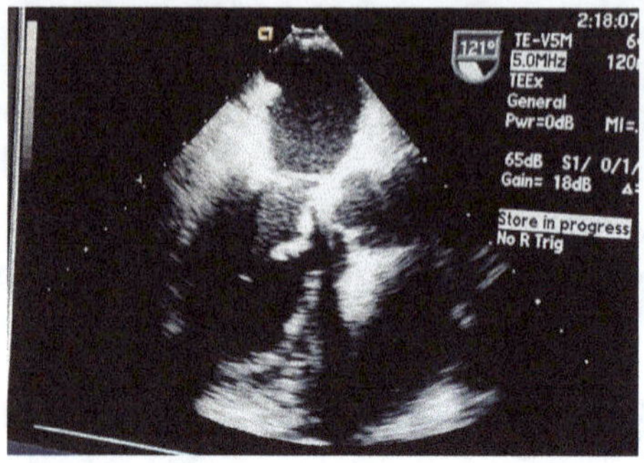

FIGURE 4: Postop ECHO showing mitral annulus after mitral annuloplasty with an EF of 49%.

Given his poor exercise tolerance, the patient was taken for mitral valve annuloplasty. Intraoperative findings included mitral valve prolapse (MVP), thickened fibrous mitral valve, and MR (Figure 3). The pathology of the fibrous band showed a cardiac valve/vascular wall-like tissue with focal degenerative changes. Three months after the repair, patient's symptoms improved significantly with good exercise tolerance. There were no audible murmurs. ECHO showed no mitral regurgitation about 3 months after mitral annuloplasty, with an EF of 49% (Figure 4).

4. Literature Review

To the best of our knowledge, fourteen cases of left atrial fibrous band have been described in the literature that met our inclusion criteria. These do not include those found incidentally on autopsy.

Table 1 summarizes the baseline demographics and associated clinical significance of these bands. There were ten males, four females, and one of undetermined sex. The mean age was 52.

Figure 5 represents a graphical presentation of these left atrial bands and their clinical significance.

The most common complication resulting from a left atrial fibrous band was MR which was present in about 37.5% of the cases. Most of the patients with MR progressed to congestive heart failure (CHF). 25% of cases were noted to have cryptogenic stroke and cardiac embolism. 18.7% of cases were noted to have atrial fibrillation (A. Fib) while 6.25% were from supraventricular tachycardia and myocardial infarction. The high incidence of stroke in these patients is likely due to increased incidence of patent foramen ovale (PFO) and A. Fib associated with left atrial fibrous band.

A graph showing the incidence of complications associated with left atrial fibrous bands is presented.

5. Discussion

Intracavitary muscle bands have been well described in all four chambers of the heart. It can be congenital, with no reported gender or racial predilection. Lev (1953) described three forms of abnormal partitioning of the left atrium which are distinguished by the location of the entrance of the venae cava and pulmonary veins [4]. The likely embryological explanation could be that the abnormal septum is likely to

Table 1: Basic demographics and the clinical presentation of these patients.

Study	Age and sex	Complications
Irwin et al., Shin et al.	75-year-old male	Mitral regurgitation
Won Young Jang et al.	76-year-old male	Persistent atrial fibrillation
Olsen et al.	54-year-old male	Acute myocardial infarction
Saade et al.	49-year-old female	MR and palpitations
Sherif et al.	72-year-old male	MR leading to CHF
Bergaglio et al.	30-year-old male	SVT
Bergaglio et al.	67-year-old female	Ischemic right hemispheric stroke
Shunsuke Uetake et al.	72-year-old male	Paroxysmal atrial fibrillation
Ozer et al.	34-year-old male and 56-year-old female	Cryptogenic stroke
James Ker et al.	29-year-old male and 43-year-old male	Cardioembolic events leading to TIA
Okajima K. et al.	65-year-old male	Persistent AF
Barant T. et al.	Age and sex unknown	MR, MVP
Vlassak et al.	20-year-old female	Dyspnea and MR
Dawson D. et al.	33-year-old female	MR

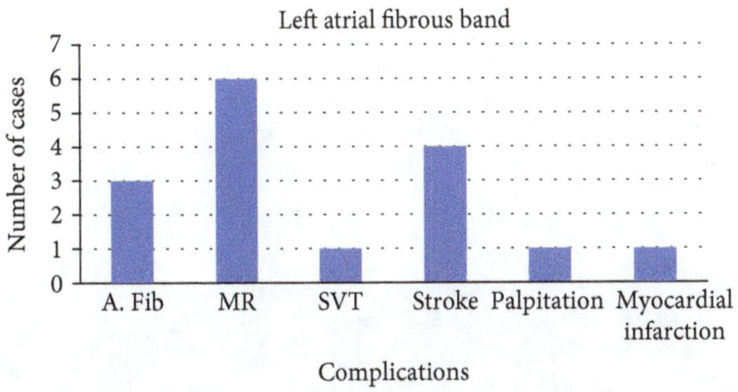

Figure 5: Incidence of complications in patients with atrial fibrous band.

be part of the septum primum, which is deviated to the left side to form an extra subdivision of the left atrium [4].

Left atrial fibrous bands are said to be a very rare cause of MR. Yamashita et al. reported 22 cases of left atrial fibrous bands from 1,100 patient autopsies [5]. The mechanism of MR associated with left atrial fibrous bands can be due to prolapse (Carpentier type II) or restricted movement (Carpentier type IIIa or b). The incidence of Chiari's network was 27% in patients with left atrial fibrous band vs. 8% in people without ($P < 0.01$) while 23% had PFO as compared to 8% in people without left atrial fibrous band ($P < 0.05$). The increased amount of PFO in this group of patients predisposes them to an increased incidence of cardioembolic phenomenon [5]. Also, about 18% of the patients with left atrial fibrous band had A. Fib; this also predisposes them to increased risk of strokes.

There have also been four reported cases of cardioembolic events from left atrial bands [6], making up about 25% of cases reported. Most of these bands are either fibrous or fibromuscular. In our patient, the fibrous band may have originated from the atrial septum. These bands are usually congenital and can be found incidentally. The clinical significance of these bands is uncertain [7]; they are mostly asymptomatic. They are however relevant since they can be associated with mitral regurgitation [3, 8], valve cardiomyopathies, atrial fibrillation, conduction disorders, and infectious endocarditis and can interfere with the manipulation of the catheter during invasive procedures [9]. As noted above, these bands are mostly associated with mitral regurgitation, which can lead to heart failure if not treated early.

Definite diagnosis of these bands can be done through cardiac imaging modality (transthoracic echocardiography, transesophageal echocardiography, cardiac MRI, and 3D live imaging which allow for complete visualization of the band attaching to the mitral valve).

In our case, the band was not an incidental finding; the fibrous band likely originated from the atrial septum and produced significant symptom requiring surgical treatment which is the definite treatment. No PFO was noted in our patient.

6. Conclusion

Fibrous bands in the left atrium are rare and extremely rare causes of MR. When they do produce symptoms, they either can be managed medically or surgically depending on the symptoms and severity of MR. Surgery should be deferred in patients who are asymptomatic. Such patients should be followed up closely with scheduled echocardiography. We recommend that PFO be ruled out in these patients given a high associated incidence rate. Anticoagulation should be considered in those with A. Fib and PFO due to increased risk of cardioembolic strokes in these patients until a definite treatment is carried out.

Authors' Contributions

All authors contributed significantly to this manuscript.

References

[1] W. Saade, F. Baldascino, A. De Bellis et al., "Left atrial anomalous muscular band as incidental finding during video-assisted mitral surgery," *Journal of Thoracic Disease*, vol. 10, no. 7, pp. E538–E540, 2018.

[2] R. B. Irwin, M. Schmitt, and S. Ray, "Left atrial fibrous band, an unexpected mechanism of mitral regurgitation," *European Heart Journal - Cardiovascular Imaging*, vol. 12, no. 7, p. 552, 2011.

[3] T. Baran, M. S. Kucukoglu, B. Okcun, G. Cetin, A. C. Hatemi, and S. Uner, "A rare cause of mitral insufficiency:. left atrial anomalous band," *Echocardiography*, vol. 20, no. 1, pp. 83–85, 2003.

[4] E. G. Olsen and J. C. Valentine, "Anomalous bands in the heart," *British Heart Journal*, vol. 34, no. 2, pp. 210–212, 1972.

[5] T. Yamashita, S. Ohkawa, T. Imai, H. Ide, C. Watanabe, and K. Ueda, "Prevalence and clinical significance of anomalous muscular band in the left atrium," *The American Journal of Cardiovascular Pathology*, vol. 4, no. 4, pp. 286–293, 1993.

[6] J. Ker, "Congenital left atrial bands and cardioembolic events," *International Journal of Cardiology*, vol. 170, no. 3, pp. e72–e73, 2014.

[7] O. Ozer, I. Sari, V. Davutoglu, R. Yıgıter, and C. Akkoyun, "Cryptogenic stroke in two cases with left atrial band: coincidence or cause?," *European Heart Journal - Cardiovascular Imaging*, vol. 10, no. 2, pp. 360-361, 2009.

[8] D. Dawson, P. Mankad, P. Bloomfield, and N. A. Boon, "An unusual cause of severe mitral regurgitation: aberrantly inserted chordae tendineae," *Journal of the American Society of Echocardiography*, vol. 21, no. 1, pp. 90.e3–90.e4, 2008.

[9] A. Alsaid, P. J. Cawley, T. D. Bauch, and C. W. Good, "Hanging by a thread, severe mitral regurgitation due to accessory left atrial cord," *European Heart Journal – Cardiovascular Imaging*, vol. 17, no. 8, p. 943, 2016.

5

A Rare but Real Necessity: Case Report of Coronary Artery Stenting in an Infant

José D. Martins,[1] **Guilherme Lourenço**,[1] **Lídia Sousa**,[2] **and Fátima F. Pinto**[1]

[1]*Pediatric Cardiology Department, Hospital de Santa Marta, Centro Hospitalar de Lisboa Central EPE, Lisbon, Portugal*
[2]*Cardiology Department, Hospital de Santa Marta, Centro Hospitalar de Lisboa Central EPE, Lisbon, Portugal*

Correspondence should be addressed to José D. Martins; jdferreiramartins@gmail.com

Academic Editor: Manabu Shirotani

Percutaneous coronary intervention (PCI) is an extremely common and well-established procedure in adults which is rarely performed in children. We present a case of a successful left main coronary artery stenting in a small infant with a congenital coronary artery anomaly. We highlight the technical challenges of performing a PCI in a small patient, the risks of antithrombotic prophylaxis in this age group, and the importance of the combined work of the adult and pediatric interventional cardiologist.

1. Introduction

Percutaneous coronary intervention (PCI) is a very common procedure in adults, but extremely rare in children. In the latter, coronary artery stenosis requiring intervention is exceptional, particularly in infancy, where we found only seven such cases [1–6]. Older children or adolescents may also present with coronary compromise requiring PCI, such as after percutaneous pulmonary valve implantation [7], Kawasaki disease [8], or heart transplantation [9].

Congenital coronary anomalies are sporadic findings that occur either as an isolated anomaly of the coronary origin or course (such as ALCAPA) or in association with other heart anomalies (such as transposition of the great arteries). These patients are managed surgically, usually with coronary reimplantation. The incidence of coronary artery stenosis requiring PCI in infancy occurs only as a rare complication after these coronary artery surgeries [1–6].

We present a successful case of coronary artery stenting in an infant with ALCAPA with a significant postoperative stenosis.

2. Case Report

Our patient was born overseas, in São Tomé and Principe, a small island nation off the western coast of Africa. Despite early symptoms of overt heart failure, she was only evacuated to our country at the age of 18 months, weighing 8.9 kg. Upon arrival, we made the echocardiographic-based diagnosis of an anomalous left coronary artery (LCA) from the pulmonary artery (ALCAPA) with a dilated and poorly functioning left ventricle (LV). The patient underwent uneventful left coronary artery implantation in the left-facing aortic sinus. Due to persistent postoperative hemorrhage around the site of LCA reimplantation, biological glue was used, with success. However, in the postoperatory period, there was no improvement of the LV function and size, and the patient remained in low cardiac output. The CT scan showed a significant left main coronary stenosis and ruled out intracoronary thrombosis.

On the 4th postoperative day, the patient underwent cardiac catheterization (Figure 1). It ruled out left coronary artery ostial narrowing at the anastomosis site but showed

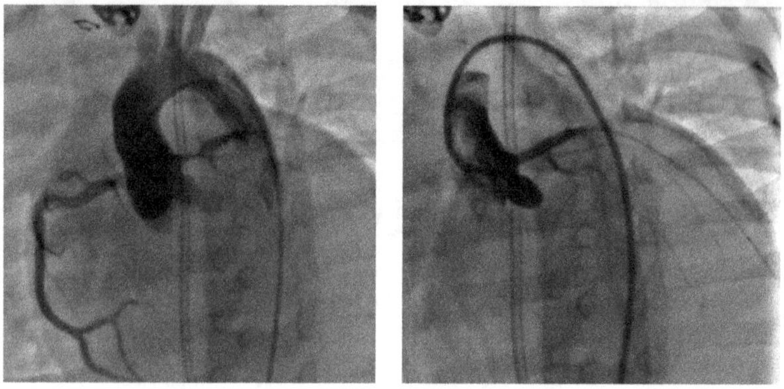

(a) (b)

FIGURE 1: On the left-hand-sided panel (a), the angiography reveals a significant stenosis of the left main coronary artery. The right-hand-sided panel (b) depicts an excellent angiographic result after stent implantation in the left main coronary artery, which is now widely patent.

a severe rosary-bead-like stenosis (minimum diameter 1.1 mm) that involved the whole left main coronary artery and extended into the ostia of the left anterior descending and circumflex arteries. The heart team discussed the case on-site, and the patient was refused for surgical reintervention, and therefore, a PCI was attempted. Informed consent was obtained prior to the procedure.

We were unable to selectively catheterize the left coronary artery with several guiding catheters, which proved too large for the patient size. Therefore, we used a 4Fr diagnostic Judkins left 2.5 catheter to catheterize the left coronary artery with a 0.014″ hydrophilic coronary guidewire, a Runthrough NS Hypercoat (Terumo Interventional Systems, Somerset, NJ, USA), which was placed distally in a diagonal artery. We exchanged over-the-wire the diagnostic catheter for a 5Fr Judkins left 3.5 guiding catheter, which was left in the left-sided sinus of Valsalva. The coronary stenosis was inframillimetric, and the normal anterior descending coronary artery measured 3 mm. We implanted a 3 × 12 mm Xience Sierra everolimus drug-eluting coronary stent system (Abbott Vascular, Santa Clara, CA, USA). The immediate postinterventional coronarography showed an optimal angiographic result, with adequate distal flow to both the anterior descending and circumflex coronary arteries.

The patient was placed under dual antiplatelet therapy with aspirin (5 mg/kg/day) and clopidogrel (0.2 mg/kg/d). Despite a widely patent flow in the coronary stent, well seen in serial transthoracic echocardiograms, the left ventricle function and size did not recover. The patient required a left-ventricular assist device due to persistent low cardiac output syndrome. She eventually died, seven days later, with sepsis.

3. Discussion

Postoperative LCA occlusion and persistent LV dysfunction after ALCAPA surgery are not uncommon [10, 11]. In our case, we speculate that external compression (due to the biological glue, blood clots, or other mechanisms) or coronary artery kinking due to surgical proximal segment mobilization may have caused the LCA stenosis. Another contributing factor could be the presence of intracoronary (so-called "steal") collaterals that may exist in ALCAPA and result in competitive flow to the normal coronary artery system [12].

We are aware that coronary artery stenting in this situation is only tolerable as a bailout technique in a critically ill infant, especially considering the risks of stent thrombosis and dual antiplatelet antiaggregation in a small infant and the fixed stent diameter which will not accompany the patient's somatic growth.

There are many challenges associated with coronary artery stenting in infants which make this a high-risk procedure. All seven published case reports were technically successful but carried significant acute and short-term complications, including myocardial ischemia, need for extracorporeal membrane oxygenator support, early in-stent thrombosis, and premature death. Several factors contributed to these findings, including the adverse baseline clinical situation that leads to the cardiac catheterization, the small patient weight, the diminutive coronary diameter, and the multiple anatomic variants in a postoperative situation. Additionally, there is a limited availability of adequate coronary catheterization hardware, which is designed for adult-sized coronary arteries and vessels, that can be cumbersome to manage in small patients. The choice of bare metal stent (BMS) vs. drug-eluting stent (DES) is also up for debate, due to concerns about potential deleterious side effects of systemic circulation of antiproliferative drugs in small patients [13]. In the previous reports, only 2/7 stents were DES, the remainder were BMS. Considering preliminary safety data of neonatal DES in the ductus arteriosus, we opted for a recent generation of DES. There is also debate about the optimal thromboprophylaxis regimen, which was dual-antiplatelet therapy in 5/7 and single-antiplatelet (aspirin) in the remainder. We chose a dual-antiplatelet regimen, which is the recommended thromboprophylaxis for DES. We had no hemorrhagic complications. Finally, there is a challenge due to the understandable lack of coronary artery expertise of the pediatric interventionalists. In our case, it was crucial to perform a four-hand procedure with an experienced adult congenital heart disease interventionalist.

Our case highlights the importance of collaborative work between adult and pediatric cardiologists that allows a patient-focused treatment and some technical challenges of this challenging interventional technique in infants.

Supplementary Materials

Supplementary Material (video legend): available at: preintervention aortic root angiogra-phy, showing a right dominant system and a severe stenosis of the left main coronary artery. Part 2: 4Fr diagnostic Judkins left 2.5 catheter is used to catheterize the left coronary artery

with a 0.014″ hydrophilic coronary guidewire. Part 3: preintervention selective left coronary artery angiography, showing a severe rosary-bead-like stenosis that involved the whole left main coronary artery and extended into the ostia of the left anterior descending and circumflex arteries. Parts 4 and 5: postintervention selective angiographies, showing an adequately placed stent in the left main coronary artery, with a good angiographic result. *(Supplementary Materials)*

References

[1] A. Bratincsak, A. Salkini, H. G. El-Said, and J. W. Moore, "Percutaneous stent implantation into coronary arteries in infants," *Catheterization and Cardiovascular Interventions*, vol. 79, no. 2, pp. 303–311, 2012.

[2] A. Hallbergson and J. J. Rome, "Percutaneous left main coronary artery stent for acute myocardial ischemia after repaired ALCAPA," *Catheterization and Cardiovascular Interventions*, vol. 85, no. 6, pp. 1017–1020, 2015.

[3] M. Schneider, W. Wiebe, V. Hraska, and P. Zartner, "Coronary interventions in congenital heart diseases: from preterm to young adult patients," *Journal of Interventional Cardiology*, vol. 26, no. 3, pp. 287–294, 2013.

[4] J. S. de Lezo, M. Pan, and C. Herrera, "Combined percutaneous revascularization and cell therapy after failed repair of anomalous origin of left coronary artery from pulmonary artery," *Catheterization and Cardiovascular Interventions*, vol. 73, no. 6, pp. 833–837, 2009.

[5] G. S. Chrysant, D. Balzer, and M. Taniuchi, "Left main stem coronary artery stenting in a 3-month-old child after anomalous left coronary artery from pulmonary artery repair," *Pediatric Cardiology*, vol. 26, no. 5, pp. 734–736, 2005.

[6] A. E. Schneider, J. N. Johnson, N. W. Taggart et al., "Percutaneous coronary intervention in pediatric and adolescent patients," *Congenital Heart Disease*, vol. 9, no. 3, pp. 228–234, 2014.

[7] A. A. Divekar, J. J. Lee, W. J. Tymchak, and J. M. Rutledge, "Percutaneous coronary intervention for extrinsic coronary compression after pulmonary valve replacement," *Catheterization and Cardiovascular Interventions*, vol. 67, no. 3, pp. 482–484, 2006.

[8] H. Muta and M. Ishii, "Percutaneous coronary intervention versus coronary artery bypass grafting for stenotic lesions after Kawasaki disease," *The Journal of Pediatrics*, vol. 157, no. 1, pp. 120–126, 2010.

[9] R. E. Shaddy, J. A. Revenaugh, G. S. Orsmond, and L. Y. Tani, "Coronary interventional procedures in pediatric heart transplant recipients with cardiac allograft vasculopathy," *The American Journal of Cardiology*, vol. 85, no. 11, pp. 1370–1372, 2000.

[10] A. Secinaro, H. Ntsinjana, O. Tann et al., "Cardiovascular magnetic resonance findings in repaired anomalous left coronary artery to pulmonary artery connection (ALCAPA)," *Journal of Cardiovascular Magnetic Resonance*, vol. 13, no. 1, p. 27, 2011.

[11] B. Castaldi, V. Vida, E. Reffo et al., "Speckle tracking in ALCAPA patients after surgical repair as predictor of residual coronary disease," *Pediatric Cardiology*, vol. 38, no. 4, pp. 794–800, 2017.

[12] M. A. Frommelt, E. Miller, J. Williamson, and S. Bergstrom, "Detection of septal coronary collaterals by color flow Doppler mapping is a marker for anomalous origin of a coronary artery from the pulmonary artery," *Journal of the American Society of Echocardiography*, vol. 15, no. 3, pp. 259–263, 2002.

[13] V. Aggarwal, G. S. Dhillon, D. J. Penny, S. T. Gowda, and A. M. Qureshi, "Drug-eluting stents compared with bare metal stents for stenting the ductus arteriosus in infants with ductal-dependent pulmonary blood flow," *The American Journal of Cardiology*, vol. 124, no. 6, pp. 952–959, 2019.

6

Cocaine-Induced Pneumopericardium: Safe for Discharge?

Xavier Galloo,[1] **Jan Stroobants**,[2] **David Yeo**,[3] **and Esmael El-Abdellati**[2]

[1]*Department of Cardiology, ZNA Middelheim, Antwerp, Belgium*
[2]*Emergency Department, ZNA Middelheim, Antwerp, Belgium*
[3]*Emergency Department, University Hospital Birmingham, Birmingham, UK*

Correspondence should be addressed to Xavier Galloo; xgalloo@vub.ac.be

Academic Editor: Aiden Abidov

A 29-year-old male presented at the Emergency Department (ED) with chest pain and neck tenderness after intranasal cocaine usage. Physical exam of the patient demonstrated moderate subcutaneous emphysema on the right side of his neck. The ECG did not demonstrate any changes associated with cocaine-induced cardiac ischemia, and blood analysis was normal (negative troponins). A chest X-ray revealed subtle evidence of pneumomediastinum. Subsequent thoracic CT confirmed the presence of subcutaneous emphysema with a pneumopericardium and a large pneumomediastinum along with a small pneumothorax. The patient was managed conservatively and kept overnight for observation. He was discharged from the ED the following day with ambulatory follow-up. A repeat thoracic CT performed two weeks later demonstrated that the findings identified in the first CT had resolved. Pneumopericardium, -mediastinum, and -thorax are rare conditions reported after cocaine abuse. A conservative approach with a period of observation in a suitable ambulatory unit is acceptable, as current literature suggests that the condition is usually self-limiting.

1. Introduction

The widespread abuse of cocaine has led to an increase in the frequency of Emergency Department (ED) visits worldwide. The respiratory and cardiovascular effects associated with cocaine abuse are well established with increasing numbers reported in the literature. The most common complaint reported by patients is chest pain [1, 2].

Cocaine activates the sympathetic nervous system leading to vasoconstriction, elevated arterial blood pressure, tachycardia, and arrhythmias. The most frequent cardiovascular complications reported are acute myocardial infarction and cardiac tachyarrhythmias. Pneumomediastinum and -thorax after cocaine abuse are reported infrequently, and of note, pneumopericardium is very rare [1, 3].

2. Case Report

A 29-year-old male (weight: 58 kg, length: 178 cm, BMI: 18.3 kg/m^2; BMI normal range: 18.5 kg/m^2 – 25 kg/m^2), without significant past medical history, presented at the ED with chest pain and localised neck tenderness. He presented with sudden onset retrosternal chest pain. The pain was described as "mild and continuous" with no radiation or any other associated symptoms (i.e., no dyspnea or cough; no nausea or vomiting). There was no history of preceding trauma, and the patient had no previous medical history of note. Apart from a 5 pack-year history of smoking cigarettes, there were no other cardiovascular risk factors.

The patient did not take regular medication but admitted to marijuana use on a weekly basis as a teenager until the age of 25. He then only used marijuana infrequently (on average once a month). With regard to cocaine, he admitted he had used it twice—the first being a year ago, and the second time a day prior to attending the ED. There was no history of any other recreational drug use.

Following intranasal cocaine inhalation at an evening social gathering, he suffered chest pain and palpitations. In an attempt to ease the chest pain, he smoked a premixed marijuana/tobacco joint (approximately 0.32 grams marijuana

[4]). The joint was smoked as per a normal cigarette technique without prolonged inhalation or Valsalva manoeuvres.

The following morning, he continued to experience retrosternal chest pain, which had since increased in intensity. He now noticed the presence of right-sided neck pain but without muscle tenderness, throat pain, or dyspnea. Despite taking 1 gram of paracetamol, the symptoms were no better and he therefore presented to the ED.

His vital signs were within normal parameters (temperature: 36.1°C, heart rate: 65 bpm, blood pressure: 125/75 mmHg, equal bilaterally with no pulsus paradoxus, respiratory rate: 13/min, oxygen saturation 100% on room air with a GCS of 15/15).

On physical examination, respiratory auscultation was normal without additional sounds; cardiac sounds were unremarkable with no murmurs or clear "Hamman's sign" (*a crunching sound synchronous with the heartbeat. It is best heard over the precordium and is suggestive for pneumopericardium or -mediastinum*) [5–7]. A moderate amount of subcutaneous emphysema on the right side of the neck was noted. The rest of the physical exam was unremarkable.

Blood analysis was normal (normal haematology and biochemical analysis, normal inflammatory markers and troponins <0.012 ng/mL). Arterial blood gas on room air demonstrated a respiratory alkalosis without metabolic compensation (pH 7.50, pCO_2 29.3 mmHg, pO_2 119.7 mmHg, base excess 0.3 mmol/L, HCO_3^- 22.2 mmol/L, saturation 98.2%, and lactate 1.3 mmol/L). ECG demonstrated normal sinus rhythm without ST-elevation with normal repolarisation. A chest X-ray showed subtle evidence of pneumomediastinum and right-sided mild subcutaneous emphysema in the neck (Figure 1(a), thick arrow) with air tracking in the centre of the mediastinum (Figure 1(a), thin arrow). There is a small denser line along the right cardiomediastinal margin (Figure 2) that is often present in normal X-rays and is attributed to an optical illusion known as the *Mach Band effect* (a visual pattern due to edge enhancement manifesting as a region of lucency adjacent to convex surfaces). Although it can be normal, taken in association with subcutaneous emphysema and air tracking in the centre of a mediastinum, this is suggestive of a pneumomediastinum [8].

As subcutaneous emphysema along with the suggestion of pneumomediastinum was identified on the chest X-ray, further workup with thoracic CT-scan was performed. This confirmed the presence of subcutaneous emphysema with a pneumopericardium, a large pneumomediastinum, and a small pneumothorax (Figure 1(b), Figure 3). The patient was managed conservatively and kept overnight for observation (continuous cardiac and pulse oximetry monitoring with two-hourly blood pressure measurement in addition to pain control titrated to a pain Visual Analogue Scale). A combination of paracetamol and tramadol was sufficient to keep the patient pain free. The following day, his clinical parameters remained within normal limits along with the resolution of chest pain and a largely unremarkable physical examination. He was discharged the next day with expectative approach, oral analgesics, and ambulatory follow-up. Repeat CT after two weeks revealed complete resolution of the free intrathoracic air.

3. Discussion

Spontaneous pneumopericardium, -mediastinum, and -thorax are rare conditions that have been reported following cocaine abuse, but diagnostic and therapeutic guidelines remain open to debate. The current ESC (European Society of Cardiology) guidelines for pericardial diseases do not describe the management of pneumopericardium in this context [9, 10]. Pneumopericardium is an extremely rare complication of cocaine abuse with only 9 published cases to the best of our knowledge [11–18]. It is unclear what the incidence, or indeed the relationship, between the use of cocaine and spontaneous pneumopericardium is. A study with a systematic toxicology screening in patients presenting with spontaneous pneumopericardium/pneumothorax might shed some light on this.

Pneumopericardium, -mediastinum, and -thorax are defined as the presence of "free" air in the pericardium, the mediastinum, or the pleural cavity, respectively [7, 19]. Where there is no clear aetiology, it is referred to as spontaneous/primary, and secondary when a specific pathologic event (trauma, infection, and iatrogenic) is thought to be causative [6]. Cocaine-related pneumopericardium, -mediastinum, and -thorax are considered as spontaneous or primary as determining the precise aetiology of "free" air is challenging and its mechanism remains unanswered.

It is unclear whether the pathophysiology of pneumopericardium is that of pulmonary barotrauma or microscopic tracheal/oesophageal tear due to the solid contaminants in the crystalline mass inhaled or snorted by the patient [11, 15]. Pulmonary barotrauma, also known as the *Macklin effect*, can be explained by a three-step process: alveolar rupture due to an abrupt increase in intra-alveolar pressure leading to air dissection along bronchovascular sheaths, with eventual spread to the pulmonary interstitium and the mediastinal and pericardial cavity [7, 20–22]. This is thought to be the result of either a sudden increase in intrathoracic pressure due to rapid nasal inhalation, coughing, sneezing, and vomiting or deep, forced, and prolonged inhalation with a Valsalva's manoeuvre [1, 3].

The patient denied any coughing, vomiting, prolonged inhalation, or Valsalva's manoeuvre. Our hypothesis is that the pneumopericardium, -mediastinum, and -thorax in this patient were the result of a sudden rise in intra-alveolar pressure due to cocaine inhalation. As the chest pain preceded the smoking of marijuana, it is believed that marijuana was far less likely to be the cause of the pneumopericardium, -mediastinum, and -thorax.

In the published literature, the majority of the patients presenting with spontaneous pneumopericardium and/or pneumomediastinum are young thin males without previous medical history, much like this patient. The most frequent complaint described is chest pain, followed by neck pain, dyspnea, and cough. Less frequent symptoms are odynophagia, hoarseness, and feeding problems [7, 9, 15, 17]. Emergency physicians should be alert for patients presenting with these symptoms as they have a considerable higher risk of developing pneumopericardium and/or pneumomediastinum.

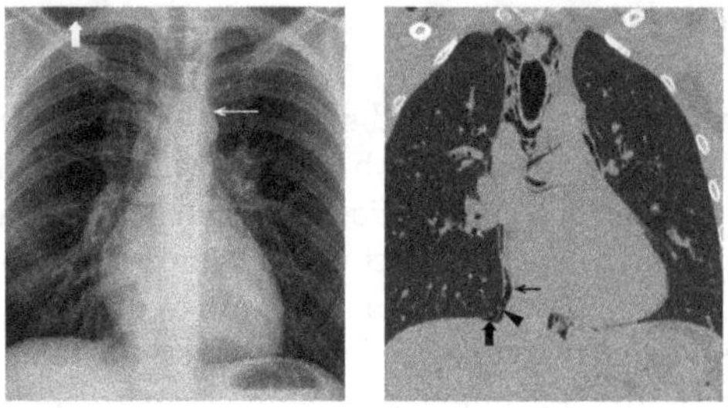

(a) (b)

Figure 1: Chest X-ray (a) and chest CT (b). On both pictures, subcutaneous emphysema is apparent at the right side of the neck (thick white arrow) as well as air tracking in the centre of the mediastinum indicative for mediastinal emphysema or pneumomediastinum (thin white arrow). Chest CT reveals a pneumopericardium (thin black arrow) and a small pneumothorax (thick black arrow). The pericardium can be seen between the pneumopericardium and pneumothorax (black triangle).

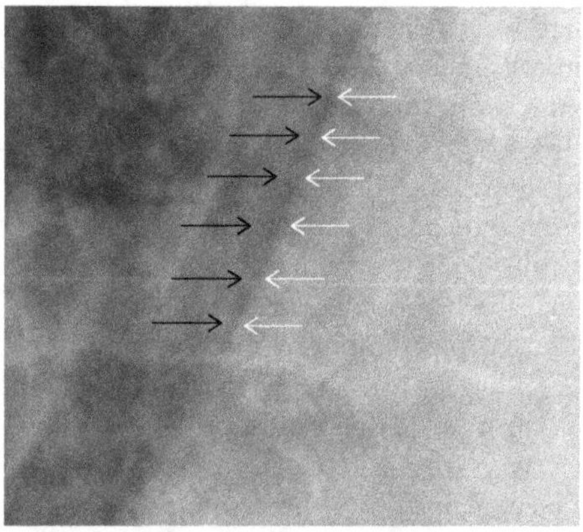

Figure 2: Mach band effect versus pneumomediastinum. Zoom in on the right cardiomediastinal border showing the edge enhancement along the cardiac margin. White arrows depicting the right cardiac border and black arrows depicting the mediastinal border of the right lung.

Spontaneous pneumopericardium and -mediastinum can be diagnosed on plain chest X-ray; although, thoracic CT remains the gold standard for radiological investigations. A CT-scan can also be helpful in excluding secondary/other causes of pneumopericardium. Further invasive diagnostic studies are not normally needed in spontaneous pneumomediastinum and should only be performed in highly suspicious cases of oesophageal or tracheal rupture [9]. There have been no reports of oesophageal rupture (Boerhaave syndrome) associated with cocaine-induced pathology. As our patient did not complain of gastrointestinal symptoms, there was no indication for invasive diagnostics such as oesophagoscopy/gastroscopy or bronchoscopy. Where tamponade due to the pneumopericardium is suspected bedside, echocardiography may be useful in evaluating such patients. As our patient remained stable throughout the entire observation with no evidence of pulsus paradoxus, echocardiography was not required.

Some guidelines for spontaneous pneumothorax and pneumomediastinum recommend a conservative approach

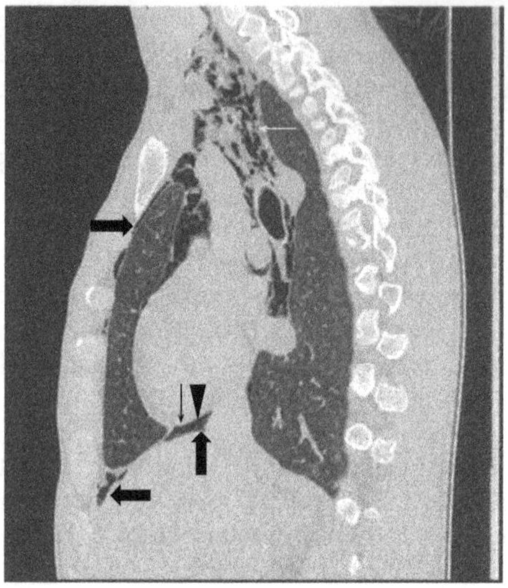

Figure 3: Chest CT showing extensive subcutaneous and mediastinal emphysema compatible with a large pneumomediastinum (white arrow), a pneumopericardium (thin black arrow, with pericardium marked by the black triangle), and a small pneumothorax (thick black arrows).

with outpatient follow-up in selected patients with minimal or no symptoms. These patients should receive clear advice to return in case of worsening dyspnea, chest pain, or fever [19, 23]. The treatment of spontaneous pneumopericardium is not clearly defined due to the rarity of its presentation. It is generally considered a benign condition, which responds well to conservative treatment, consisting of bed rest, oxygen therapy, and analgesia. All reported cases treated conservatively have resulted in complete resolution over a period of one to two weeks. Oxygen therapy should be considered as its use increases the diffusion pressure of nitrogen in the interstitium, promoting the absorption of free air in the mediastinum and possibly in the pericardium [7, 9]. In the referenced literature, there were no reports of patients developing pericarditis or mediastinitis. Antibiotic treatment should only be considered in patients at risk for infective pericarditis (presenting with fever, blood sample showing elevated inflammatory parameters, or pneumopericarditis secondary to oesophageal rupture) and should not normally be given empirically [9].

4. Conclusion

Cocaine-related complaints are increasingly seen in the ED as cocaine abuse increases in the community. The most common complaint of cocaine abuse is chest pain. Although pneumomediastinum and pneumothorax after cocaine abuse has been reported, they are infrequent complications; pneumopericardium is even less common and poorly documented. Whilst the emergency physician is familiar with the most common causes (acute myocardial ischemia or arrhythmia) of chest pain after cocaine abuse, they should be aware of other rarer causes. Patients meeting the criteria of a young thin male with no previous medical history are at increased risk of developing pneumopericardium and/or pneumomediastinum. When the ECG shows no signs of cardiac ischemia or arrhythmia and serial cardiac marker testing are negative in asymptomatic, or mildly symptomatic, patients with spontaneous pneumopericardium, a short observation with monitoring in a Chest Pain Unit is advised to follow-up or promptly exclude and treat life-threatening complications (i.e. tension pneumothorax or tamponade) early, followed by an expectative approach, since most patients will have spontaneous resolution within one or two weeks.

Each case needs to be managed on its own merits based upon the history, physical examination, investigations, clinical course of the patient, and clinical judgment of the treating physician. In some cases, prolonged observation may be necessary.

Authors' Contributions

Xavier Galloo contributed in the acquisition and analysis/interpretation of data, drafting, and revision of the article. Jan Stroobants contributed in the critical revision of the article and supervising. David Yeo contributed in the critical and grammatical revision of the article. Esmael El-Abdellati contributed in the analysis/interpretation of data, drafting, revision of the article, and supervising. All authors approved the final version of the article to be published.

References

[1] L. L. Cregler and H. Mark, "Medical Complications of Cocaine Abuse," *The New England Journal of Medicine*, vol. 315, no. 23, pp. 1495–1500, 1986.

[2] C. S. Restrepo, J. A. Carrillo, S. Martinez, P. Ojeda, A. L. Rivera, and A. Hatta, "Pulmonary complications from cocaine and cocaine-based substances: imaging manifestations," *RadioGraphics*, vol. 27, no. 4, pp. 941–956, 2007.

[3] M. Underner, J. Perriot, and G. Peiffer, "Pneumomédiastin et consommation de cocaïne," *La Presse Médicale*, vol. 46, no. 3, pp. 249–262, 2017.

[4] G. Ridgeway and B. Kilmer, "10.1016/j.drugalcdep.2016.06.004," *Drug and Alcohol Dependence*, vol. 165, pp. 175–180, 2016.

[5] L. Hamman, "Spontaneous interstitial emphysema of the lungs," *Tr Assoc Am Physicians.*, vol. 52, pp. 311–319, 1937.

[6] M. Caceres, S. Z. Ali, R. Braud, D. Weiman, and H. E. Garrett, "Spontaneous pneumomediastinum: a comparative study and review of the literature," *The Annals of Thoracic Surgery*, vol. 86, no. 3, pp. 962–966, 2008.

[7] S. Sahni, S. Verma, J. Grullon, A. Esquire, P. Patel, and A. Talwar, "Spontaneous pneumomediastinum: time for consensus," *North American Journal of Medical Sciences*, vol. 5, no. 8, pp. 460–464, 2013.

[8] C. M. Zylak, J. R. Standen, G. R. Barnes, and C. J. Zylak, "Pneumomediastinum revisited," *RadioGraphics*, vol. 20, no. 4, pp. 1043–1057, 2000.

[9] K. S. Kim, H. W. Jeon, Y. Moon et al., "Clinical experience of spontaneous pneumomediastinum: diagnosis and treatment," *Journal of Thoracic Disease*, vol. 7, no. 10, pp. 1817–1824, 2015.

[10] Y. Adler, P. Charron, M. Imazio et al., "2015 ESC Guidelines for the diagnosis and management of pericardial diseases: the Task Force for the Diagnosis and Management of Pericardial Diseases of the European Society of Cardiology (ESC) endorsed by: the European Association for Cardio-Thoracic Surgery (EACTS)," *European Heart Journal*, vol. 36, no. 42, pp. 2921–2964, 2015.

[11] C. A. Albrecht, A. Jafri, L. Linville, and H. V. Anderson, "Cocaine-induced pneumopericardium," *Circulation*, vol. 102, no. 22, pp. 2792–2794, 2000.

[12] D. Katzir, E. Klinovsky, V. Kent, A. Shucri, and Y. Gilboa, "Spontaneous pneumopericardium: case report and review of the literature," *Cardiology*, vol. 76, no. 4, pp. 305–308, 1989.

[13] B. S. Leitman, A. Greengart, and H. J. Wasser, "Pneumomediastinum and pneumopericardium after cocaine abuse," *American Journal of Roentgenology*, vol. 151, no. 3, p. 614, 1988.

[14] S. J. Savader, M. Omori, and C. R. Martinez, "Pneumothorax, pneumomediastinum and pneumopericardium: complications of cocaine smoking," *Journal of the Florida Medical Association*, vol. 75, no. 3, pp. 151-152, 1988.

[15] A. Adrouny and P. Magnusson, "Pneumopericardium from cocaine inhalation," *The New England Journal of Medicine*, vol. 313, no. 1, pp. 48-49, 1985.

[16] F. J. Garcipérez de Vargas, J. J. Gómez Barrado, S. Luis Moyano Calvente, M. J. Amaya García, and G. Marcos, "Pneumopericardium and pneumomediastinum in a diabetic and cocaine user patient," *Endocrinología y Nutrición*, vol. 60, no. 8, pp. e3–e4, 2013.

[17] L. Brander, D. Ramsay, D. Dreier, M. Peter, and R. Graeni, "Continuous left hemidiaphragm sign revisited: a case of spontaneous pneumopericardium and literature review," *Heart*, vol. 88, no. 4, article e5, 2002.

[18] V. G. Schweitzer, "Osteolytic sinusitis and pneumomediastinum: deceptive otolaryngeologic complications of cocaine abuse," *The Laryngoscope*, vol. 96, no. 2, pp. 206–210, 1986.

[19] A. MacDuff, A. Arnold, and J. Harvey, "Management of spontaneous pneumothorax: British Thoracic Society pleural disease guideline 2010," *Thorax*, vol. 65, Supplement 2, pp. -ii18–ii31, 2010.

[20] C. C. Macklin, "Transport of air along sheaths of pulmonic blood vessels from alveoli to mediastinum," *Archives of Internal Medicine*, vol. 64, no. 5, pp. 913–926, 1939.

[21] M. Wintermark and P. Schnyder, "The Macklin effect: a frequent etiology for pneumomediastinum in severe blunt chest trauma," *Chest*, vol. 120, no. 2, pp. 543–547, 2001.

[22] S. Murayama and S. Gibo, "Spontaneous pneumomediastinum and Macklin effect: overview and appearance on computed tomography," *World Journal of Radiology*, vol. 6, no. 11, pp. 850–854, 2014.

[23] J.-M. Tschopp, O. Bintcliffe, P. Astoul et al., "ERS task force statement: diagnosis and treatment of primary spontaneous pneumothorax," *European Respiratory Journal*, vol. 46, no. 2, pp. 321–335, 2015.

7

A Rare Case of Pericardial Effusion in a Patient with Silicosis

Kosuke Saku, Keisuke Yamamoto, Hironori Inoue, and Masahiro Ueno

Department of Cardiovascular Surgery, Tenyokai Central Hospital and Central Clinic, Kagoshima, Japan

Correspondence should be addressed to Kosuke Saku; saku_kosuke@yahoo.co.jp

Academic Editor: Ming-Ren Chen

Silicosis is an occupational lung disorder caused by inhalation of silica dust. It not only causes respiratory disorders but also affects other organs. We report an extremely rare case of silicosis complicated by pericarditis in an 83-year-old male. He had been working as a coal miner and was diagnosed with silicosis at the age of 63. Because he had experienced repeated pericardial effusions, he was referred for a surgical pericardial biopsy to elucidate the cause of his repeated pericardial effusion and to perform pericardial fenestration. Thoracoscopic surgery was performed. The pericardium was resected, and a drain was placed in the left thoracic cavity. Histopathological examination revealed the pericardial degeneration due to silicosis, suggesting that pericarditis and pericardial effusion are related to silicosis. The operation was successful, and he experienced no recurrence of pericardial effusion at the 7-month follow-up.

1. Introduction

Silicosis is an irreversible and incurable lung disease caused by inhalation of dust containing crystalline silica particles [1] and is one of the most important occupational diseases in the world [1, 2]. Occupations such as mining, stone work, and sandblasting are associated with an increased risk of silicosis in individuals [2]. Silicosis is a form of pneumoconiosis and can be associated with lung cancer and disorders of other organs [3]. Here, we report an extremely rare case of silicosis complicated by pericarditis and pericardial effusion.

2. Case Presentation

The patient was an 83-year-old male who had been working as a coal miner and was diagnosed with silicosis at another hospital at the age of 63. He had experienced repeated pericardial effusions 5 years ago and had undergone pericardiocentesis twice; however, the cause of pericardial effusion remained unclear, and he was referred to our hospital for surgical pericardial biopsy and pericardial fenestration.

He presented with general fatigue and exhibited stable vital signs. Fine crackles were heard during inspiration, and a restrictive pattern was observed on pulmonary function testing (vital capacity 2040 mL (71% predicted) and forced expiratory volume in 1 s 1550 mL (81.2% predicted)). We noted peripheral vein swelling and mild limb edema. Laboratory testing showed a white blood cell count of 4900/μL, hemoglobin levels of 11.3 g/dL, platelet count of $18.2 \times 10^3/\mu$L, and C-reactive protein levels of 0.06 mg/dL. No obvious liver or renal insufficiency (aminotransferase levels of 17 U/I, alanine transaminase levels of 6 U/I, total bilirubin levels of 0.2 mg/dL, total protein levels of 6.6 g/dL, albumin levels of 3.9 g/dL, blood urea nitrogen levels of 30.3 mg/dL, and creatinine levels of 0.8 mg/dL) was detected. His brain natriuretic peptide levels were 104.0 pg/mL. Low QRS voltage was observed on electrocardiography. A chest radiograph revealed cardiomegaly; his cardiothoracic ratio was 61.0% (Figure 1(a)). Opaque nodules measuring ~30 mm were observed bilaterally in the upper lung, and diffuse, small nodules were observed throughout the lung field and hilar region (Figure 1(a)). Transthoracic echocardiography and chest computed tomography both revealed massive pericardial effusion (Figures 1(b) and 1(c)). Additional findings on echocardiography included not only a right atrium collapse but also a hyperechoic pericardium and pericardial thickening (Figure 1(b)). In addition, there were no significant valvular disease and signs of heart failure (ejection fraction value of 84.0%, left ventricular end diastolic/systolic

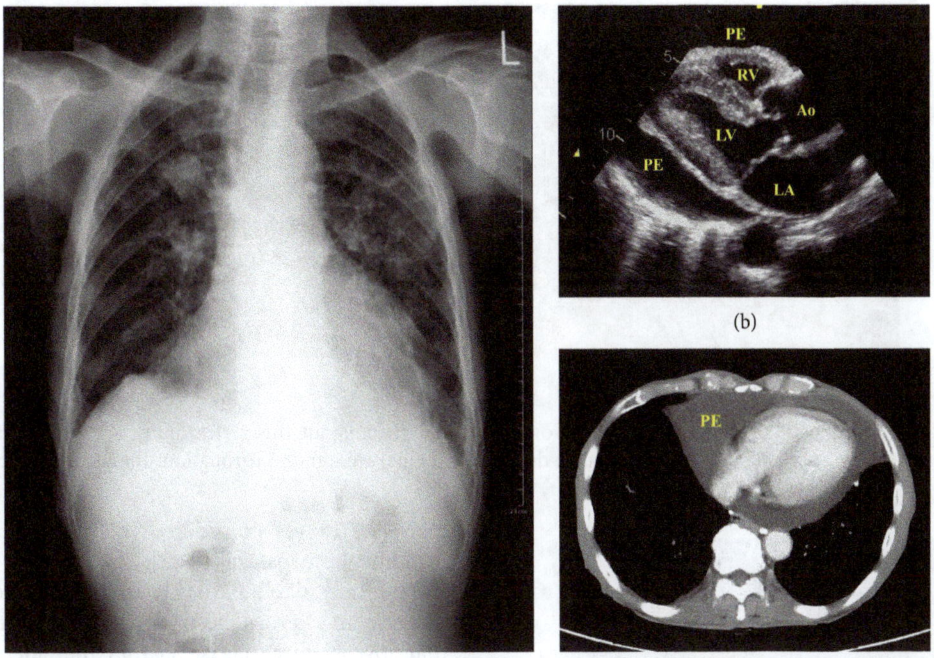

(a) (b) (c)

Figure 1: (a) Chest radiograph showing nodular opacities in the bilateral upper lung and diffuse small nodules throughout the lung field. (b) Transthoracic echocardiogram revealing a massive pericardial effusion. PE: pericardium effusion; LA: left atrium; LV: left ventricle; Ao: aorta; RV: right ventricle. (c) Computed tomography revealing a massive pericardial effusion. PE: pericardium effusion.

diameter of 39/18 mm, inferior vena cava diameter during inspiration of 18 mm, right ventricular systolic pressure of 29 mmHg, and E/e' value of 15.1). The patient was referred for a surgical pericardial biopsy to elucidate the cause of his repeated pericardial effusion and to perform pericardial fenestration.

Thoracoscopic surgery was performed using a 3 cm incision through the 8th intercostal space. Thoracoscopic examination again revealed serous pleural effusion and multiple nodular opacities throughout the pleura and pericardium (Figures 2(a) and 2(b)). A small incision was made on the pericardium (Figure 2(b)), taking care to preserve the left phrenic nerve, through which approximately 1200 mL of the effusion fluid was drained. We resected the pericardium largely of a 4×6 cm section using the Harmonic Scalpel® (Ethicon, US) and placed a drain in the left thoracic cavity.

Cytological examination of the pericardial biopsy sample was unremarkable; however, histopathological examination revealed inflammatory cell (mainly lymphocytes) infiltration and hyalinized fibrosis within the nodular tissue (Figures 3(a) and 3(b)), consistent with a diagnosis of silicosis. Lastly, polymerase chain reaction (PCR) results were negative for tuberculosis.

The patient's fatigue was resolved after surgery, and he experienced no recurrence of pericardial effusion at the 7-month follow-up.

3. Discussion

Silicosis is a well-known occupational respiratory disease [1], which causes lung inflammation and fibrosis. Silicosis is caused by inhalation and deposition of large amounts of crystalline silica over time [4]. Although protective measures such as dust control and respirators have reduced deaths attributable to silicosis in developed countries, new outbreaks still occur [5].

When silica dust is inhaled, the particles deposit within the distal airways. Macrophages ingest these particles and initiate an inflammatory response by releasing proinflammatory molecules such as tumor necrosis factor, interleukin-1, and other cytokines. These often lead to tissue fibrosis and formation of nodular lesions [5]. Thus, silicosis is characterized by fibrotic nodules with concentrically arranged collagen fibers, central hyalinization, and fibrotic lesions [5]. In our case, white nodules were showed on the pericardial surface, and inflammatory cell infiltration and hyalinized fibrosis within the nodular tissue were found by the histopathological examination. It was diagnosed as silicosis nodules.

Although the deposition of silica is common in lung tissues, it can also accumulate in other organs like the brain, peritoneum, bone marrow, liver, and spleen [6]. Our patient presented with an extremely rare condition as silica affected the pericardium on evoking a chronic inflammatory response; these processes could be involved in pericarditis and recurrent pericardial effusion.

There are a few reports on silica involved in pericardial degeneration [2, 6]. Jiang and Shao reported a male stone miner patient having both silicosis and constrictive pericarditis [2]. Mohebbi et al. reported a pericardial plague seen in a patient with silicosis and pathology findings of the pericardial specimen which had a typical basket-weave collagen pattern suggesting silica deposits [6]. The mechanisms through which silica causes pericarditis are unclear; however, one potential cause is immune reactions [2]. Individuals with

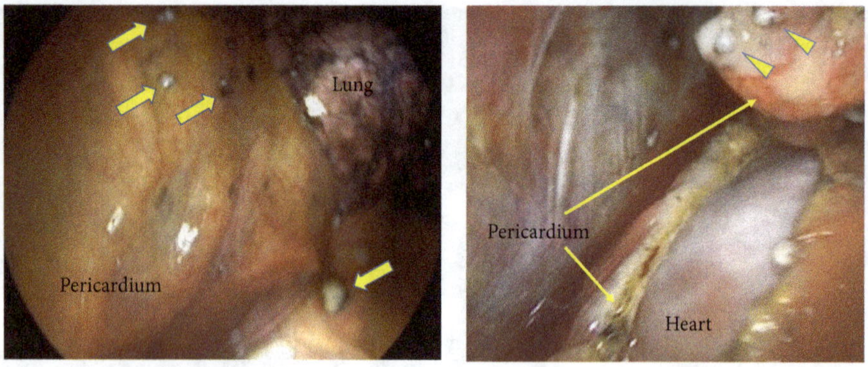

(a) (b)

FIGURE 2: (a) Multiple white, nodular deposits (yellow arrows) observed throughout the pericardium. (b) Pericardial fenestration was performed using the Harmonic Scalpel®. White nodular-like deposits (triangle) were found throughout the pleura and pericardium.

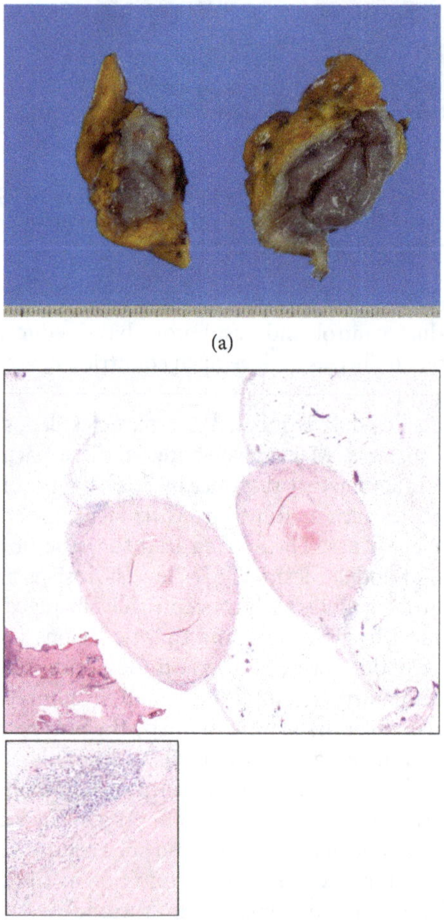

(a)

(b)

FIGURE 3: (a) Macroscopic findings of the resected pericardium. (b) Hematoxylin and Eosin staining revealed chronic infiltration of inflammatory cells and hyalinized fibrosis within the white nodular tissue of the resected pericardium.

silicosis manifest a significantly increased risk for autoimmune diseases such as rheumatoid arthritis, progressive systemic sclerosis, systemic lupus erythematosus, ANCA-associated small vessel vasculitis, and Wegener's granulomatosis [7]. It was considered that silica deposits broke the immune homeostasis [2, 7]. In addition, silica which has the nondegradable nature leads to saturation of the macrophages, and it has been demonstrated that macrophages that ingest silica release factors that increase biosynthesis by fibroblasts [7, 8]. Zeren et al. have reported that lymphatic and venous spread of the dust is thought to be responsible for extrapulmonary disease, because silica particles cannot be destroyed with phagocytosis and enzymatic reactions [3]. These immune responses may have affected not only the lungs but also the pericardium in our case. Another possibility is unrelated, yet concurrent, infections leading to pericarditis [2]. Exposure to silica dust is a potent risk factor for tuberculosis, as demonstrated by multiple studies [9]. However, the PCR result for tuberculosis was negative in our patient.

Because pericardial fenestration provides continuous drainage into the pulmonary cavity, absorption from the pleura is expected [10]. Consequently, pericardial fenestration carries a lower risk of pericardial effusion recurrence than temporary drainage methods like pericardiocentesis. A previous study has described that pericardial fenestration or pericardial biopsy via thoracoscopy is a safe and minimally invasive technique [10] and that the thoracoscopy approach can excise a larger window of the pericardium to prevent a recurrent effusion [10]. Our patient also achieved good outcomes following pericardial fenestration via thoracoscopy.

4. Limitations

This case report has some limitations. (1) Although histopathological examination has revealed that the degeneration of the pericardium is due to silicosis, the silica itself has not been identified from the pericardium. In addition, histopathological examination revealed chronic inflammatory cell (mainly lymphocytes) infiltration and hyalinized fibrosis within the nodular tissue, and it was diagnosed as a consistent finding as silicosis nodules. (2) The mechanisms through which silica causes pericarditis are still unclear. Further studies are needed in the future.

5. Conclusion

We reported an extremely rare case of silicosis complicated by pericarditis and pericardial effusion. The precise mechanisms through which silica deposits affect the pericardium are unclear; however, pericarditis and pericardial effusion could be the products of immune reactions induced by silica and/or translocation of silica dust via lung tissue. Although the pathological condition in which silicosis is involved in pericarditis as this case is very rare, we should be aware of such a pathological condition in the clinical practice.

References

[1] T. Sato, T. Shimosato, and D. M. Klinman, "Silicosis and lung cancer: current perspectives," *Lung Cancer: Targets and Therapy*, vol. 9, pp. 91–101, 2018.

[2] Y. Jiang and F. Shao, "A stone miner with both silicosis and constrictive pericarditis: case report and review of the literature," *BMC Pulmonary Medicine*, vol. 13, no. 1, p. 71, 2013.

[3] E. H. Xeren, T. V. Colby, and V. L. Roggli, "Silica-induced pleural disease: an unusual case mimicking malignant mesothelioma," *Chest*, vol. 112, no. 5, pp. 1436–1438, 1997.

[4] B. Hutyrová, P. Smolková, M. Nakládalová, T. Tichý, and V. Kolek, "Case of accelerated silicosis in a sandblaster," *Industrial Health*, vol. 53, no. 2, pp. 178–183, 2015.

[5] C. C. Leung, I. T. S. Yu, and W. Chen, "Silicosis," *The Lancet*, vol. 379, no. 9830, pp. 2008–2018, 2012.

[6] I. Mohebbi, A. Lameei, B. Booshehri, N. Aslanabadi, R. Maasomi, and M. Dehghani, "Pericardial plaque: a unique complication of silicosis," *Industrial Health*, vol. 49, no. 1, pp. 122–125, 2011.

[7] N. Ghahramani, "Silica nephropathy," *The International Journal of Occupational and Environmental Medicine*, vol. 1, no. 3, pp. 108–115, 2010.

[8] O. J. Stone, "Autoimmunity as a secondary phenomenon in scleroderma (and so-called human adjuvant disease)," *Medical Hypotheses*, vol. 34, no. 2, pp. 127–130, 1991.

[9] International Commission on Occupational Health (ICOH), "Preventing tuberculosis among silica dust exposed workers," *Occupational & Environmental Medicine*, vol. 75, no. 11, pp. 765-766, 2018.

[10] M. I. A. Muhammad, "The pericardial window: is a video-assisted thoracoscopy approach better than a surgical approach?," *Interactive CardioVascular and Thoracic Surgery*, vol. 12, no. 2, pp. 174–178, 2011.

8

A Case of an Abdominal Aortic Dissection in a Hemodynamically Stable Marfan Syndrome Patient Presenting without Pain

Hussein Al-Mohamad,[1] Kara Stout,[2] Taryn Bolling,[2] and Ronald Walsh[1]

[1]*Department of Cardiology, Largo Medical Center, Largo, FL, USA*
[2]*Department of Internal Medicine, Largo Medical Center, Largo, FL, USA*

Correspondence should be addressed to Hussein Al-Mohamad; halmohamad@vcom.vt.edu

Academic Editor: Assad Movahed

Introduction. Marfan syndrome (MFS) is a rare connective tissue disorder attributed to a defect in the fibrillin-1 gene. Aortic aneurysms and dissection are common causes of morbidity and mortality in Marfan syndrome. *Case Report.* A 43-year-old female with a history of MFS and a 4.0 cm dilated ascending aorta presented to her cardiologist reporting that since a C-section two years prior, the left side of her abdomen painlessly protruded when standing. An outpatient CT scan of the abdomen/pelvis noted a 5.5 cm abdominal aortic dissection, and she was directed to the hospital. Repeat CT scan of the abdomen/pelvis revealed a 5.6 cm dissecting aneurysm of the infrarenal abdominal aorta. The patient was admitted to the ICU and started on a nitroglycerin drip to maintain systolic blood pressure less than 110 mmHg. The patient underwent repair of her abdominal aortic dissection via a retroperitoneal approach, and she tolerated the procedure well. She was started on metoprolol tartrate 12.5 mg BID and aspirin 81 mg postoperatively. She was safely discharged with follow-up care. *Conclusion.* This case stresses the importance of having a low threshold to obtain imaging in a MFS patient with protruding abdomen, even though the patient may not have pain and be hemodynamically stable.

1. Introduction

Marfan syndrome (MFS) is a rare connective tissue disorder with an estimated incidence of about 1 in 5,000 persons in the United States; it is generally inherited in an autosomal dominant pattern [1, 2]. The pathogenesis involves a defect in the fibrillin-1 (FBN-1) gene located on chromosome 15 [2–4]. The role of FBN-1 is to provide structural support to tissues and to regulate elastogenesis [5]. Defects in this gene can lead to mitral valve prolapse (MVP), joint laxity, and ectopia lentis [5]. More serious clinical findings include aortic root dilatation and thoracoabdominal aortic aneurysms and dissections [2]. Annual echocardiograms are recommended for patients with known MFS to monitor for aortic root dilatation [6].

Several cases have been reported about abdominal aortic aneurysms, dissections, and ruptures [2, 3, 7–9]. In review of the literature, it is rare to find a case of a hemodynamically stable and fairly asymptomatic abdominal aortic dissection in a patient with MFS. We present such a case to increase awareness about this rare, yet severe complication.

2. Case Report

We present a case of a 43-year-old nonsmoking female with a past medical history of MFS, MVP, and a 4.0 cm dilated ascending aorta who presented to her cardiologist after being diagnosed with an abdominal aortic dissection by her OB-GYN. The patient noted that since a C-section 2 years prior, the left side of her abdomen protruded more when standing compared to the right. She denied associated abdominal, chest, or back pain. The patient was told that she may have a hernia in the past.

Because she was concerned about the asymmetry of her abdomen, she went to a new OB-GYN who ordered an abdominal CT scan of the abdomen/pelvis with IV contrast which showed a 5.5 cm abdominal aortic dissection. The patient was reluctant to go to the hospital until she saw her

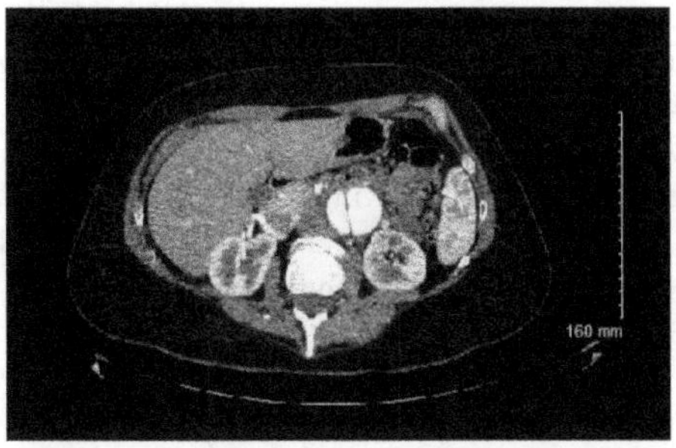

Figure 1: CT scan of the abdomen/pelvis with IV contrast demonstrating dissection of the abdominal aorta.

cardiologist a few days later, who recommended hospitalization and a consult for cardiothoracic surgery.

Interestingly, when the patient was seen in the hospital, she again denied chest pain, back pain, abdominal pain, dyspnea, nausea, vomiting, and dizziness. She only mentioned that her left side of the abdomen protrudes more than the right side when standing. On physical exam, patient had several features typical to MFS: she was tall, had a high arched palate, arachnodactyly, pectus excavatum, and her arm span was greater than her height. Her abdomen was soft, nontender, nondistended, had normal bowel sounds, and no pulsatile mass was appreciated. However, when the patient stood up, it was clear that the left side of her abdomen was bulging out in comparison to the right. A repeat CT scan of the abdomen/pelvis revealed a dissecting aneurysm of the infrarenal abdominal aorta measuring up to 5.6 cm (Figure 1); the false lumen supplied the left common iliac artery and the true lumen supplied the right common iliac artery. There was no evidence of thoracic aortic dissection.

The patient was admitted to the ICU and started on a nitroglycerin drip to maintain a systolic blood pressure less than 110 mmHg. Cardiothoracic surgery was consulted and recommended the patient to undergo open surgical repair of the abdominal aortic dissection. In order to risk stratify the patient prior to the procedure, the patient underwent a regadenoson nuclear medicine stress test, which was low risk for ischemia. The patient underwent successful repair of her abdominal aortic dissection via a minimally invasive open retroperitoneal approach. She tolerated the procedure well without postoperative complications.

The patient came into the hospital with no home medications. As she has reported in the past, she was tried on nebivolol but had failed it due to syncope. Given this, metoprolol tartrate 12.5 mg PO BID was started cautiously to provide long-term benefits for the patient's abdominal and thoracic aorta. The patient tolerated this medication well and was safely discharged home with close cardiovascular follow-up.

3. Discussion

Aortic root disease leading to aneurysmal dilation, regurgitation, and dissection is the most common cause of morbidity and mortality in MFS [10]. Aortic aneurysms and dissections arise due to the fragility of the aortic tissues, which are responsible for the rise of cystic medial necrosis [11].

Class I screening guidelines by the American College of Cardiology (ACC) include an echocardiogram at the time of diagnosis of MFS to determine the diameter of the aortic root and ascending aorta. Repeat imaging is recommended at six months and then annually to follow the rate of enlargement. If the aorta is greater than 4.5 cm or has significantly changed from baseline, more frequent screening is recommended [12].

Pregnancy in women with MFS can be challenging and is associated with an increased risk of aortic dissection. Recommendations include preconception counseling, TTE, and initiation of a protective beta blocker to slow the growth of the aortic root [13]. Serial TTE's are performed every 4-12 weeks to monitor aortic size, and C-section is recommended for aortic root dilation over 4 cm [13]. For aortic root dilatations over 4.5 cm, prophylactic aortic root and ascending aorta replacement is recommended prior to pregnancy [13]; but, even after successful root replacement, these patients remain at high risk for future events [14]. In our case, the patient followed the pregnancy guidelines and delivered her child via a C-section.

While MFS commonly leads to aortic root aneurysm and descending thoracic aortic aneurysms, the presence of an abdominal aortic aneurysm (AAA) and abdominal aortic dissection is rarely reported [3, 4, 7–9]. Up to 20% of patients with infrarenal AAAs have a family history of AAAs, suggesting there is a likely inherited component. Routine spiral thin-slice CT angiography or magnetic resonance angiography imaging of the entire aorta is recommended if there is enlargement of the descending thoracic aorta and abdominal aorta or if there is aortic dissection [6, 15].

Strategies to combat the increased risk of dissection include life-long β-blockade and elective aortic root replacement at 5 cm [2]. In addition, low-dose aspirin therapy helps to reduce major coronary events, cardiovascular-related mortality, and ischemic stroke risk [16]. Blood pressure management with a beta blocker up titrated to a goal heart rate less than 100 beats per minute with exercise is initiated to reduce cardiovascular mortality [15]. In our case, the patient was started on metoprolol tartrate and low-dose aspirin to maximize risk reduction for future events.

A decision to repair an AAA is also not MFS specific. It is based on size greater than or equal to 5.5 cm in males, 5 cm in females, or expansion of more than 5 mm in 6months or 1 cm over one year [16]. Risk factors for rupture include advanced age, male sex, Caucasians, smoking, other large vessel aneurysms, and atherosclerosis [16, 17].

The decision to repair a dissection depends on the type of dissection but is also not specific to MFS. Stanford Type A dissections are a surgical emergency [18]. For Stanford Type B dissections, medical treatments are initially attempted with esmolol or labetalol to keep systolic blood pressure between 100 and 120 mmHg and nitroprusside for vasodilation [18]. In Type B dissections, indications for surgery include the evidence of end-organ malperfusion, refractory pain, a rapidly expanding false lumen, impending or frank rupture, or a chronic aneurysmal dilation with a diameter of greater than or equal to 5 cm [18]. In our case, the patient met the final criteria of chronic aneurysmal dilation over 5 cm. Nitroprusside was used for both blood pressure management and vasodilation. Perioperative management includes an assessment for underlying coronary artery disease and ischemia if needed [6]. In this case, our patient underwent a regadenoson nuclear medicine stress test prior to her surgical procedure.

In general, endovascular techniques were not initially intended for thoracic and abdominal aorta pathology in patients with connective tissue diseases [14, 19]. Patients specifically with MFS were not included in initial endograft studies due to the fragile nature of the marfanoid aorta and concern for the predictive ability of the long-term radial force of the endograph to provide a seal without adversely damaging the vessel [14, 19]. Furthermore, as patients are typically young and with unclear long-term durability of current stent grafts, these should be avoided [14]. The European Society of Vascular Surgery guidelines recommend an open surgical procedure, with considerations for EVAR only if the patient is deemed too high of a risk for the open intervention [14] or if EVAR is a life-saving bridging procedure until definitive open repair can be safely performed [19]. In accordance, a minimally invasive retroperitoneal approach for open AAA repair was performed for our patient, and she tolerated the procedure without major complications.

4. Conclusion

In conclusion, this case stresses the importance of having a low threshold to obtain imaging in a MFS patient with bulging or protruding abdomen, even though, the patient may not have pain and be hemodynamically stable.

Consent

The patient provided informed consent.

Acknowledgments

We would like to thank Dr. Furqan Haq for his assistance in reviewing and helping to prepare this manuscript. Secondly, we would like to thank Dr. Christopher Stone of cardiothoracic surgery for his clinical input and surgical expertise. This research was supported (in whole or in part) by HCA Healthcare and/or an HCA Healthcare-Affiliated Entity.

References

[1] S. Westaby, "Aortic dissection in Marfan's syndrome," *The Annals of Thoracic Surgery*, vol. 67, no. 6, pp. 1861–1863, 1999.

[2] B. Wolfgarten, I. Kruger, and M. Gawenda, "Rare manifestation of abdominal aortic aneurysm and popliteal aneurysm in a patient with Marfan's Syndrome," *Vascular Surgery*, vol. 35, no. 1, pp. 81–84, 2001.

[3] A. Verstraeten, M. Alaerts, L. van Laer, and B. Loeys, "Marfan syndrome and related disorders: 25 years of gene discovery," *Human Mutation*, vol. 37, no. 6, pp. 524-531, 2016.

[4] T. Takayama, T. Miyata, and H. Nagawa, "True abdominal aortic aneurysm in Marfan syndrome," *Journal of Vascular Surgery*, vol. 49, no. 5, pp. 1162–1165, 2009.

[5] B. L. Loeys, H. C. Dietz, A. C. Braverman et al., "The revised Ghent nosology for the Marfan syndrome," *Journal of Medical Genetics*, vol. 47, no. 7, pp. 476–485, 2010.

[6] D. M. Milewicz, H. C. Dietz, and D. C. Miller, "Treatment of aortic disease in patients with Marfan syndrome," *Circulation*, vol. 111, no. 11, pp. e150–e157, 2005.

[7] T. Hagerty, P. Geraghty, and A. C. Braverman, "Abstract 12688: abdominal aortic aneurysm in Marfan syndrome: time for screening guidelines?," *Circulation*, vol. 132, Supplement 3, 2015.

[8] K. Lafferty, L. McLean, J. Salisbury, and L. T. Cotton, "Ruptured abdominal aortic aneurysm in Marfan's syndrome," *Postgraduate Medical Journal*, vol. 63, no. 742, pp. 685–687, 1987.

[9] S.-M. Yuan and H. Jing, "Cystic medial necrosis: pathological findings and clinical implications," *Brazilian Journal of Cardiovascular Surgery*, vol. 26, no. 1, pp. 107–115, 2011.

[10] J. N. Adams and R. J. Trent, "Aortic complications of Marfan's syndrome," *The Lancet*, vol. 352, no. 9142, pp. 1722-1723, 1998.

[11] D. P. Zipes, P. Libby, B. O. Bonow, D. L. Mann, G. F. Tomaselli, and E. Braunwald, *Braunwald's Heart Disease: A Textbook of Cardiovascular Medicine*, Elsevier, Philadelphia, PA, USA, Eleventh edition, 2019.

[12] L. F. Hiratzka, G. L. Bakris, J. A. Beckman et al., *ACC/AHA pocket guideline: guidelines for the diagnosis and Management of Patients with thoracic aortic disease*, The American College of Cardiology Foundation and the American Heart Association, 2010, https://www.acc.org/~/media/clinical/pdf-files/approvedpdfs/2015/01/13/11/13/thoracic%20aortic%20disease%202010%20pocket%20guide.pdf.

[13] S. Goland and U. Elkayam, "Pregnancy and Marfan syndrome," *Annals of Cardiothoracic Surgery*, vol. 6, no. 6, pp. 642–653, 2017.

[14] L. G. Svensson, N. T. Kouchoukos, D. C. Miller et al., "Expert consensus document on the treatment of descending thoracic aortic disease using endovascular stent-grafts," *The Annals of Thoracic Surgery*, vol. 85, no. 1, Supplement, pp. S1–S41, 2008.

[15] Marfan Foundation, "Overview of cardiac management of Marfan syndrome," 2014, https://www.marfan.org/resource/fact-sheet/cardiac-management-marfan-syndrome#.XbtVtEVKhE4.

[16] F. L. Moll, J. T. Powell, G. Fraedrich et al., "Management of abdominal aortic aneurysms clinical practice guidelines of the European society for vascular surgery," *European Journal of Vascular and Endovascular Surgery*, vol. 41, no. 1, pp. S1–S58, 2011.

[17] E. L. Chaikof, R. L. Dalman, M. K. Eskandari et al., "The Society for Vascular Surgery practice guidelines on the care of patients with an abdominal aortic aneurysm," *Journal of Vascular Surgery*, vol. 67, no. 1, pp. 2–77.e2, 2018.

[18] R. Erbel, V. Aboyans, C. Boileau et al., "2014 ESC guidelines on the diagnosis and treatment of aortic diseases: document covering acute and chronic aortic diseases of the thoracic and abdominal aorta of the adult: the Task Force for the Diagnosis and Treatment of Aortic Diseases of the European Society of Cardiology (ESC)," *European Heart Journal*, vol. 35, no. 41, pp. 2873–2926, 2014.

[19] D. Böckler, K. Meisenbacher, A. S. Peters, C. Grond-Ginsbach, and M. S. Bischoff, "Endovascular treatment of genetically linked aortic diseases," *Gefasschirurgie*, vol. 22, no. S1, Supplement 1, pp. 1–7, 2017.

9

A Case of Profound Bradycardia in Endurance Athlete with Severe Anorexia Nervosa

John Pueringer[1] **Joseph Cinderella**[2] **and M. Greg Treuth**[2]

[1]*Philadelphia College of Osteopathic Medicine, Philadelphia, Pennsylvania, USA*
[2]*TidalHealth, Salisbury, Maryland, USA*

Correspondence should be addressed to John Pueringer; jp8464@pcom.edu

Academic Editor: Takatoshi Kasai

We present a case of a 54-year-old woman with asymptomatic bradycardia who was referred for consideration of a pacemaker for profound chronic sinus bradycardia (heart rate is 33 beats per minute). Further, history and physical revealed a self-described endurance athlete with severe anorexia nervosa (AN). *Background.* Anorexia nervosa and endurance training are known contributors to bradycardia; however, profound asymptomatic sinus bradycardia in the 20-30 beats per minute is underdocumented in the literature and not a common presentation in any setting. The decision to implant a permanent pacemaker could potentially lead to further physical and psychological repercussions in such a frail patient.

1. Case Report

A 54-year-old female is presented to the emergency department (ED) with altered mental status. The patient had a history of anorexia nervosa (AN), treated with Mirtazapine and Hashimoto's thyroiditis, for which she took levothyroxine. The patient was compliant with medications. A week prior, she had a seizure-like episode attributed to hypoglycemia. Her admission blood glucose was 24 mg/dl. This was felt to be the etiology of her altered mental status, and following administration of 50% dextrose, she became responsive. Computed tomography (CT) scan of the head was unremarkable. The patient was found to be hypothermic at 89 degrees F, for which she was placed on bear hugger. She was markedly cachectic, weighting 88 pounds with a body mass index (BMI) of 14.12. The patient was a self-described endurance athlete and claimed to workout 4 hours per day, 7 days per week. She also followed a calorie deficient diet, which was evidenced by her extensive muscle wasting and cachectic state. In addition, she had chronic sinus bradycardia noted on previous records. She denied any purging or laxative use and was under the care of a psychiatrist for the AN; however, her condition has not improved much over the last few months. The patient was admitted for unexplained fugue, profound bradycardia, hypoglycemia, and hypothermia.

Cardiology was consulted regarding heart rate dipping into the 30 s; the thought, being this, could potentially also account for her altered mentation. Electrocardiogram (EKG) showed pronounced sinus bradycardia at 33 beats per minute (Figure 1). A week earlier, EKG in the ED showed sinus bradycardia at 36 beats per minute. In October 2019, EKG showed sinus bradycardia at 29 beats per minute (Figure 2). The oldest EKG noted was 2017, with a sinus bradycardia at 44 beats per minute (Figure 3). A Holter monitor had been ordered in the past, but the patient never carried it through. CT scan of the head showed no acute intracranial abnormality. Transthoracic echocardiogram revealed an ejection fraction (EF) of 55% but was otherwise unremarkable. Exercise tolerance test (ETT) was performed to look for chronotropic incompetence; however, there was no evidence to suggest chronotropic intolerance. The stress test was a regular "Bruce Protocol" ETT. She went $5'50''$ and achieved a heart rate of 141 beats per minute, and the test was reportedly stopped due to fatigue. She reached 7 metabolic equivalents (METs). The study was read and reported

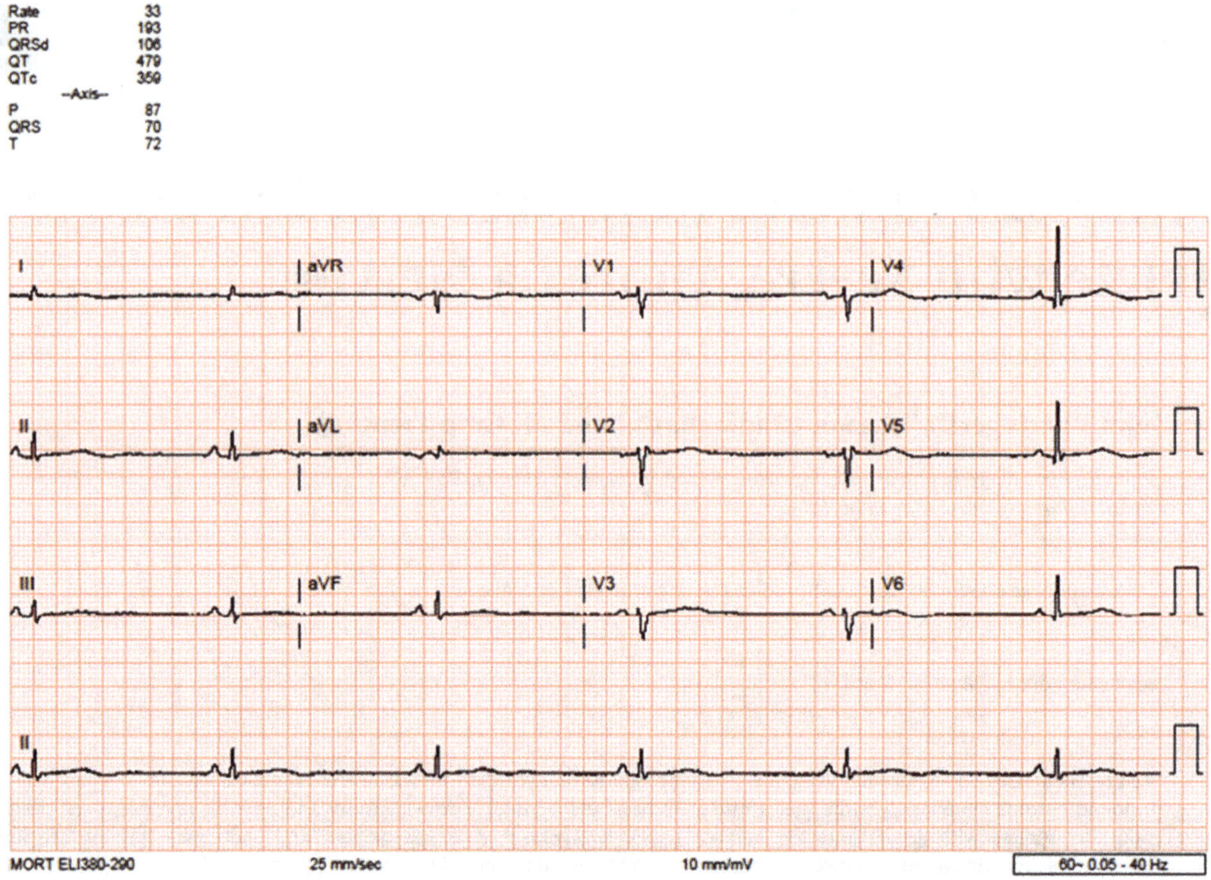

Figure 1: ECG from 11/2021 showing sinus bradycardia of 33 bpm.

that her heart rate accelerated as expected. She also reportedly achieved 85% of her predicted maximum heart rate (PMHR). Chest radiograph was unremarkable. Workup for adrenal insufficiency was negative. She did have a cortisol level of 30.1 mcg/dl and a prolactin level of 6.0 ng/dl; both of which are normal. Female sex hormone or growth hormone levels were not obtained.

2. Treatment

The patient was placed on telemetry on admission with no sign of heart block as evidenced on the EKG in Figure 1. The presumptive explanation for her symptoms was her profound hypoglycemia. She had Hashimoto's thyroiditis, although current labs revealed, essentially, the euthyroid state (Table 1). Electrophysiology (EP) was consulted for evaluation of treatment of sinus bradycardia with possible pacemaker implantation. Exercise tolerance test showed no evidence of chronotropic intolerance. In the absence of symptoms, ventricular arrhythmia or structural heart disease, and owing to normal ventricular function, no permanent pacemaker implantation was undertaken. The etiology of her chronic sinus bradycardia is likely multifactorial but related to her AN. The heart rate increased to 60 s during her stay. Refeeding was gradual to prevent refeeding syndrome and further heart damage. The patient would continue treatment with her psychiatric team in the outpatient setting, who currently had her on Mirtazapine 7.5 mg daily, with no current plans for a permanent pacemaker. A Holter monitor was considered but not done due to her past medical history of noncompliance. She was discharged home with arrangements for a life alert bracelet, glucose monitoring devices, and glucose tablets.

3. Case Discussion

Anorexia nervosa (AN) is a psychiatric disorder characterized by low body weight (e.g, BMI $< 18.5\,kg/m^2$) caused by disordered energy intake relative to requirements. It can also be secondary to endocrine and metabolic changes in the body. Anorexia nervosa has the highest mortality rate of any of the psychiatric disorders [1]. Weight loss and chronic malnutrition lead to dysfunction in multiple organ systems, notably cardiac dysfunction, where sudden cardiac death accounts for 60% of deaths associated with the disorder [2].

There are many documented cardiovascular complications of anorexia, including bradycardia, dilated cardiomyopathy, electrolyte-induced arrhythmias, hypotension, mitral valve prolapse, and pericardial effusion [3]. Anorexia nervosa can affect the structure and size of the heart by causing left ventricular atrophy and sometimes annular changes leading to mitral valve prolapse, possibly secondary to

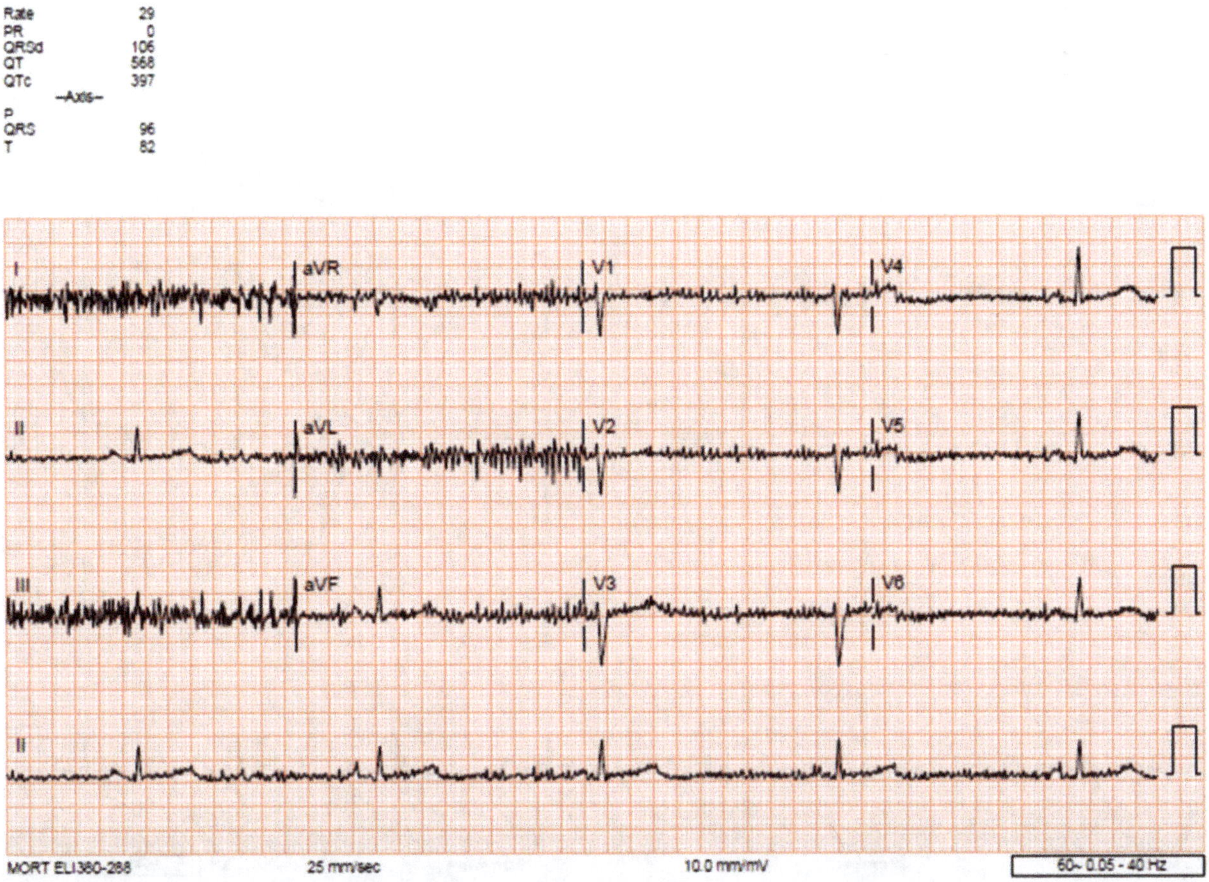

Figure 2: ECG from 10/2019 showing sinus bradycardia of 29 bpm.

reduced blood volume [2]. An autopsy study showed left ventricular atrophy with endocardial and interstitial fibrosis in a patient with AN [4]. It is plausible that bradycardia may be the hearts physiologic response to myocardial atrophy to prevent heart failure.

Effects of anorexia on the electrical activity of the heart include a heightened vagal tone in the setting of substantial weight loss. The mechanism of bradycardia in AN is thought to be due to cardiac vagal hyperactivity and decreased metabolism of energy utilization, due to low caloric intake [5]. It was reported that patient with AN had a 30% increase in vagal activity [5, 6]. A resting heart rate of less than 50 bpm was found in 70% of patients in a consecutive series [7]; however, most of the individuals were under the age of 25, compared to our 54-year-old patient. Furthermore, as we present here, a resting heart rate of 20-30 beats per minute is not as well documented. Patients may also present with prolonged QT_c interval secondary to electrolyte disturbances (such as hypokalemia, hypomagnesemia, and hypophosphatemia), which is thought to be the root of sudden cardiac death in patients with AN [1].

Anorexia can cause alterations in cardiac conduction and repolarization and thus result in a range of arrythmias. Sinus bradycardia has been described as the most common cardiovascular physical finding and the most common arrhythmia in patients with anorexia nervosa [7].

Resting bradycardia is a known physiologic change in endurance athletes. Studies have shown that endurance training is able to enhance vagal control of the heart and to reduce the resting HR by more than 8% in older adults who trained for more than 30 weeks [8]. Interestingly, D'Souza et al. posit that training-induced bradycardia may be the result of widespread remodeling of pacemaker ion channels, notably a downregulation of funny channel HCN4 and the corresponding ionic current [9]. In addition, the HERITAGE family study found that after 20 weeks of endurance training, resting heart rate is reduced by approximately 5 bpm, with greater reductions occurring in female than males [10]. Sinus bradycardia and first-degree atrioventricular block are common arrhythmias documented in endurance athletes, among other [11]. Therefore, it is probable that her aerobic training and AN had an additive effect on her vagal hyperactivity, or possible synergistic effect, although that would need to be studied further. However, her athletic training was self-described as a rigorous 4 hour, 7 days-a-week running schedule, but there was no real data in her chart that she participated in any sports or athletics other than her self-described running.

It is important to consider what led a 54-year-old female athlete to anorexia nervosa. She claimed to be physically active, although not well supported on chart review. We do not think she was an athlete who somehow decided to

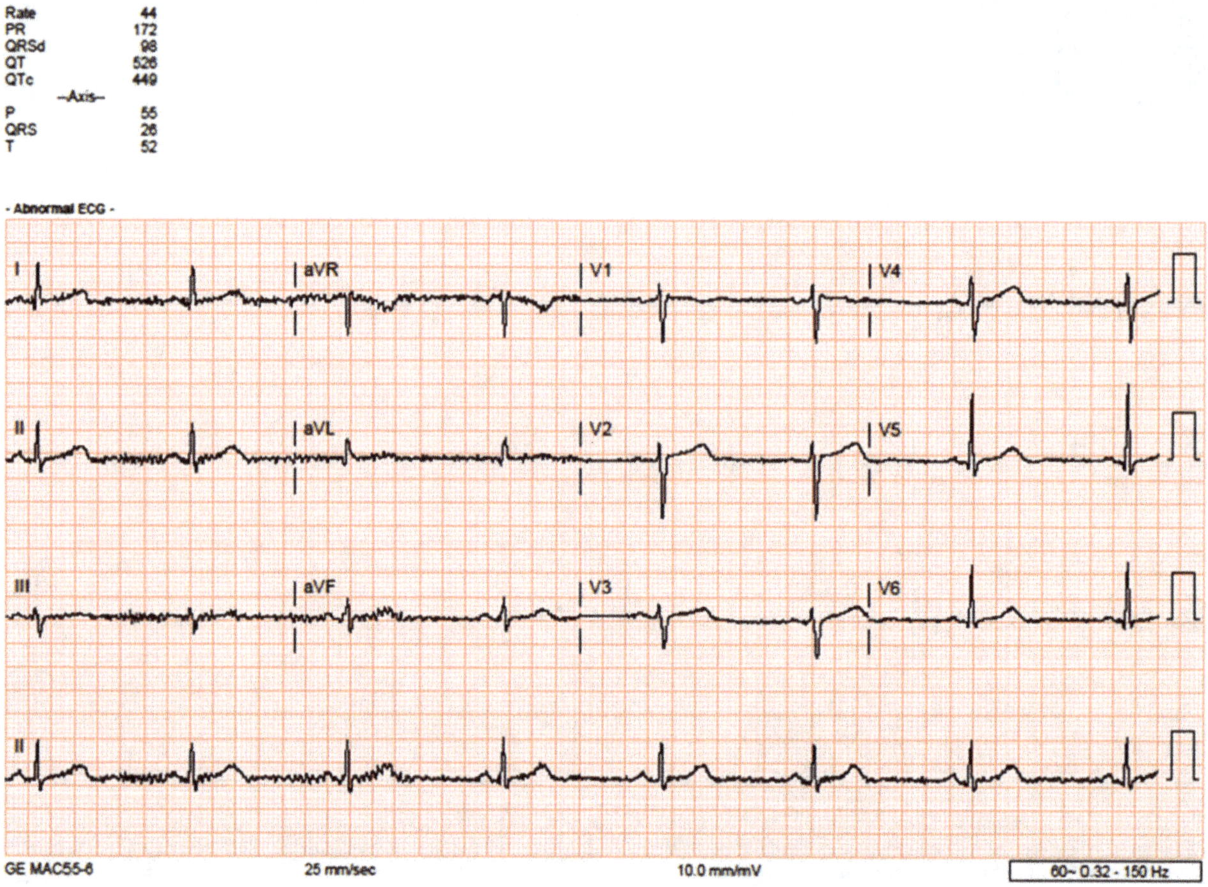

FIGURE 3: ECG from 09/2017 showing sinus bradycardia of 44 bpm.

TABLE 1: Notable vitals and laboratory values.

Vitals		Chemistries		CBC		Endocrinology	
Temp	89.6 F	Na	133 mEq/L	WBC	5.5/mm3	TSH	8.5 mU/L
Heart rate	33 bpm	K	3.7 mEq/L	Hb	12.5 g/dl	T3, free	1.9 ng/dl
Respiratory rate	10-14 bpm	Cl	99 mEq/L	Hct	36.20%	Free T4	1.12 ng/dl
Blood pressure	94-99/73-78	CO2	24 mEq/L	Plt	203/mm3	Cortisol	30.1 mcg/dl
Sp02	100%	BUN	47 mg/dl			Prolactin	6.0 ng/dl
POCT Glucose	47 mg/dl	Cr	0.75 mg/dl				
BMI	14.12	Glu	24 mg/dl				
		Calcium	8.3 mg/dl				
		Mg	2.1 mg/dl				
		ALT	81 U/L				
		AST	65 U/L				
		ALP	43 U/L				
		Bili total	0.6 mg/dl				
		Troponin	0.03 ng/ml				

become anorexic. It would appear that her primary issue was anorexia, and running helped her maintain what she felt was a desirable body weight. We would argue that she was not in particularly good shape for a runner, as documented by her limited functional capacity on the stress test. However, the importance of her proclaimed 28-hour per week training schedule is that it parallels prolific endurance athletes who typically perform 15 to 40 hours of training per week. Cycling, triathlon, cross-country skiing, rowing, and endurance running are examples of sports in which intensive training has been associated with the highest exercise capacities and the most profound cardiac remodeling [12]. Thus, any history of this prolific endurance training is likely contributing to her cachectic anorexic state in addition to exacerbating her presenting arrythmia through chronic remodeling and enhanced vagal tone. We notably did not consult psychiatry, because our patient was being treated in the outpatient setting with Mirtazapine 7.5 mg. On further chart review, our patient was unable to tolerate Fluoxetine and Sertraline due to side effects. In addition, she had a history of denying or creating excuses to eat or get intravenous nutrition when hospitalized for recurrent syncope, hypoglycemia, and unresponsive states. She understood that she had anorexia nervosa but minimized and denied the connection between her recurrent symptoms and her urgent medical status. Therefore, it would appear that her resistance to proper nutrition may be the primary culprit. Of note, Mirtazapine can cause orthostatic hypotension, hyponatremia, serotonin syndrome, increased QTc interval, and torsades de pointes, which is relevant in this patient with these symptoms and workup for syncope. Furthermore, bradycardia increases the risk for torsades de pointes. The combination of AN-induced bradycardia and Mirtazapine could put her at increased risk for torsades de pointes. However, based on her history of present illness and clinical findings, we do not feel like this influenced her syncopal episode.

A study by Mehler and Brown reported bradycardia in greater than 95% of anorexic patients, and hypotension likewise is quite common [13]. Our patient had both. The article then goes on to state that many of these patients attribute their bradycardia to what they perceive as an "athletic heart" and often attempt exercise to maintain or lose weight. Our patient was put on a treadmill to document chronotropic competence and avoid a pacemaker. She only went 5 minutes and 50 seconds on a Bruce protocol treadmill before stopping due to fatigue. That protocol would be 2.5 miles per hour (mph) at a 12-degree incline, hardly what an "athlete" would be capable of. The average person her age can go approximately 9 minutes, and an athlete should be able to go 12-15 minutes. Her systolic blood pressure (SBP) during the treadmill stress test remained in the 85-105 mmHg range, consistent with the chronic hypotension of anorexia. This posits that the bradycardia is related to heightened parasympathetic tone, as the body tries to conserve energy due to limited energy reserves from chronic starvation.

Low energy availability is a relatively common complaint among female athletes. Energy availability is defined as the difference between energy obtained through oral nutrition and energy expended with exercise. It is reasonable to conclude that low energy may result as a consequence of increased energy expenditure, decreased oral nourishment, or both. Chronic energy deficit in the female athlete can result in musculoskeletal and reproductive dysfunction. Low energy in combination with menstrual disorder and altered mineral bone density is known as the classic "female athlete triad". In individual cases, the patient may require multidisciplinary care from an endocrinologist, an orthopedic surgeon, a psychiatrist, an exercise physiologist, and in some cases, a cardiologist. Many female athletes, however, fail to maintain adequate energy intake. When this energy deficit is intentional, it is described as disordered eating. The energy deficit in anorexia nervosa causes a heightened parasympathetic tone that is part of the body's compensatory mechanism to conserve energy when faced with limited caloric reserves. Bradycardia and hypotension are the consequences.

Our indication for "treatment" would be a recognition that bradycardia is very common in anorexia, and understanding that pacing is rarely or never required. The most common indications for permanent pacemaker implantation are sinus node dysfunction (SND) and high-grade atrioventricular (AV) block [14]. For our patient, the absence of symptoms, ventricular arrhythmia or structural heart disease, and owing to normal ventricular function, we felt that permanent pacemaker implantation was unnecessary. According to the American College of Cardiology (ACC), the American Heart Association (AHA), and the Heart Rhythm Society (HRS) Guidelines on the Evaluation and Management of Patients with Bradycardia, in patients with sinus node dysfunction with minimal or infrequent symptoms without hemodynamic compromise, temporary transcutaneous or transvenous pacing should not be performed [15]. Furthermore, in asymptomatic patients with sinus bradycardia or sinus pauses that are secondary to physiologically elevated parasympathetic tone, permanent pacing should not be performed. Thus, unless the patient shows symptomatic bradycardia, a pacemaker is generally not indicated.

Accordingly, treatment should be directed at the underlying psychiatric issues and not for unnecessary pacemaker or other procedures. The stress test was done to confirm chronotropic competence, or the ability to appropriately raise one's heart rate with activity. Alternatively, a Holter monitor or another monitor could have been done. The problem with relying on a monitor is the difficulty in teasing out bradycardia as the cause of her recurrent near syncopal spells. In retrospect, the syncopal spells appear to be due to anorexia associated hypoglycemia, but confirming a lack cardiac syncope in light of the concerns related to her bradycardia.

Other possible etiologies of syncopal episodes and sinus bradycardia could be underlying heart disease, heart block, toxic ingestion of medication, electrolyte derangements (hyperkalemia), hypothyroidism, hypothermia, hypoxemia, hypovolemic shock, infection, and intracranial hypertension, but there was no clinical or lab evidence of this, and the echocardiogram revealed no structural or functional abnormalities to her heart. The EKG was able to rule out heart block or any underlying arrythmias.

Additionally, since this patient showed up bradycardic, hypoglycemic, hypotensive, mild hyponatremic, and with a syncopal episode, there was a concern for thyroid dysfunction as the etiology. She was diagnosed 3 months ago, initially with subclinical hypothyroid, but the patient was compliant with meds and in a euthyroid state. She was treated with Levothyroxine 50 mcg and 0.5 mg of Dexamethasone, and we also ordered an adrenocorticotropic hormone (ACTH) stimulation test, which was benign, helping us rule out adrenal insufficiency. The patient did present in a hypothermic state, but correction of her temperature did not affect her underlying heart rhythm. The patient did not present with a hypoxemic or hypovolemic picture.

4. Conclusions

Anorexia nervosa can cause profound sinus bradycardia due to cardiac vagal hyperactive and decreased caloric intake. In the presence of asymptomatic bradycardia secondary to severe anorexia nervosa, an implantable pacemaker did not appear necessary as it may cause more physical and psychological harm than good. Severe anorexia in combination with long-term aerobic training may have a synergistic effect on vagal tone and its effects on resting heart rate; however, that needs to be studied further.

Acknowledgments

This project is funded by the Richard A. Henson Student Research Awards provided by TidalHealth Richard A. Henson Research Institute.

References

[1] D. Casiero and W. H. Frishman, "Cardiovascular complications of eating disorders," *Cardiology in Review*, vol. 14, no. 5, pp. 227–231, 2006.

[2] P. Westmoreland, M. J. Krantz, and P. S. Mehler, "Medical complications of anorexia nervosa and bulimia," *The American Journal of Medicine*, vol. 129, no. 1, pp. 30–37, 2016.

[3] C. A. Moore and B. R. Bokor, "Anorexia Nervosa," in *StatPearls*, StatPearls Publishing Copyright © 2021, StatPearls Publishing LLC, Treasure Island (FL), 2021.

[4] I. Lamzabi, S. Syed, V. B. Reddy, R. Jain, A. Harbhajanka, and P. Arunkumar, "Myocardial changes in a patient with anorexia nervosa: a case report and review of literature," *American Journal of Clinical Pathology*, vol. 143, no. 5, pp. 734–737, 2015.

[5] M. Kollai, I. Bonyhay, G. Jokkel, and L. Szonyi, "Cardiac vagal hyperactivity in adolescent anorexia nervosa," *European Heart Journal*, vol. 15, no. 8, pp. 1113–1118, 1994.

[6] B. Ekblom, A. Kilbom, and J. Soltysiak, "Physical training, bradycardia, and autonomic nervous system," *Scandinavian Journal of Clinical and Laboratory Investigation*, vol. 32, no. 3, pp. 251–256, 1973.

[7] M. Yahalom, M. Spitz, L. Sandler, N. Heno, N. Roguin, and Y. Turgeman, "The significance of bradycardia in anorexia nervosa," *International Journal of Angiology*, vol. 22, no. 2, pp. 83–94, 2013.

[8] G. Huang, X. I. A. N. G. R. O. N. G. Shi, J. A. Davis-Brezette, and W. H. Osness, "Resting heart rate changes after endurance training in older adults: a meta-analysis," *Medicine and Science in Sports and Exercise*, vol. 37, no. 8, pp. 1381–1386, 2005.

[9] A. D'Souza, A. Bucchi, A. B. Johnsen et al., "Exercise training reduces resting heart rate via downregulation of the funny channel HCN4," *Nature Communications*, vol. 5, no. 1, p. 3775, 2014.

[10] J. H. Wilmore, P. R. Stanforth, J. Gagnon et al., "Heart rate and blood pressure changes with endurance training: the heritage family study," *Medicine and Science in Sports and Exercise*, vol. 33, no. 1, pp. 107–116, 2001.

[11] M. Abela and S. Sharma, "Electrocardiographic interpretation in athletes," *Minerva Cardioangiologica*, vol. 69, no. 5, pp. 533–556, 2021.

[12] A. L. Gerche and H. Heidbuchel, "Can intensive exercise harm the heart?," *Circulation*, vol. 130, no. 12, pp. 992–1002, 2014.

[13] P. S. Mehler and C. Brown, "Anorexia nervosa - medical complications," *Journal of Eating Disorders*, vol. 3, no. 1, p. 11, 2015.

[14] T. Dalia and B. S. Amr, "Pacemaker Indications," in *StatPearls*, StatPearls Publishing Copyright © 2021, StatPearls Publishing LLC, Treasure Island (FL), 2021.

[15] F. M. Kusumoto, M. H. Schoenfeld, C. Barrett et al., "2018 ACC/AHA/HRS guideline on the evaluation and management of patients with bradycardia and cardiac conduction delay: executive summary: a report of the American College of Cardiology/American Heart Association task force on clinical practice guidelines, and the Heart Rhythm Society," *Journal of the American College of Cardiology*, vol. 74, no. 7, pp. 932–987, 2019.

10

Aortic Valve Replacement and Penicillin Desensitization in a Patient with *Abiotrophia defectiva* Aortic Valve Endocarditis

S. Kumar,[1] **S. Mahmood,**[2] **A. Madras,**[3] **and A. Iyer**[4]

[1]*St. George Hospital, Sydney, Australia*
[2]*Hornsby Hospital, Sydney, Australia*
[3]*North Manchester General Hospital, Manchester, UK*
[4]*Northern Beaches Hospital, Sydney, Australia*

Correspondence should be addressed to S. Kumar; shejil_kumar@hotmail.com

Academic Editor: Assad Movahed

Abiotrophia defectiva is an uncommon and insidious yet destructive cause of infective endocarditis preferentially treated with penicillin/gentamicin and often requiring surgical treatment. A 60-year-old man with penicillin anaphylaxis history presented with fevers and a nonspecific constellation of symptoms. He was ultimately diagnosed with bicuspid aortic valve infective endocarditis based on blood cultures growing *A.defectiva* and echocardiographic evidence of bicuspid aortic valve, severe valvular regurgitation, and 5 × 7 mm vegetation. Aortic valve replacement and culture yielded penicillin-sensitive *A.defectiva*. After successful penicillin desensitization, antibiotic therapy was switched from vancomycin/gentamicin to benzylpenicillin. This is the first published case of penicillin desensitization in a patient with *A.defectiva*-associated infection. Penicillin desensitization, optimal antibiotic therapy, prompt aortic valve replacement, and close collaboration between cardiology and various other specialties were essential in achieving a positive outcome.

1. Introduction

Abiotrophia defectiva is a coccobacillus bacterium which is part of the normal flora of the intestinal tract, oral cavity, and urogenital tract [1]. *A.defectiva* has been reported to cause various deep-seated infections such as bacteremia, endocarditis, osteomyelitis, and endophthalmitis [2–6]. *A.defectiva* is an uncommon (<1%) but aggressive and potentially devastating cause of infective endocarditis with high rates of complications, surgery, treatment failure, and mortality [2, 7]. Penicillin is the preferred antibiotic therapy and patients often require surgical valvular replacement. We present the case of a 60-year-old man with fevers and nonspecific symptoms diagnosed with bicuspid aortic valve, *A.defectiva* bacteraemia, and aortic valve infective endocarditis with severe aortic regurgitation at presentation necessitating surgical aortic valve replacement. This is the first reported case where penicillin desensitization was utilized in a patient with *A.defectiva*-associated infection to facilitate optimal antimicrobial therapy. Written informed consent was obtained from the patient for publication.

2. Case Presentation

A 60-year-old man was referred to hospital by his general practitioner with fevers. He had 3-month history of lower back pain, night sweats, fatigue, and 13-kilogram weight loss. He had no significant past medical history or recent dental procedures, denied intravenous drug use, and was not taking any regular medications (including immunosuppressants). He reported a history of anaphylaxis to penicillin at 6 months of age.

On examination, he was tachycardic (102 bpm), normotensive (153/64 mmHg), and afebrile. He exhibited a grade 3/6 diastolic murmur in the aortic region and midlumbar spinal tenderness. He lacked signs of cardiac failure, neurological deficits, or peripheral stigmata of infective endocarditis. Systems review did not reveal any other infective source for his fevers. There was no clinical lymphadenopathy,

TABLE 1: Initial results of serum laboratory investigations.

Study	Result	Normal range (units)
C-reactive protein	88.1^{H}	<3 (mg/L)
Erythrocyte sedimentation rate	95^{H}	<21 (mm/h)
White cell count	7.7	4-11 ($\times 10^9$/L)
Neutrophils	6.2	2-8 ($\times 10^9$/L)
Platelets	302	150-450 ($\times 10^9$/L)
Hemoglobin	105^{L}	130-180 (g/L)
Mean corpuscular volume	91	80-99 (fL)
Creatinine	111^{H}	60-110 (μmol/L)
Urea	7.5	3-9 (mmol/L)
Estimated glomerular filtration rate	62	>59 (mL/min/1.73m^2)
Bicarbonate	28	22-32 (mmol/L)
Albumin	28^{L}	35-50 (g/L)
Corrected calcium	2.47	2.15-2.55 (mmol/L)
Phosphate	1.05	0.75-1.50 (mmol/L)
Thyroid-stimulating hormone	0.79	0.50-5.00 (mIU/L)
Free thyroxine	22.4	9-25 (pmol/L)

H: high; L: low. Initial full blood count and biochemistry revealed elevated inflammatory markers such as C-reactive protein and erythrocyte sedimentation rate. Other abnormalities included mild renal impairment, hypoalbuminemia, and normocytic anemia, all likely secondary to subacute infection. Thyroid function was normal.

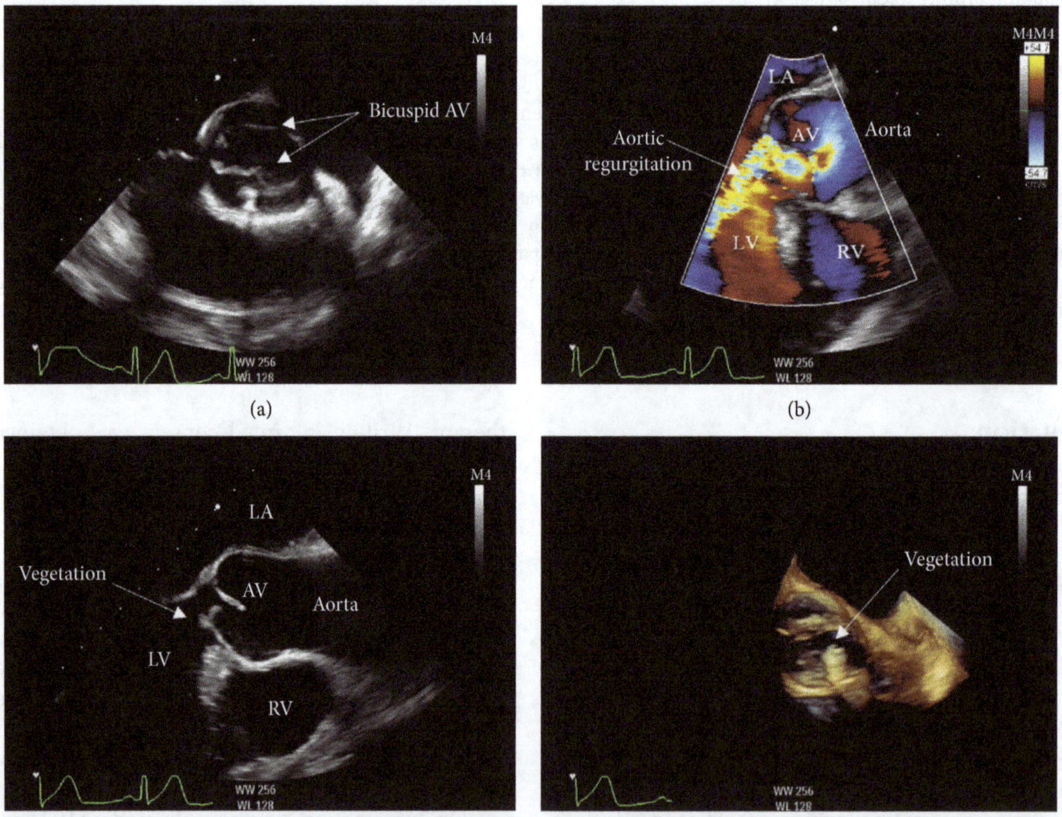

FIGURE 1: Transoesophageal echocardiogram images suggestive of bicuspid native aortic valve infective endocarditis. AV: aortic valve; LV: left ventricle; RV: right ventricle; LA: left atrium. Transoesophageal echocardiogram demonstrates the classical "fish mouth" appearance of aortic bicuspid valve during systole (a), severe aortic regurgitation (b), 5 × 7 mm vegetation adherent to the ventricular aspect of the aortic valve seen in two-dimensional echocardiogram (c), and three-dimensional echocardiogram (d).

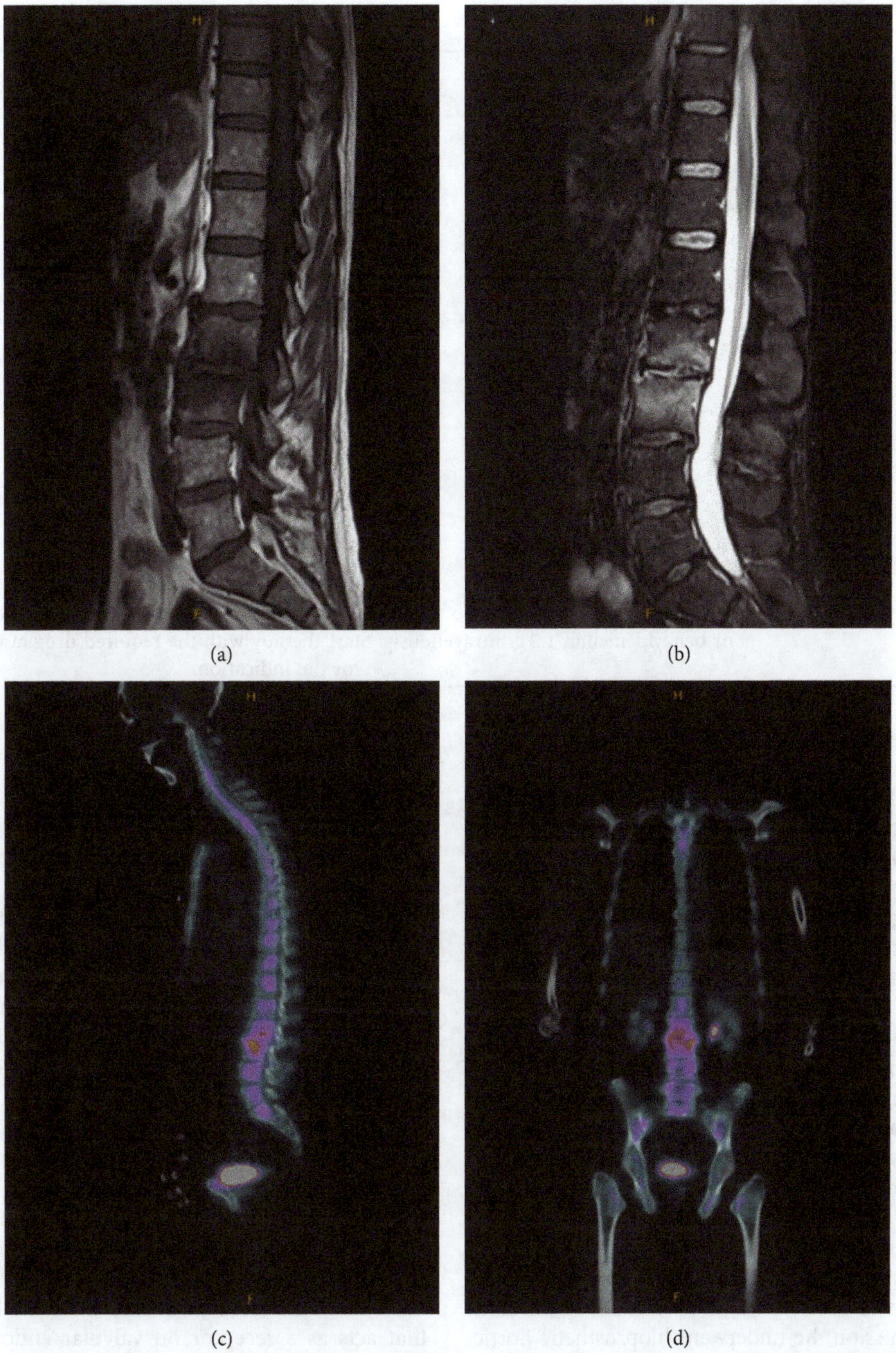

FIGURE 2: Magnetic resonance imaging (MRI) and single-photon emission computed tomography-computed tomography (SPECT-CT) images of the spine suggestive of L3/L4 discitis. Sagittal-view MRI whole spine demonstrates hypointense T1-weighted signal (a) and hyperintense short tau inversion recovery- (STIR-) weighted signal (b) surrounding the L3/L4 vertebral disc consistent with edema, with no evidence of collection. SPECT-CT whole spine shows increased uptake surrounding the L3/L4 vertebral disc in both sagittal view and coronal view consistent with L3/L4 discitis.

abdominal masses, or organomegaly or palpable purpura. Twelve lead electrocardiogram (ECG) demonstrated sinus tachycardia.

Initial biochemistry (Table 1) revealed elevated C-reactive protein (CRP) and erythrocyte sedimentation rate (ESR), mild renal impairment, hypoalbuminemia, and normocytic anemia. Inpatient blood culture yielded gram-positive coccobacilli in aerobic and anaerobic bottles after 18 hours of incubation deemed to be *A.defectiva*. Transthoracic echocardiogram (TTE) showed bicuspid aortic valve with moderate regurgitation and small vegetation, normal biventricular size and function, and mildly dilated ascending aorta (3.9 cm). *A. defectiva* was sensitive to vancomycin but not to penicillin (mean inhibitory concentration (MIC)

TABLE 2: Rapid oral phenoxymethylpenicillin desensitization protocol for adults.

Step (at 15-minute intervals)	Phenoxymethylpenicillin suspension (mg/mL)	Volume (mL)	Dose (mg)	Cumulative dose (mg)
1	0.5	0.1	0.05	0.05
2	0.5	0.2	0.1	0.15
3	0.5	0.4	0.2	0.35
4	0.5	0.8	0.4	0.75
5	0.5	1.6	0.8	1.55
6	0.5	3.2	1.6	3.15
7	0.5	6.4	3.2	6.35
8	5.0	1.2	6	12.35
9	5.0	2.4	12	24.35
10	5.0	4.8	24	48.35
11	50	1	50	98.35
12	50	2	100	198.35
13	50	4	200	398.35
14	50	8	400	798.35
15	Observe for 30 minutes; if no reaction occurs, administer phenoxymethylpenicillin 500 mg orally or benzylpenicillin 1.2 g intravenously. Start therapy with the required drug at the standard dosage for the indication.			

0.25-2.0 μg/mL). Three subsequent blood cultures were negative. Viral hepatitis, tuberculosis, human immunodeficiency virus (HIV), vasculitis, and malignancy screens were negative.

Transoesophageal echocardiogram (TOE) revealed severe aortic regurgitation with significant destruction and a 5×7 mm vegetation (Figure 1). Magnetic resonance imaging (MRI) scan of the whole spine and bone scan localized with single photon emission computed tomography (SPECT)/CT both suggested L3/L4 discitis (Figure 2). Orthopantomogram did not yield an abscess or dental caries. Cardiothoracic surgical referral prompted CT angiograms of coronary arteries (calcium score 0, no coronary artery disease) and thoracic aorta (4.2 cm ascending aorta aneurysm).

Empiric treatment of intravenous cephazolin (2 g three times daily), vancomycin 1.5 g twice daily, and gentamicin 80 mg twice daily was recommended by infectious diseases. On day 16 of admission, he underwent bioprosthetic aortic valve replacement followed by routine 48-hour intensive care admission. At 1 week postoperatively, TTE showed a well-seated and functioning bioprosthetic aortic valve with no vegetations. Aortic valve culture grew *A.defectiva* sensitive to penicillin (MIC 0.016 μg/mL). As per infectious and allergy specialist recommendations, he underwent oral desensitization to penicillin on postoperative day 7 in intensive care. He then switched to intravenous benzylpenicillin 1.8 g four hourly for 6 weeks from operation date, completed by 3 months of oral phenoxymethylpenicillin 750 mg six hourly.

At treatment completion, he regained 9 kilograms of weight and CRP normalized. He will follow up with an allergy specialist for penicillin skin testing to guide future endocarditis prophylaxis.

3. Discussion

Abiotrophia defectiva is an uncommon (<1%) yet aggressive cause of infective endocarditis with high rates of complications, surgery, and mortality [2, 7]. Patients experience fever, fatigue, and sometimes significant weight loss for a median 3 months prior to diagnosis [2]. Complications are frequent at presentation, such as valvular regurgitation, heart failure, and septic embolization, with surgery indicated in >50% of cases [2]. Delays in diagnosis occur due to the insidious and nonspecific nature of symptoms and difficulties in culturing the bacteria with fastidious growth requirements and gram-stain pleomorphism [2, 7]. Similarly, our patient had undiagnosed subacute infection for 3 months during which his aortic valve was destroyed to the point of severe regurgitation. *A.defectiva* has a particular predilection for abnormal aortic and mitral valves [2, 7] due to its moderate ability to bind fibronectin, an extracellular matrix protein that acts as a receptor on valvular endothelium [7]. Once diagnosed, treatment failure is common due to emerging penicillin resistance [8] and inadequate response to antibiotics that demonstrate in-vitro sensitivity [7]. In our case, despite 2 weeks of culture- and sensitivity-guided vancomycin therapy, his aortic valve culture still grew *A.defectiva.* Delayed diagnosis and treatment failure often necessitate urgent surgical valvular replacement due to valvular regurgitation causing heart failure [2, 7]. On presentation, despite our patient having severe aortic regurgitation, the vegetation was not large, and he lacked evidence of heart failure and so did not meet criteria for emergency surgery. However, given the destructive nature of *A.defectiva,* we proceeded with aortic valve replacement after a period of stabilization with intravenous antibiotics.

Penicillin is the most common cause of drug-induced anaphylaxis [9]. Penicillin desensitization is indicated in patients with penicillin anaphylaxis history when penicillin is the preferred antibiotic [9, 10]. Penicillin is first-line therapy for *A.defectiva* endocarditis [10], although due to intermediate penicillin-sensitivity, desensitization was not pursued initially. However, given aortic valve culture that showed penicillin-sensitive *A.defectiva* and was still positive despite 2 weeks of vancomycin, we performed oral desensitization in consultation with infectious diseases and local protocols (Table 2) [10]. Due to his new bioprosthetic valve and history of endocarditis, he is at high risk of future endocarditis and will require antibiotic prophylaxis prior to high-risk dental procedures [10]. Desensitization develops short-term tolerance however does not determine the presence of true allergy [9] and therefore, he will follow up with an allergy specialist for penicillin skin testing to determine if ampicillin can be used for future endocarditis prophylaxis.

4. Conclusion

Abiotrophia defectiva is an uncommon yet important and potentially destructive cause of subacute infective endocarditis and presents insidiously and nonspecifically, which can lead to delayed diagnosis and significant complications at presentation. Preferred antibiotic treatment is with penicillin/gentamicin, and surgical treatment is often required. We have described the first reported case of penicillin desensitization in *A.defectiva* endocarditis management. Valve culture proved a useful adjunct to blood culture testing in this patient and led to a meaningful change in management. Penicillin desensitization (which facilitated appropriate antibiotic therapy), prompt aortic valve replacement, and close collaboration between multiple specialties including cardiologists, cardiothoracic surgeons, intensivists, infectious, allergy, and microbiology specialists were essential in achieving a positive outcome. Cardiologists and other physicians should be made more aware of *A.defectiva* as a cause for subacute endocarditis and the need for earlier diagnosis and treatment to reduce the high rates of complications, surgery, and mortality.

References

[1] J. J. Christensen and R. R. Facklam, "Granulicatella and Abiotrophia species from human clinical specimens," *Journal of Clinical Microbiology*, vol. 39, no. 10, pp. 3520–3523, 2001.

[2] A. Téllez, J. Ambrosioni, J. Llopis et al., "Epidemiology, clinical features, and outcome of infective endocarditis due to Abiotrophia species and Granulicatella species: report of 76 cases, 2000-2015," *Clinical Infectious Diseases*, vol. 66, no. 1, pp. 104–111, 2018.

[3] P. C. Woo, A. M. Fung, S. K. Lau et al., "Granulicatella adiacens and Abiotrophia defectiva bacteraemia characterized by 16S rRNA gene sequencing," *Journal of Medical Microbiology*, vol. 52, no. 2, pp. 137–140, 2003.

[4] M. O. Alberti, J. A. Hindler, and R. M. Humphries, "Antimicrobial susceptibilities of Abiotrophia defectiva, Granulicatella adiacens, and Granulicatella elegans," *Antimicrobial Agents and Chemotherapy*, vol. 60, no. 3, pp. 1411–1420, 2015.

[5] C. Puzzolante, G. Cuomo, M. Meschiari et al., "Granulicatella adiacens and Abiotrophia defectiva Native Vertebral Osteomyelitis: Three Cases and Literature Review of Clinical Characteristics and Treatment Approach," *Case Reports in Infectious Diseases*, vol. 2019, 8 pages, 2019.

[6] M. A. Horstkotte, S. Dobinsky, H. Rohde et al., "Abiotrophia defectiva endophthalmitis with retinal involvement and infiltrative keratitis: case report and review of the literature," *European Journal of Clinical Microbiology & Infectious Diseases*, vol. 29, no. 6, pp. 727–731, 2010.

[7] M. A. Carleo, A. del Giudice, R. Viglietti, P. Rosario, and V. Esposito, "Aortic valve endocarditis caused by *Abiotrophia defectiva*: case report and literature overview," *In Vivo*, vol. 29, no. 5, pp. 515–518, 2015.

[8] K. Prasidthrathsint and M. A. Fisher, "Antimicrobial susceptibility patterns among a large, Nationwide cohort of Abiotrophia and Granulicatella clinical isolates," *Journal of Clinical Microbiology*, vol. 55, no. 4, pp. 1025–1031, 2017.

[9] D. Reynoso and A. C. White, "Penicillin allergy," *The New England Journal of Medicine*, vol. 382, no. 14, pp. 1379-1380, 2020.

[10] eTG complete by Therapeutic Guidelines [Internet], "Melbourne (Vic):Therapeutic Guidelines Ltd," 2020, https://tgldcdp.tg.org.au/etgcomplete.

11

Saphenous Vein Graft Aneurysm after Drug-Eluting Stent Implantation: Treatment by Covered Stent

Kyriacos Papadopoulos and Panayiotis Avraamides

Cardiology Department, Nicosia General Hospital, Nicosia, Cyprus

Correspondence should be addressed to Kyriacos Papadopoulos; kyriacospap@hotmail.com

Academic Editor: Ertugurul Ercan

Saphenous vein graft aneurysms (SVGAs) occur as a rare complication of coronary artery bypass graft but increases the risk of morbidity and mortality. Atherosclerosis is considered to be the most common cause of saphenous vein graft aneurysms. Other etiologies include infections, varicosities of vein grafts, and surgical technical issues. These aneurysms usually present as an incidental finding of a mediastinal or cardiac mass on chest radiograph. Symptomatic aneurysms may present with a wide variety of clinical manifestations such as chest pain/angina, shortness of breath, and myocardial infarction. Treatment options of SVG aneurysms include surgery, percutaneous intervention (including vascular plugs, covered stents, and embolization coils), and conservative management. Herein, we describe a case of a saphenous vein graft aneurysm that developed after percutaneous intervention, which has never been described, to our knowledge, in the previous literature. The aneurysm was treated with polytetrafluoroethylene covered stent implantation.

1. Introduction

Coronary artery bypass grafting (CABG) has become one of the most common surgical procedures performed across the world since Favaloro first described it in 1967. Aneurysmal dilatation of aorto-coronary SVGs (saphenous vein grafts) was first reported in 1975 by Riahi and associates [1].

Saphenous vein graft aneurysms (SVGAs) occur as a rare complication of coronary artery bypass graft but increases the risk of morbidity and mortality. Atherosclerosis [2] is considered to be the most common cause of saphenous vein graft aneurysms. Other etiologies include infections, varicosities of vein grafts, and surgical technical issues [3–5].

Treatment options include surgery, percutaneous intervention such as such as coil embolization and deployment of a polytetrafluoroethylene- (PTFE-) covered stent and conservative medical management [6, 7]. Herein, we describe a case of a saphenous vein graft aneurysm that developed after percutaneous intervention, which has never been described, to our knowledge, in the previous literature. The aneurysm was treated with polytetrafluoroethylene covered stent implantation.

2. Case Report

A 70-year old man with previous history of three vessel coronary artery bypass graft surgery (left anterior descending to left internal mammary artery (LIMA to LAD), SVG to posterior descending artery (PDA), and SVG to obtuse marginal (OM)) was admitted to the Cardiology Department of Nicosia General Hospital with unstable angina. The patient complained of tight precordial pain (lasting for 15-20 minutes), radiating to the left arm, and accompanied by sweating. Other medical problems include type 2 diabetes, dyslipidaemia, and hypertension.

On physical examination, the blood pressure was 115/78 mmHg, the heart rate 87 beats per minute, and the respiratory rate 16 breaths per minute.

His auscultation revealed normal first and second heart sounds with no murmurs. No third or fourth heart sounds were heard.

Electrocardiogram on admission showed normal sinus rhythm with T-wave inversions in leads II, III, aVF.

Chest X-ray was clear, and serial cardiac enzymes were negative.

The transthoracic echocardiogram revealed normal left ventricular size with mildly reduced ejection fraction (LVEF: 45%) and severe hypokinesis of the inferior wall. The aortic valve was trileaflet with mildly thickened leaflets. The mitral valve annulus was calcified with no mitral stenosis or regurgitation.

The patient underwent coronary angiography which demonstrated total occlusion of mid LAD after giving rise to the first diagonal branch that had a separate severe stenosis at its origin. LCx (left circumflex) was totally occluded from its proximal part after giving off the first obtuse marginal artery that was subtotally occluded at the ostium. RCA (right coronary artery) had a severe stenosis in the proximal segment and was totally occluded at the midportion. The LIMA to LAD graft was patent and flowing into distal native artery. The SVG to OM was occluded ostially, and the SVG to PDA had two consecutive critical stenoses located in the distal segment (Figure 1).

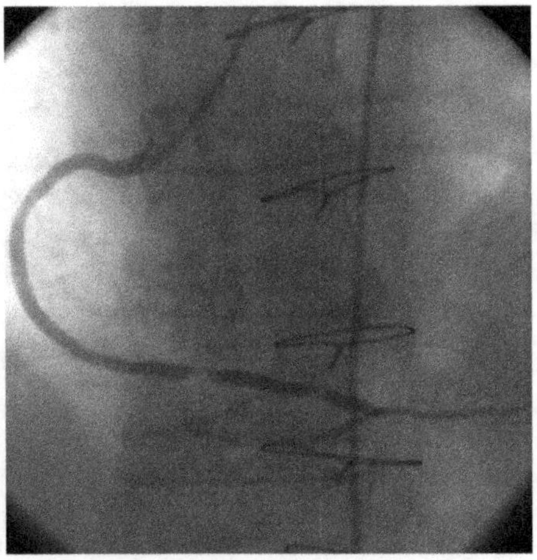

FIGURE 1: Coronary angiography revealed two consecutive critical stenosis of the SVG to PDA.

Ad hoc PCI to SVG to PDA was performed using a Judkin's right 4 (JR4) guiding catheter and a 0.014" balanced middleweight (BMW) guide wire. An everolimus eluting-stent (Xience Pro 4.0 × 33 mm) was directly deployed at the lesion site in the distal segment of the SVG (Figure 2(a)). Subsequent contrast injection revealed a focal aneurysm formation at the site of the stent implantation (Figure 2(b)). The patient maintained a stable hemodynamic condition with a BP = 132/72 and HR = 92. Considering the potential risk of rupture, we decided to seal the aneurysm with a PTFE-covered stent. A Graft Master 4.0 × 26 mm covered stent was deployed within the aneurysmal segment of the stented SVG at an inflation pressure of 10 atmospheres (Figure 3(a)). Postcovered stent angiogram showed total exclusion of the aneurysmal sac with good distal flow (Figure 3(b)). After the procedure, the patient remained hemodynamically stable and a control echocardiogram excluded pericardial effusion. The postoperative period was uneventful, and the patient was discharged after 2 days on 75 mg of aspirin and 75 mg of clopidogrel for at least one year. The patient was planned to have a control coronary angiogram at 6 months.

3. Discussion

SVGA is defined as a focal dilation of the vessel to 1.5 times greater than the proximal reference diameter [8].

The etiology of aneurysm formation remains unclear. Late aneurysm formation (i.e., >5 years after CABG) is thought to result from atherosclerotic degeneration leading to structural to weakening of the vessel and subsequent graft dilation [9]. Early aneurysms <12 months after surgery may be related to intrinsic weakness of the vessel wall [10], infections [11], and technical problems.

Although percutaneous coronary intervention-induced aneurysms of the coronary arteries have been increasingly reported over the past few years, formation of SVG aneurysm after stent implantation has never been described. In our case, the development of the aneurysm occurred after everolimus-eluting stent placement. Mechanical factors responsible for aneurysm formation include oversized balloons/stents or high-pressure balloon inflations, all of which can cause dissection and vascular wall injury with weakening and stretching of the vessel [12–14]. After drug-eluting stents implantation, the elution of antiproliferative drugs in combination with the presence of a polymer may result in delayed reendothelialization and incomplete healing, local hypersensitivity reactions, inflammation, and incomplete stent apposition, eventually leading to aneurysm formation [15].

CABG aneurysms can be divided into true aneurysms and pseudoaneurysms. Pseudoaneurysm is a rare postoperative complication, most frequently appearing within the first 6 months of surgery [16]. They usually occur often occur near sites of surgical anastomosis. Potential causes of pseudoaneurysms include surgical technical issues and infections.

True aneurysms commonly occur at the body of the graft [17, 18] and involve the entire vessel wall. They appear as a late complication [15] (>5 years after CABG) and are considered to be atherosclerotic in origin.

These aneurysms usually present as an incidental finding of a mediastinal or cardiac mass on chest radiograph [19–21]. Symptomatic aneurysms may present with a wide variety of clinical manifestations such as chest pain/angina, shortness of breath, and myocardial infarction.

Reported complications of SVG aneurysms include rupture, cardiac tamponade, hemothorax, distal embolization, myocardial infarction, compression of adjacent structures, and fistula formation [8, 22].

The most frequently affected grafts are those directed to the right coronary arteries, followed by the left anterior descending coronary artery.

Most aneurysms can be detected as mediastinal masses on plain chest X-rays. Computed tomography can demonstrate the size of the aneurysm and its relation to surrounding structures. Cardiac MRI is another noninvasive imaging modality with no risk of exposure to ionizing radiation which can define the content and mass effect of SVG aneurysm. Transesophageal echocardiography provides additional information about the size and intraluminal

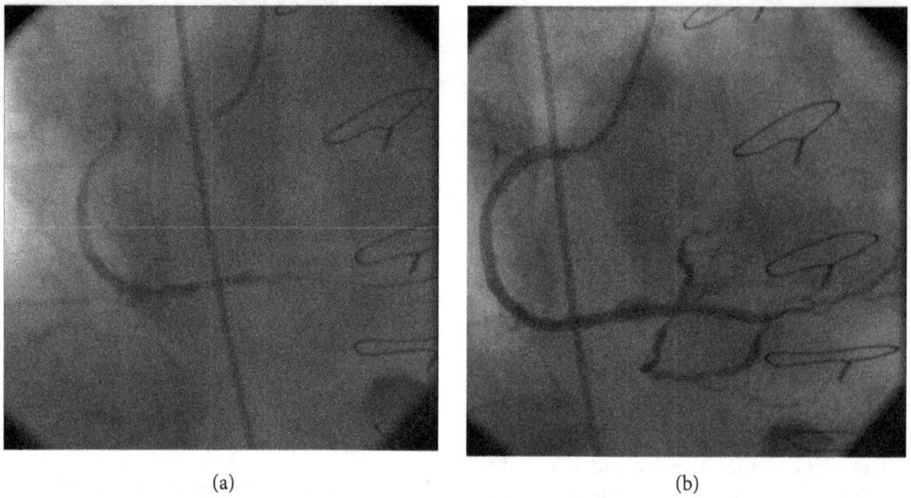

FIGURE 2: (a) An everolimus eluting-stent was implanted to cover the entire diseased segment of the SVG. (b) Check angiogram showed a focal aneurysm formation at the site of the stent implantation.

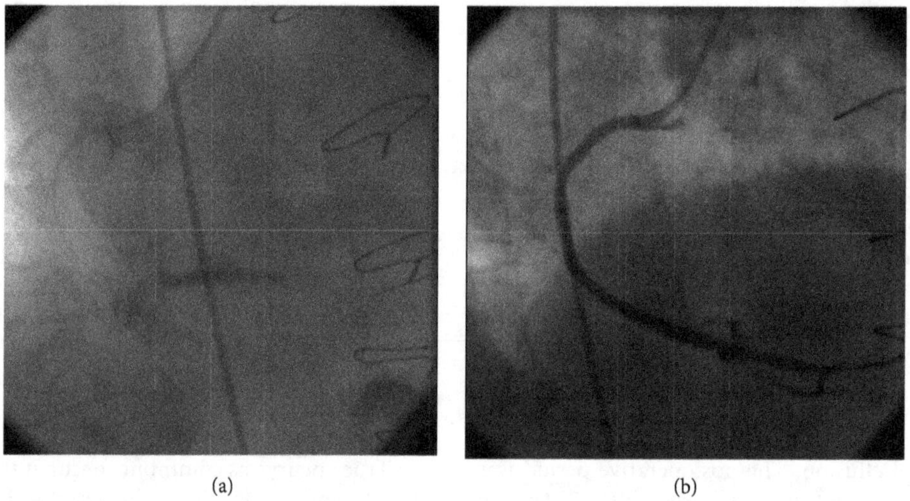

FIGURE 3: (a) A covered stent was deployed across the aneurysmal segment of the vessel. (b) Completion angiogram showed complete exclusion of the aneurysm.

pathology. Two-dimensional echocardiography can provide diagnostic information about the cardiac function [23]. Coronary angiography is definitive in confirming the graft dilatation and can detect other lesions in the native coronary circulation. Intravascular ultrasound (IVUS) has become the "gold standard" for providing critical diagnostic information regarding the morphology, pathogenesis, and management of SVG aneurysms. IVUS is useful to differentiate true aneurysm from pseudoaneurysm which is important in choosing the optimal strategy.

No consensus exists on the optimal treatment of patients SVG aneurysms. Currently, there are no evidence-based guidelines to direct patient management. Treatment options of SVG aneurysms include surgery, percutaneous intervention (including vascular plugs, covered stents, and embolization coils), and conservative management. In asymptomatic patients with small SVGAs (less than 1 cm in diameter), conservative medical management may be reasonable. Operative therapy may include aneurysmal resection or ligation followed by bypass grafting when the native coronary artery requires further revascularization. In patients with other indications for cardiac surgery (multiple territories requiring revascularization or concomitant valve surgery) or mechanical complications, surgical treatment should be pursued. In addition, for patients with graft anatomy not amenable to stent implantation, surgery is the preferred method of treatment. Percutaneous treatment offers an alternative method of management in elderly patients where risk of repeat surgery is very high. Different approaches are used depending upon the anatomic characteristics of the aneurysm and coronary circulation. Interventions utilizing coil embolization [24] or vascular plug insertion [25] are indicated when the affected graft is occluded or the coronary territory is perfused. Covered stent implantation is considered a suitable option when continued antegrade SVG flow is required [6, 26, 27]. In our patient, the SVG was patent, so a covered stent was selected as the preferred treatment.

References

[1] M. Riahi, C. Mark Vasu, L. A. Tomatis, R. J. Schlosser, and G. Zimmermann, "Aneurysm of saphenous vein bypass graft to coronary artery," *The Journal of Thoracic and Cardiovascular Surgery*, vol. 70, no. 2, pp. 358-359, 1975.

[2] J. Mayglothling, M. P. Thomas, J. B. Nyzio, M. D. Strong, and L. E. Samuels, "Aneurysm of aortocoronary saphenous vein Graft:," *The Heart Surgery Forum*, vol. 7, no. 4, pp. E317–E320, 2004.

[3] M. B. Mitchell and D. N. Campbell, "Pulmonary artery compression by a giant aortocoronary vein graft aneurysm," *The Annals of Thoracic Surgery*, vol. 69, no. 3, pp. 948-949, 2000.

[4] M. L. Williams, E. Rampersaud, and W. G. Wolfe, "A man with saphenous vein graft aneurysms after bypass surgery," *The Annals of Thoracic Surgery*, vol. 77, no. 5, pp. 1815–1817, 2004.

[5] M. Riahi, K. S. Stone, C. L. Hanni, E. Fierens, and R. E. Dean, "Right ventricular-saphenous vein graft fistula: Unusual complication of aorta- coronary bypass grafting," *The Journal of Thoracic and Cardiovascular Surgery*, vol. 87, no. 4, pp. 626–628, 1984.

[6] D. Walters, M. Patel, and W. Penny, "Saphenous vein graft aneurysm: a case-based review of percutaneous management," *Cardiovascular Revascularization Medicine*, vol. 20, no. 12, pp. 1190–1195, 2019.

[7] R. S. Dieter, A. K. Patel, D. Yandow et al., "Conservative vs. invasive treatment of aortocoronary saphenous vein graft aneurysms: treatment algorithm based upon a large series," *Cardiovascular Surgery*, vol. 11, no. 6, pp. 507–513, 2003.

[8] F. D. Ramirez, B. Hibbert, T. Simard et al., "Natural history and management of aortocoronary saphenous vein graft Aneurysms," *Circulation*, vol. 126, no. 18, pp. 2248–2256, 2012.

[9] Z. Vlodaver and J. E. Edwards, "Pathologic changes in aortic-coronary arterial saphenous vein grafts," *Circulation*, vol. 44, no. 4, pp. 719–728, 1971.

[10] B. M. Ennis, D. M. Zientek, N. T. Ruggie, R. A. Billhardt, and L. W. Klein, "Characterization of a saphenous vein graft aneurysm by intravascular ultrasound and computerized three-dimensional reconstruction," *Catheterization and Cardiovascular Diagnosis*, vol. 28, no. 4, pp. 328–331, 1993.

[11] B. Douglas, B. Bulkley, and G. Hutchins, "Infected Saphenous Vein Coronary Artery Bypass Graft with Mycotic Aneurysm: Fatal Dehiscence of the Proximal Anastomosis," *Chest*, vol. 75, no. 1, pp. 76-77, 1979.

[12] P. A. Slota, D. L. Fischman, M. P. Savage, R. Rake, and S. Goldberg, "Frequency and Outcome of Development of Coronary Artery Aneurysm *After* Intracoronary Stent Placement and Angioplasty," *The American Journal of Cardiology*, vol. 79, no. 8, pp. 1104–1106, 1997.

[13] A. Baumbach, J. A. Bittl, E. Fleck et al., "Acute complications of excimer laser coronary angioplasty: A detailed analysis of multicenter results," *Journal of the American College of Cardiology*, vol. 23, no. 6, pp. 1305–1313, 1994.

[14] M. R. Bell, K. N. Garratt, J. F. Bresnahan, W. D. Edwards, and D. R. Holmes Jr., "Relation of deep arterial resection and coronary artery aneurysms after directional coronary atherectomy," *Journal of the American College of Cardiology*, vol. 20, no. 7, pp. 1474–1481, 1992.

[15] J. Aoki, A. Kirtane, M. B. Leon, and G. Dangas, "Coronary artery aneurysms after drug-eluting stent implantation," *JACC: Cardiovascular Interventions*, vol. 1, no. 1, pp. 14–21, 2008.

[16] R. Puri, B. K. Dundon, D. P. Leong, S. G. Worthley, and M. I. Worthley, "Giant saphenous vein graft pseudoaneurysm rupture presenting with cardiac tamponade," *Heart, Lung and Circulation*, vol. 18, no. 1, pp. 52–54, 2009.

[17] K. Pintar, J. J. Barboriak, W. D. Johnson, and E. D. Co, "Atherosclerotic aneurysm in aortocoronary artery saphenous vein graft," *Archives of Pathology & Laboratory Medicine*, vol. 102, pp. 287-288, 1978.

[18] O. Topaz, M. S. Rutherford, S. Mackey-Bojack et al., "Giant aneurysms of coronary arteries and saphenous vein grafts: angiographic findings and histopathological correlates," *Cardiovascular Pathology*, vol. 14, no. 6, pp. 298–302, 2005.

[19] H. le Breton, D. Pavin, T. Langanay et al., "Aneurysms and pseudoaneurysms of saphenous vein coronary artery bypass grafts," *Heart*, vol. 79, pp. 505–508, 1998.

[20] J. A. Quin, I. B. Cetindag, V. Mukerji, R. P. Embrey, A. L. Grasch, and S. R. Hazelrigg, "Letter to the Editor," *Angiology*, vol. 55, no. 5, pp. 587-588, 2004.

[21] S. Gupta, T. Khan, L. W. Stephenson, D. Cooley, and J. Schnader, "Clinical conference on management Dilemmas," *Chest*, vol. 118, no. 6, pp. 1769–1775, 2000.

[22] K. Nishimura, Y. Nakamura, S. Harada et al., "Saphenous vein graft aneurysm after coronary artery bypass grafting," *Annals of Thoracic and Cardiovascular Surgery*, vol. 15, no. 1, pp. 61–63, 2009.

[23] V. Dzavik, M. Lemay, and K. L. Chan, "Echocardiographic diagnosis of an aortocoronary venous bypass graft aneurysm," *American Heart Journal*, vol. 118, no. 3, pp. 619–621, 1989.

[24] A. Maroo, P. A. Rasmussen, T. J. Masaryk, S. G. Ellis, A. M. Lincoff, and S. Kapadia, "Stent-assisted detachable coil embolization of pseudoaneurysms in the coronary circulation," *Catheterization and Cardiovascular Interventions*, vol. 68, no. 3, pp. 409–415, 2006.

[25] I. Mylonas, Y. Sakata, M. H. Salinger, and T. Feldman, "Successful closure of a giant true saphenous vein graft aneurysm using the Amplatzer vascular plug," *Catheterization and Cardiovascular Interventions*, vol. 67, no. 4, pp. 611–616, 2006.

[26] S. S. El-Jack, S. Pornratanarangsi, D. C. McNab, R. A. Luke, and M. W. Webster, "Percutaneous treatment of a large vein graft aneurysm with covered and conventional stents," *Circulation*, vol. 113, no. 1, pp. 8-9, 2006.

[27] Q. Jehangir, C. Lambert, and A. Sawar, "Saphenous vein graft pseudoaneurysm repair with GraftMaster," *Cureus*, vol. 10, 2018.

12

Case Report: TAVI in a Patient with Single Coronary Artery and Bicuspid Valve

Murielle Bertin,[1] Mohamed Aboukofa,[1] Pierre Francois Laterre,[2] and Zuhair Yousif[3]

[1]*Department of Anaesthesia, Mediclinic City Hospital, Dubai Health Care City, Building 37, Dubai, UAE*
[2]*Intensive Care Department, Saint Luc University Hospital, UCL, Avenue Hippocrate 10, 1200 Brussels, Belgium*
[3]*Department of Cardiology, Mediclinic City Hospital, Dubai Health Care City, Building 37, Dubai, UAE*

Correspondence should be addressed to Murielle Bertin; murielle.bertin@mediclinic.ae

Academic Editor: Assad Movahed

A single coronary artery is a rare congenital abnormality which consists of one coronary artery arising from the aortic trunk by a single coronary ostium and providing the perfusion of the entire myocardium. Its prevalence is approximately 0.024-0.066% of the population undergoing coronary angiography. A bicuspid aortic valve is the most common congenital cardiac abnormality and is found in 0.4-2.25% of the population. The coexistence of these two abnormalities together with severe aortic stenosis is extremely rarer. We report a patient who underwent transcatheter aortic valve implantation (TAVI) with a single coronary artery and a bicuspid valve. The procedure was successful, and the patient was discharged home without complication. To the best of our knowledge, this is the first report of these combined abnormalities and TAVI.

1. Introduction

A single coronary artery is at a high risk of coronary obstruction during a TAVI procedure. The bicuspid aortic valve is also at a high risk of coronary obstruction. In addition, there is an increased risk of paravalvular leakage and the need for operative pacemaker device placement.

Patients with bicuspid aortic valves have previously been excluded from clinical trials involving TAVI, and this abnormality continues to be a relative contraindication for the use of TAVI.

However, a recent success in the placement of new-generation valves means that a bicuspid aortic valve is no longer a contraindication to TAVI and this technique may offer a viable alternative to open-heart surgery in the elderly population.

2. Case Presentation

A 65-year-old woman with severe, symptomatic aortic stenosis was admitted to a hospital for a TAVI. Her past medical history included type 2 diabetes mellitus, hypertension, diabetic chronic kidney disease, and dyslipidemia. The patient was well known to have a bicuspid aortic valve and had been followed up by echocardiography for 20 years. She complained of exertional dyspnea for the last three months and was admitted with severe pulmonary edema. Following careful assessment, it did appear that the primary precipitant for refractory pulmonary edema is severe aortic stenosis. The aortic valve area of a heavily calcified valve was only 0.3 cm^2. Aortic valve replacement was a necessary therapeutic strategy to achieve hemodynamic stability and reduce in-hospital mortality.

Contrast-enhanced computed tomography (CT) scan was contraindicated because of her renal impairment. Noncontrast computed tomography would not have added significant diagnostic information to influence the treatment plan. Catheterization with limited contrast injections for coronaries, aortic root, and peripheral bed had provided the required details to plan the procedure with less contrast than computed tomography with contrast. In addition, noninvasive imaging with echocardiography has been used pre and postprocedure.

Coronary angiography was normal but revealed a single right coronary artery, with the left main coronary artery arising from the proximal right coronary artery (Figure 1). This is a very rare congenital malformation which can be a lethal obstruction of the orifice of the right coronary artery occurring secondary to stenosis or because of coronary emboli during the deployment of a new aortic valve.

The distance of the single coronary artery to the bicuspid aortic valve was >12 mm and to the annulus of the valve was >20 mm, and to S5 was 25 mm (Figure 2).

Echocardiography showed a severe bicuspid aortic valve stenosis with a gradient of 80/50 and a valve area of 0.3 cm (Figure 3). Mild mitral regurgitation was observed, but there is no aortic regurgitation.

An electrocardiogram showed a normal sinus rhythm.

The patient was informed by the cardiac team, and it was agreed to proceed with an urgent TAVI procedure.

A direct implantation of Evolut Pro, 26 mm valve from Medtronic, was performed using a right femoral artery approach. Close monitoring of the single coronary artery with coronary angiography revealed no complications (Figure 4). The left main coronary artery took its origin from the proximal right coronary artery. 2Proglide was used on the right-hand side, with 6F Angioseal on the left side; a hundred mL contrast medium was used.

The procedure was performed in the cardiac catheter laboratory under local anaesthesia plus sedation, and the patient remained hemodynamically stable throughout.

The patient was then transferred to the intensive care unit for observation and was discharged to the ward the following day. The patient remained in sinus rhythm and did not require a pacemaker postoperatively.

The post TAVI echocardiography showed a well-functioning aortic valve with trivial paravalvular leakage and no pericardial effusion. Ejection fraction was 70% with a peak and mean gradient after TAVI of 10/4. The mild mitral valve regurgitation apparent before the procedure remained unchanged.

The patient was asymptomatic and consequently discharged home after 3 days. The two-week follow-up showed a well-functioning valve with similar echocardiography. The electrocardiogram confirmed normal sinus rhythm, and the patient remained asymptomatic.

3. Case Discussion

Single coronary artery is a very rare congenital artery anomaly. It is found in approximately 0.03 to 0.05% of the population undergoing coronary angiography [1].

Lipton and coworkers propose a very useful angiographic classification and describe "R" as the right type and "L" as the left type according to the site of origin of the single coronary artery in the right or left sinus of Valsalva [2].

The etiology of a single coronary artery is unclear. This anomaly can be asymptomatic or may lead to angina, syncope, myocardial infarction, cardiac arrhythmia, congestive heart failure, or sudden death in case of stenosis or blockage of the only coronary artery ostium.

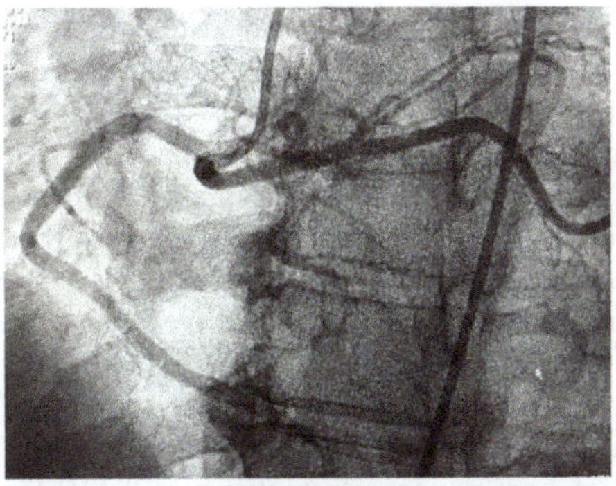

Figure 1: Single coronary artery with the left main coronary artery coming from the right coronary artery.

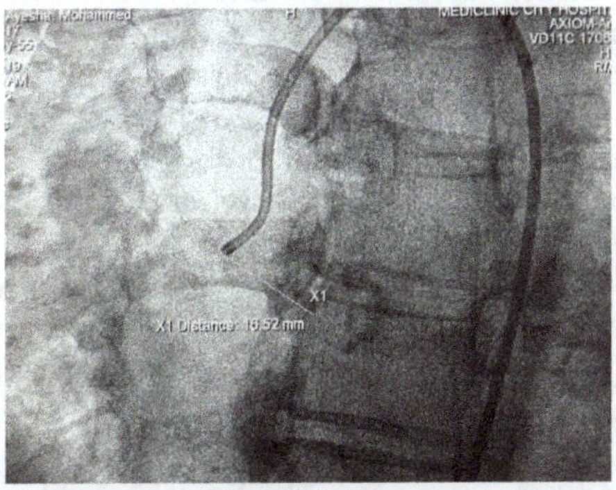

Figure 2: Calculation of the distance between the single coronary artery and the aortic valve.

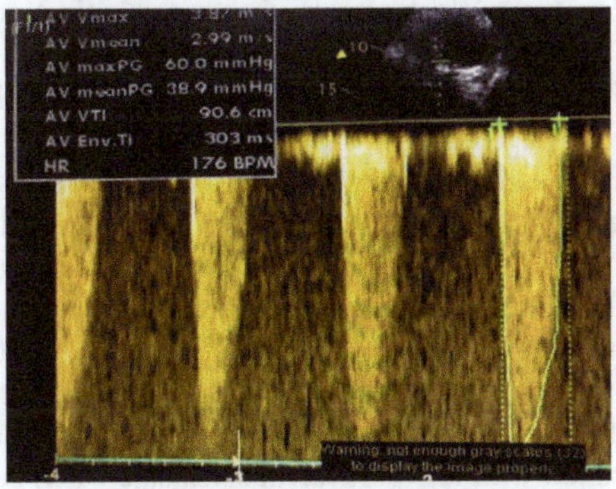

Figure 3: Echography done just before TAVI.

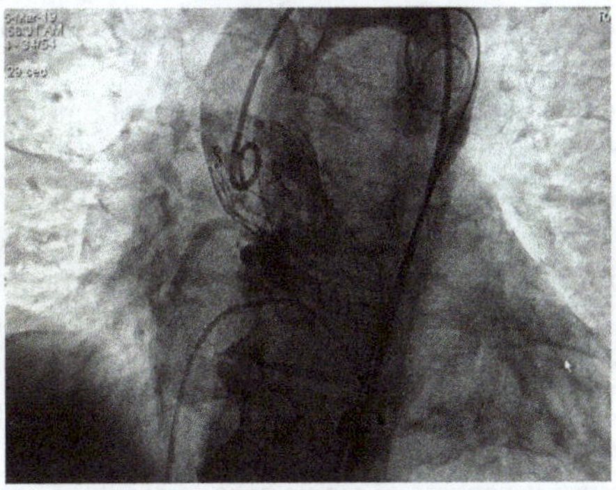

Figure 4: 26 mm Evolut Pro valve in place.

In the case of TAVI, valve deployment should be extremely cautious because any obstruction of this only coronary artery could be proven fatal.

Another challenge for the operator in this case was the bicuspid aortic valve as it resulted in a smaller opening with heavy calcification which bulged down close to the interventricular node. Hence, passing the wire from the femoral artery through the valve took longer time and was more technically challenging and the procedure could be expected to be more proarrhythmogenic than usual. In cases of the bicuspid aortic valve, the literature commonly reports the need for insertion of a permanent pacemaker post-TAVI [3].

The asymmetric nature of the bicuspid valve orifice and heavy regional calcification has been a challenge for adequate valve positioning and expansion for TAVI operators. There is an increased risk of coronary occlusion, aortic dissection, and annular rupture in these patients.

A careful evaluation of the aorta is compulsory as a bicuspid aortic valve is often associated with coarctation of the aorta, aortic dissection, and aortic aneurysm. These aortic pathologies may necessitate surgical intervention, rather than TAVI.

An additional challenge for the operator is correct valve selection. Nowadays, the use of a CT angiography may improve the selection of the valve size and device [4]. This minimizes the risk of complications including aortic annulus rupture, perivalvular leak, and coronary occlusion.

A large study comparing CT scans of bicuspid and tricuspid valves showed that aortic valve ellipticity indices were smaller in patients with bicuspid valves (1.24 vs 1.29) but the annular area was larger (5.21 vs. 4.63 cm^2) than that with tricuspid valves. We know that more calcification of the annulus and eccentric leaflets in the bicuspid valve give a higher chance of paravalvular leakage and higher chance of the need for pacemaker implantation after TAVI.

Compared to the tricuspid valve, TAVI operators will pay extra attention to the angiographic visualization of the annulus level and selection of proper projection for implantation of the valve. There is a risk of elliptic distortion or noncircular expansion, and it seems that risks are less when the valve is placed deeper below the annulus level than exactly at the level of the annulus. Self-expanding valves seem safer and are associated with less paravalvular leakage when compared to balloon mounted prostheses.

There are different classifications of the bicuspid valve, and the most widely used is that of Sievers and Schmidtke [5], based on the number of cusps, presence of raphes, and the position and symmetry of the cusps.

There is a relatively higher proportion of patients requiring pacemaker implantation after TAVI if they have bicuspid aortic valves.

Risk factors for coronary obstruction are low origin of the coronary arteries, bulky calcifications, a small sinus of Valsalva and valve misplacement, or coronary emboli.

Patients so afflicted will present with severe hypotension immediately after the balloon valvuloplasty or bioprosthesis implantation.

In previous reports of single coronary artery with TAVI, operators performed angiography during balloon valvuloplasty to anticipate the risk of coronary obstruction [6]. In one case, the operator placed a coronary wire to serve as a protection of the single coronary during balloon valvuloplasty and bioprosthesis implantation [7].

Another team did not perform any protective intervention during TAVI for the single coronary but used a self-expandable valve because of the recapturable property of the valve.

A Medtronic Core Valve can be recaptured up to 2/3 of the bioprosthesis deployment. In the case of any complication during TAVI, e.g., coronary obstruction, the valve can then be recaptured by the operator [8].

In our case, the operator spent time localizing precisely the single coronary artery origin before positioning and deploying the new valve very cautiously. The position of the valve was carefully adjusted, guided by intraoperative imaging with aortic root injections. The ample cusp to coronary ostia distance did not mandate the need for dedicated coronary protection procedures. There was no need to recapture the new valve which was perfectly positioned on the first attempt. No arrhythmia occurred, and no pacemaker was required. Very good valve functioning with only a trivial leakage was demonstrated on the echocardiogram performed immediately after the placement of the Medtronic valve. The patient was stable hemodynamically and did not require any inotropic support.

All data generated or analyzed during this study are included in the case presentation of this article: Figures 1–4.

4. Conclusion

We describe here a successful case of TAVI in a patient presenting with a combination of two rare abnormalities: a single coronary artery and a bicuspid aortic valve. The coexistence of a single coronary artery with severe aortic stenosis is extremely rare. The most feared complication of TAVI is a lethal obstruction of the single coronary artery origin. There are limited reports in the literature of TAVI associated with single coronary artery and no case of a bicuspid valve with a single coronary artery and TAVI. To our knowledge, this is the first reported case of TAVI with a self-expandable bioprosthesis. The procedure used the new Medtronic valve which can be recaptured in case of misplacement.

References

[1] F. Fengli, H. Jin, and Y. A. Feng, "A rare case of single right coronary artery with congenital absence of left coronary artery in an adult: a case report," *Journal of Cardiothoracic Surgery*, vol. 10, p. 57, 2015.

[2] M. J. Lipton, W. H. Barry, I. Obrez, J. F. Silverman, and L. Wexler, "Isolated single coronary artery: diagnosis, angiographic classification, and clinical significance," *Radiology*, vol. 130, no. 1, pp. 39–47, 1979.

[3] R. Das and R. Puri, "Transcatheter treatment of bicuspid aortic valve disease: imaging and interventional considerations," *Frontiers in Cardiovascular Medicine*, vol. 5, p. 91, 2018.

[4] A. H. Frangieh and A. M. Kasel, "TAVI in bicuspid aortic valves 'made easy," *European Heart Journal*, vol. 38, no. 16, pp. 1177–1181, 2017.

[5] H. H. Sievers and C. Schmidtke, "A classification system for the bicuspid aortic valve from 304 surgical specimens," *Journal of Thoracic and Cardiovascular Surgery*, vol. 133, pp. 1226–1233, 2007.

[6] E. Sorbets, M. Choby, and D. Tchetche, "Transcatheter aortic valve implantation with either CoreValve or SAPIEN XT devices in patients with a single coronary artery," *Journal of Invasive Cardiology*, vol. 24, no. 7, pp. 342–344, 2012.

[7] J. Giri, W. Y. Szeto, J. Bavaria, and H. C. Herrmann, "Transcatheter aortic valve replacement with coronary artery protection performed in a patient with an anomalous left main coronary artery," *Journal of the American College of Cardiology*, vol. 60, no. 6, p. e9, 2012.

[8] H. Dursun, J. Z. Gonencer, O. Karabay, A. C. Erdal, and D. Kaya, "TAVI in a patient with single Coronary Artery: the choice of self-expandable valve may be reasonable," *Balkan Medical Journal*, vol. 33, no. 3, pp. 357–359, 2016.

13

Mechanical Circulatory Support in Management of Cardiogenic Shock and Myxedema Coma

Jelena Z. Arnautovic,[1] **Randi Connor-Schuler**,[2] **and Randy Ip**[1]

[1]*Division of Cardiovascular Medicine, St. John Providence Ascension Health System, Warren, MI, USA*
[2]*Department of Emergency Medicine, Henry Ford Health System, Detroit, MI, USA*

Correspondence should be addressed to Jelena Z. Arnautovic; jzarnautovic@gmail.com

Academic Editor: Manabu Shirotani

The cardiovascular system is a major target of thyroid hormone action and the two systems are closely interlinked. It can be greatly impacted even with subtle alterations in thyroid function. Caution is needed when implementing thyroid hormone replacement in patients with severe hypothyroidism, especially in the setting of ischemic coronary artery disease. If not properly treated, myxedema may ensue. Given the high mortality of myxedema coma, supportive care may not always suffice and patients may require more invasive interventions. We present a challenging case of a patient with overt hypothyroidism with concurrent acute coronary syndrome which subsequently lead to myxedema coma and cardiogenic shock. A transcaval approach for the delivery of an Impella 5.0 (Abiomed Inc., Danvers, MA) was utilized in supporting this patient. To our knowledge, this is the first reported case that describes the use of a mechanical circulatory support in treating myxedema-induced cardiovascular collapse.

1. Introduction

Thyroid function and the cardiovascular (CV) system have an intricate relationship as patients with untreated thyroid dysfunction may develop an accelerated onset of symptomatic CV disease [1]. Modifiable atherosclerotic risk factors, including hypercholesterolemia, diastolic hypertension, increased carotid intimal-media thickness, and reduced endothelial nitric oxide, accompany overt hypothyroidism and could be reversible with proper TH replacement [2]. Although there is a close relationship between thyroid function and cardiovascular health, there have been no interventional studies of TH replacement in patients with acute myocardial infarction that have been published to date, therefore making a causal relationship between thyroid dysfunction and outcomes difficult to ascertain [1].

We present a challenging case of a patient with overt hypothyroidism complicated by myxedema with concomitant ischemic heart disease. This case is also remarkable for the use of a transcaval access for the delivery of an Impella 5.0 (Abiomed Inc., Danvers, MA) in supporting myxedema-induced cardiovascular collapse, which to our knowledge has not been previously documented.

2. Case Report

A 41-year-old male, without regular medical care, initially presented in the outpatient setting with progressive fatigue, weight gain, shortness of breath, and lower extremity edema over the past year. At that time, he was diagnosed with hypothyroidism (TSH 136 uIU/mL) and was started on 50 μcg PO levothyroxine daily. Two days later, he presented to the emergency room with chest pain and worsening shortness of breath. The patient was admitted for further evaluation which included an ischemic workup for coronary artery disease.

A diagnostic cardiac catheterization was performed and the patient was noted to have multivessel obstructive coronary disease with a severely reduced ejection fraction. The patient subsequently underwent stenting of the left anterior descending and left circumflex coronary arteries. However, within 24 hours, the patient developed cardiogenic shock

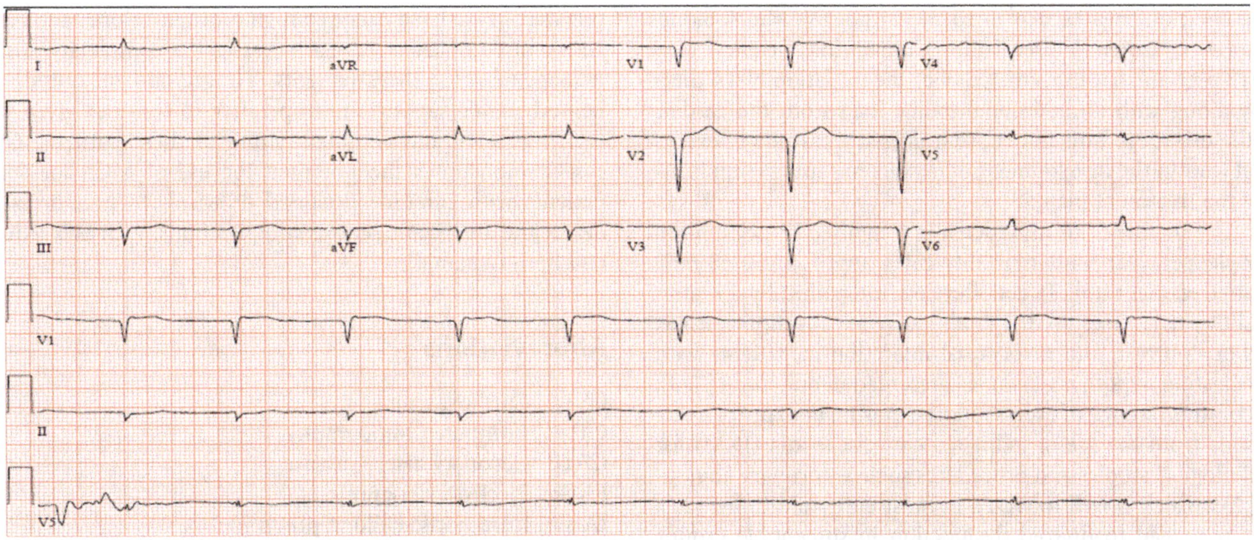

FIGURE 1: Admission electrocardiogram. Low-voltage junctional bradycardia with anteroseptal and inferior Q waves.

and a second percutaneous intervention was emergently done to address the right coronary artery lesion. Due to patient's condition, an intra-aortic balloon pump (IABP) was utilized and he was transferred to another institution for escalation of care.

Upon arrival to the second institution, vital signs demonstrated a blood pressure of 67/31 mmHg, a heart rate of 68 bpm, an oral temperature of 35.7°C, a respiratory rate of 14, and an oxygen saturation of 99% on 4 L nasal cannula. Evaluation of the patient was significant for altered mental status and signs of systemic hypoperfusion with cold extremities in the lower extremities. The physical exam also was positive for bilateral nonpitting edema in all extremities. Further pertinent positives on the physical exam were notable for thinned hair to the lateral eyebrows, macroglossia, a waxy, yellow appearance to his skin, and an absence of hair on the lower extremities.

Initial laboratory findings included hemoglobin of 7.7 g/dL, platelets of 24 K/μL, and a TSH level of 51.09 uIU/mL with free T4 of 0.26 ng/dL and free T3<1.0 pg/mL. Thyroid peroxidase was also noted to be elevated at 209 IU/mL (normal < 9 IU/mL). An electrocardiogram was obtained which showed diffuse Q waves (Figure 1). Cardiac monitoring was reviewed which demonstrated low-voltage complexes with an intermittent junctional bradycardia. Bedside echocardiogram revealed severely reduced systolic ejection fraction of 10% with mild to moderate RV dysfunction.

Patient's clinical presentation was consistent with myxedema coma, and the patient was treated with stress-dose steroids and intravenous levothyroxine. Given the refractory cardiogenic shock, the IABP was upgraded to a transcaval Impella 5.0 upon admission. Patient's clinical condition subsequently improved as his lactate cleared from 5.5 mmol/L to 1.1 mmol/L; vasopressors were discontinued; Impella wean commenced over the course of a few days. Unfortunately, his clinical course was complicated with acute ischemia of his right lower extremity on day 6 leading to acute renal failure and sepsis. Ischemia was likely multifactorial with a large 24F venous sheath from the Impella exerting pressure on the femoral artery also containing 5F arterial line; the patient also developed an aortic thrombus further impairing perfusion. Despite emergent revascularization efforts and Impella removal, the muscles were nonviable. Family was informed of the need for an above the knee amputation; however, the family decision was to proceed with comfort care and the patient died on the 8th day of hospitalization.

3. Discussion

Thyroid function plays a significant role in the health of the cardiovascular system. Thyroid hormone activates cytoprotective mechanisms, stimulates cell growth, and promotes neoangiogenesis and metabolic adaptation. In the acute myocardial infarction setting, optimal thyroid function aids in cardioprotection by reducing myocardial damage and reversing left ventricular (LV) remodeling [3]. A recent meta-analysis showed that patients with subclinical hypothyroidism are at higher risk of developing cardiovascular events, particularly with TSH levels > 10 μU/L, and patients with untreated hypothyroidism are at an increased risk of bradycardia, systolic and diastolic dysfunction, and increased peripheral vasoconstriction [3, 4].

Patients with newly diagnosed severe hypothyroidism and significant cardiovascular risk factors may present a difficult challenge for the clinician. Great caution is needed when implementing TH replacement in this subset of patients, as thyroxine (T4) therapy increases the metabolic demands of the body which can provoke myocardial ischemia. Patients at risk for ischemic heart disease may require risk stratification for coronary disease. If coronary insufficiency is apparent, prompt management should be implemented to improve the oxygen supply to the ischemic myocardium before increasing the myocardial demand with T4 [5].

It was likely that our patient infarcted prior to initial presentation to the outside facility and had a preexisting cardiomyopathy from long-standing, untreated, hypothyroidism in addition to underlying ischemic disease. Patient's presentation may be explained by cardiogenic shock alone. However, patient's preexisting cardiac insufficiency may have been further exacerbated after the initiation of T4 therapy along with an additional iodine load from the cardiac catheterization. This may have triggered a cascade of events that lead to the development of myxedema coma complicating the treatment plan.

The incidence of myxedema is roughly 0.22 per million people per year with mortality rates approaching 30-60% with treatment [6]. It can develop idiopathically or after additional stresses to the body such as infection, stroke, iodine contrast, and myocardial infarction in patients with preexisting hypothyroidism, as presented in our study [7, 8]. A common source of excess iodine exposure in many patients results from the use of iodinated contrast media (ICM) for radiological studies and procedures such as coronary angiography, which is well tolerated in most euthyroid individuals but may lead to thyroid dysfunction in susceptible groups [9, 10]. The prevalence of thyroid dysfunction after coronary angiogram contrast exposure is not very well described, and no specific guidelines exist [9]. Several studies have shown a clear and definitive association between ICM exposure and the development of overt hypothyroidism [9, 11, 12]. Case control studies suggest that ICM exposure at least doubles the risk of subsequent overt hyperthyroidism and triples the risk of overt hypothyroidism [9], and Lee et al. noted that 22% of their study population developed an abnormal TSH within one to four weeks of receiving an elective computed tomography scan [13].

The main mechanism for iodine contrast-induced hypothyroidism is known as a failure to escape the Wolff-Chaikoff effect, first described in 1948 [14]. This effect is usually transitory and does not typically lead to overt hypothyroidism. This escape process is mainly due to the downregulation and reduction in sodium/iodide symporter (NIS) expression resulting in decreased iodine transport into the thyroid and subsequent resumption of thyroid hormone synthesis, typically occurring 24 hours after excess iodine exposure [15–17].

Monitoring of thyroid function should be considered especially in at-risk patients, as there is a potential for serious complications including the development of myxedema, as presented in this case study. Traditional treatment in patients who develop myxedema includes the use of steroids and TH replacement therapy. In patients with significant risk factors for coronary disease, caution should be exercised as giving high-dose TH replacement will exert an increase in metabolic demand in an otherwise ischemic prone heart. The use of invasive therapies, such as the use of mechanical circulatory support (MCS), can be considered especially in patients with concomitant myxedema coma and cardiogenic shock as they can help support myocardial function by unloading the left ventricle and reduce diastolic volume. Multiple trials have demonstrated Impella's hemodynamic superiority when compared to IABP in shock and postarrest patients; its use in patients with concomitant myxedema has not been studied [18, 19].

Patients who develop myxedema coma and subsequent cardiovascular collapse are rarely encountered in clinical practice. Myxedema carries a high mortality alone, and concomitant coronary ischemia increases the complexity of the management for these patients. Timing and magnitude of hemodynamic support are imperative to consider given the high mortality and complex nature of these patients. Our case demonstrates the potential for use of MCS for such patients with carefully designed protocols to preemptively detect and ameliorate serious complications, such as bleeding and limb ischemia.

Abbreviations

CV: Cardiovascular
CT: Computed tomography
CAD: Coronary artery disease
EKG: Electrocardiogram
IABP: Intra-aortic balloon pump
ICM: Iodinated contrast media
LV: Left ventricle
MCS: Mechanical circulatory support
NIS: Sodium/iodide symporter
TH: Thyroid hormone
T4: Thyroxine
TSH: Thyroid-stimulating hormone.

References

[1] S. Razvi, A. Jabbar, A. Pingitore et al., "Thyroid hormones and cardiovascular function and diseases," *Journal of the American College of Cardiology*, vol. 71, no. 16, pp. 1781–1796, 2018.

[2] A. R. Cappola and P. W. Ladenson, "Hypothyroidism and atherosclerosis," *The Journal of Clinical Endocrinology & Metabolism*, vol. 88, no. 6, pp. 2438–2444, 2003.

[3] A. L. de Castro, R. O. Fernandes, V. D. Ortiz et al., "Thyroid hormones improve cardiac function and decrease expression of pro-apoptotic proteins in the heart of rats 14 days after infarction," *Apoptosis*, vol. 21, no. 2, pp. 184–194, 2016.

[4] I. Klein and S. Danzi, "Thyroid disease and the heart," *Circulation*, vol. 116, no. 15, pp. 1725–1735, 2007.

[5] I. M. Grais and J. R. Sowers, "Thyroid and the heart," *The American Journal of Medicine*, vol. 127, no. 8, pp. 691–698, 2014.

[6] J. Klubo-Gwiezdzinska and L. Wartofsky, "Thyroid emergencies," *Medical Clinics of North America*, vol. 96, no. 2, pp. 385–403, 2012.

[7] D. Byrum and P. Kirkwood, "Pituitary, thyroid, and adrenal disorders," in *Advanced Critical Care Nursing*, pp. 951–957, Saunders Elsevier Inc, St Louis, MO, USA, 2009.

[8] D. Gardner, "Endocrine emergencies," in *Greenspan's Basic & Clinical Endocrinology*, pp. 868–871, McGraw-Hill, New York, NY, USA, 8th edition, 2007.

[9] C. M. Rhee, I. Bhan, E. K. Alexander, and S. M. Brunelli, "Association between iodinated contrast media exposure and incident hyperthyroidism and hypothyroidism," *Archives of Internal Medicine*, vol. 172, no. 2, pp. 153–159, 2012.

[10] S. Y. Lee, C. M. Rhee, A. M. Leung, L. E. Braverman, G. A. Brent, and E. N. Pearce, "A review: radiographic iodinated contrast media-induced thyroid dysfunction," *The Journal of Clinical Endocrinology & Metabolism*, vol. 100, no. 2, pp. 376–383, 2015.

[11] W. Gartner and M. Weissel, "Do iodine-containing contrast media induce clinically relevant changes in thyroid function parameters of euthyroid patients within the first week?," *Thyroid*, vol. 14, no. 7, pp. 521–524, 2004.

[12] C. M. Rhee, K. E. Lynch, K. Zandi-Nejad, E. N. Pearce, E. K. Alexander, and S. M. Brunelli, "Iodinated contrast media exposure and incident hyperthyroidism and hypothyroidism in a community-based cohort," *Endocrinology Studies*, vol. 3, no. 2, article e8, 2013.

[13] S. Y. Lee, D. L. F. Chang, X. He, E. N. Pearce, L. E. Braverman, and A. M. Leung, "Urinary iodine excretion and serum thyroid function in adults after iodinated contrast administration," *Thyroid*, vol. 25, no. 5, pp. 471–477, 2015.

[14] J. Wolff and I. L. Chaikoff, "Plasma inorganic iodide as a homeostatic regulator of thyroid function," *Journal of Biological Chemistry*, vol. 174, no. 2, pp. 555–564, 1948.

[15] P. H. K. Eng, G. R. Cardona, S. L. Fang et al., "Escape from the acute Wolff-Chaikoff effect is associated with a decrease in thyroid sodium/iodide symporter messenger ribonucleic acid and protein," *Endocrinology*, vol. 140, no. 8, pp. 3404–3410, 1999.

[16] C. Serrano-Nascimento, S. da Silva Teixeira, J. P. Nicola, R. T. Nachbar, A. M. Masini-Repiso, and M. T. Nunes, "The acute inhibitory effect of iodide excess on sodium/iodide symporter expression and activity involves the PI3K/Akt signaling pathway," *Endocrinology*, vol. 155, no. 3, pp. 1145–1156, 2014.

[17] P. Pramyothin, A. M. Leung, E. N. Pearce, A. O. Malabanan, and L. E. Braverman, "A hidden solution," *New England Journal of Medicine*, vol. 365, no. 22, pp. 2123–2127, 2011.

[18] M. Seyfarth, D. Sibbing, I. Bauer et al., "A randomized clinical trial to evaluate the safety and efficacy of a percutaneous left ventricular assist device versus intra-aortic balloon pumping for treatment of cardiogenic shock caused by myocardial infarction," *Journal of the American College of Cardiology*, vol. 52, no. 19, pp. 1584–1588, 2008.

[19] D. M. Ouweneel, E. Eriksen, K. D. Sjauw et al., "Percutaneous mechanical circulatory support versus intra-aortic balloon pump in cardiogenic shock after acute myocardial infarction," *Journal of the American College of Cardiology*, vol. 69, no. 3, pp. 278–287, 2017.

14

Multimodality Imaging for the Evaluation of an Undifferentiated Pleomorphic Sarcoma Presenting as Cardioembolic Stroke

Ricardo O. Escárcega,[1] David Bailey,[1] and Michael P. DeFrain[2]

[1]*Florida Heart Associates and Heart and Vascular Institute, Lee Health System, Fort Myers, FL, USA*
[2]*Shipley Cardiothoracic Center, Lee Health System, Fort Myers, FL, USA*

Correspondence should be addressed to Ricardo O. Escárcega; orlandoe@yahoo.com

Academic Editor: Kathleen Ngu

Background. Cancer and ischemic stroke are associated with significant morbidity and mortality. Hypercoagulability, disseminated intravascular coagulation, venous-to-arterial embolism, and non-bacterial thrombotic endocarditis are among recognized mechanisms. Emboli to the brain, or to other organs, are known to occur as a consequence of liberated thrombotic debris originating from the thrombogenic surface of intracardiac neoplastic entities. The most common primary malignancy of the heart is sarcoma; however, masses that occur in the heart are 20 to 40 times more likely as a consequence of metastasis from other sites. *Case Report.* A 67-year-old woman presented to the emergency room with two brief episodes of dizziness and diplopia for 2 minutes. She had a medical history of provoked upper extremity DVT after a fracture, hypothyroidism, hyperlipidemia, and soft tissue sarcoma. The sarcoma was initially diagnosed in, and subsequently resected from, the right triceps muscle. During posttreatment surveillance, a second lesion was discovered in the left upper pulmonary lobe, and this was also completely resected 9 months following initial diagnosis. We present a case of a woman with a tertiary (cardiac) site sarcoma that presented with embolic stroke. *Conclusion.* Our case highlights the benefits of multimodality imaging, heart-team approach with oncology support to define anatomy, thereby enable surgical treatment, of a complex intracardiac lesion.

1. Introduction

Cardioembolic debris is a well-established source of ischemic stroke that has a robust clinical presence in everyday hospital practice. Of those presenting with ischemic stroke, a cardioembolic source is implicated in 15-20% of the cases [1]. Reports in the literature emphasize the importance of echocardiography determining the possibility of a cardioembolic cause [2, 3], and the most recent stroke guidelines recommend echocardiography in the evaluation of suspected ischemic stroke [4].

Cancer and ischemic stroke are associated with significant morbidity and mortality [5]. Hypercoagulability, disseminated intravascular coagulation, venous-to-arterial embolism, non-bacterial thrombotic endocarditis are among recognized mechanisms [5]. A stroke can also occur due to tumor-related embolism [6, 7]. This cardioembolic debris can consist of neoplastic material itself, or thrombus material that can form on the surface of the neoplasm when it is exposed to the bloodstream [8, 9]. Primary cardiac tumors are rare, but the most common malignant types are the sarcomas [10]. Cardiac sarcomas are also common as metastatic lesions. In one series, cardiac metastases were present in 25% consecutive autopsies in patients diagnosed with soft-tissue sarcoma, and of these, 50% had metastasis to the myocardium, 33% to the pericardium, and 17% both [11]. Metastatic lesions to the heart occur 20 to 40 times more common than primary neoplasms [12]. Metastases to the heart can occur from nearly any source, but the most common are the melanoma and carcinomas of the lung, breast, and esophagus [5]. We present a patient with a tertiary site cardiac sarcoma that experienced an embolic stroke which was successfully treated with complete resection.

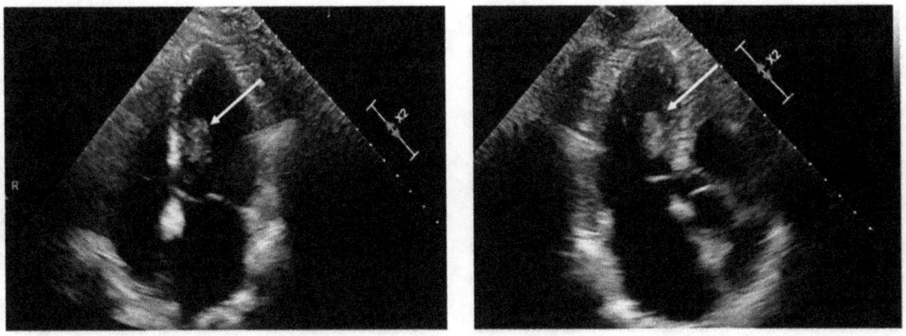

(a) (b)

FIGURE 1: Transthoracic echocardiogram. Panels (a) (apical 4-chamber view) and (b) (apical 3-chamber view) show an echogenic mass located inside the left ventricle attached to the interventricular septum.

2. Case Report

A 67-year-old healthy appearing woman experienced dizziness and 2 episodes of brief diplopia leading to an acute inpatient evaluation. The patient had a history of provoked upper extremity deep vein thrombosis (DVT) after a fracture, hypothyroidism, hyperlipidemia, and soft tissue sarcoma of the right triceps. Physical exam, including gross neurologic function, was normal at time of presentation. Laboratory analysis was normal. Magnetic Resonance Imaging (MRI) of the brain demonstrated cerebral hemispheric and cerebellar foci which were felt to represent embolic lesions.

18 months prior to presentation, the patient had undergone complete resection of a sarcoma that had arisen in the right triceps muscle. 9 months after the initial resection of the triceps sarcoma, surveillance imaging revealed a newly developed left upper lobe pulmonary mass. This lung lesion was completely resected and was a metastatic sarcoma. 9 months after the pulmonary resection, the patient presented to our institution with two episodes of acute neurologic change manifested as two brief episodes of dizziness and diplopia for 2 minutes. Subsequent imaging of the brain demonstrated two foci of acute or subacute ischemia in the superior right frontal lobe and left cerebellum, reflective of embolic lesions. Peripheral vascular imaging with carotid ultrasound did not demonstrate vascular abnormalities. Transthoracic echocardiography (TTE) revealed a large mobile mass based of the interventricular septum within the left ventricular cavity (Figure 1). Transesophageal echocardiogram (TEE) showed large mobile left ventricular sessile-appearing mass related to the interventricular septum and the subvalvular mitral apparatus (Figure 2). Finally, cardiac MRI (Figure 3) showed a mobile, oval shaped mass within the left ventricle measuring approximately 1.5 x 2.9 x 2.4 cm, in transverse anteroposterior (AP) and craniocaudal dimensions, intricately related to the chordae tendinae of the mitral valve and involving the posterior-medial papillary muscle which was continuous with, and adjacent to, the interventricular septum. The left ventricular mass was implicated by our team as the most likely source for embolic injury to the brain, and with this detailed anatomic definition, the patient was offered resection. Coronary angiography revealed no significant coronary disease. Intraoperatively, the mass appeared as a broad-based lesion originating from the tip of the posterior-medial papillary muscle and appeared to extend along the chordae tendinae toward the anterior leaflet of the mitral valve. Wide excision of the papillary muscle, the associated chordae and half of the anterior mitral leaflet, was performed in an effort to achieve negative resection margins. Initial histopathological evaluation of the resected mass revealed the lesion to be a sarcoma, and that the resection margin at the papillary muscle was positive. A wider resection of the interventricular septal tissue around the papillary muscle was performed to ultimately achieve a negative margin. Mitral valve replacement with a bovine tissue prosthesis was performed. The patient's postoperative course was complicated by atrial fibrillation and pleural effusions. She was discharged in sinus rhythm and in good health on postoperative day 10. Her histopathology was ultimately diagnosed as undifferentiated pleomorphic sarcoma (atypical spindle cell neoplasm), likely representing metastatic, rather than a primary lesion. Patient was discharged with follow-up at a regional cancer center that was originally involved with her triceps and subsequent pulmonary sarcoma resections.

3. Discussion

This case posed multiple diagnostic challenges that were relevant to, and ultimately defined her treatment options. Our patient presented with symptoms of a neurological event which prompted brain imaging. Cardiac tumors can be asymptomatic [13]. Our patient had involvement of her left ventricle. However, prior reports have indicated that although metastatic cells could be filtered by the pulmonary circulation, the level of vascularity may be the focus of metastases [13, 14].

Tumors occurring on the left side of the heart can produce symptoms due to direct contact with the systemic arterial circulation. Neoplastic or thrombotic emboli from the tumor nidus can lead to stroke or another systemic organ damage [9].

The driving impetus in the management of our patient was the prevention of further cerebrovascular embolic event. Given the relatively brief disease-free interval from her sarcoma diagnoses, as well as an initial surface echocardiographic finding suggestive of a large sessile left ventricular-

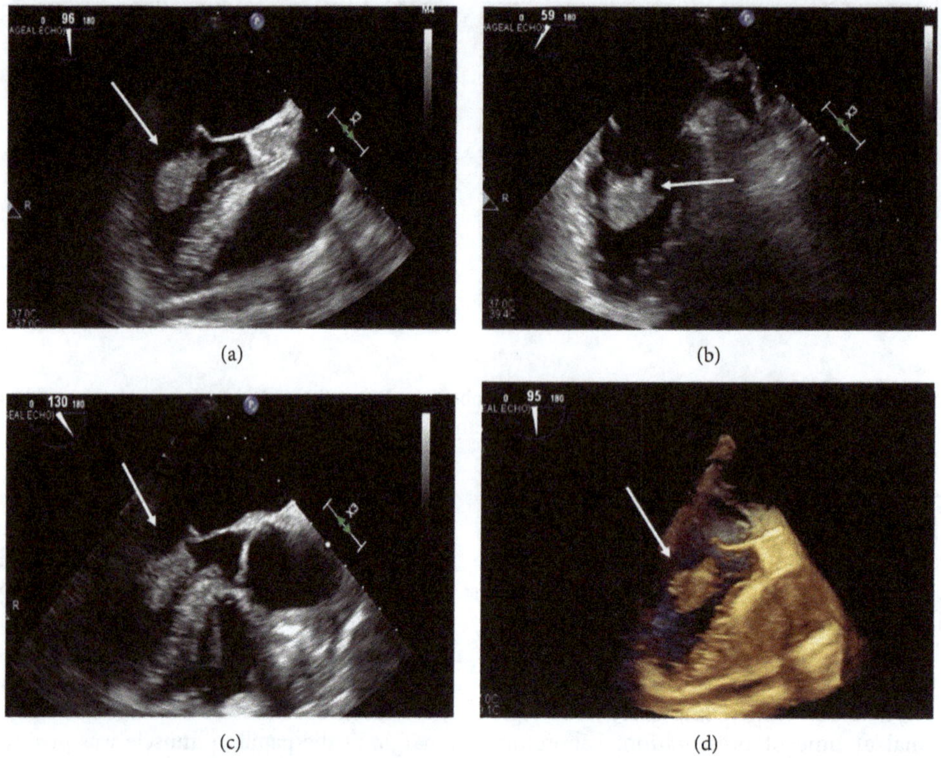

FIGURE 2: Transesophageal echocardiogram. Panels (a), (b), (c), and (d) show a large echogenic mass attached to the mitral valve apparatus and interventricular septum at different orthogonal views.

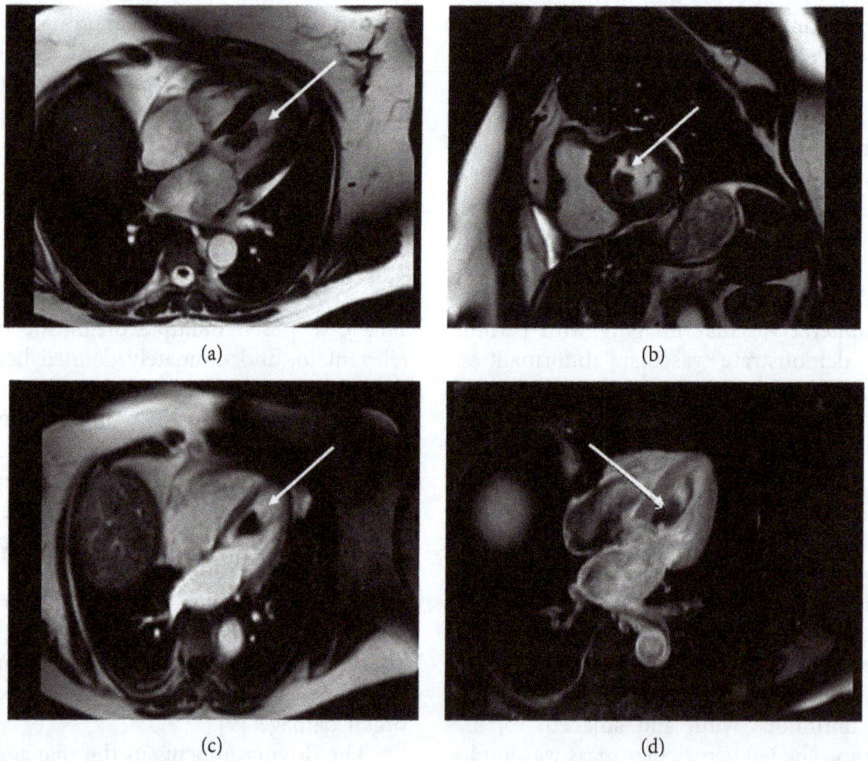

FIGURE 3: Cardiac MRI. Panels (a), (b), (c), and (d) show in different sequences a mass attached to the mitral valve apparatus and interventricular septum.

based intracardiac mass, the initial clinical impression was to offer the patient a chemo-radiotherapy treatment option. Confidence in the ability to offer resection of the mass only occurred after further anatomical characterization of the lesion with transesophageal echocardiography and cardiac MRI. Ultimately, intraoperative analysis of the anatomical extent of the lesion mirrored our estimations from imaging, and a complete resection with negative margins was achieved. This treatment modality, in contrast to the nonsurgical treatment options that were proposed prior to anatomical delineation of the mass, offered removal of the cardioembolic nidus and the hope of completely resecting the malignancy.

For patients presenting with echogenic structures located inside the heart, multimodality imaging is often required. Initial TTE is useful; however, TEE is frequently required for comprehensive and accurate assessment [15]. The multiplanar assessment of anatomy, visualization of tissue composition with high contrast, and the functional assessment of intracardiac flow dynamics afforded by cardiac MRI provide a thorough assessment of the tumor extent and to help determine respectability. MRI allows for early differentiation between a nonneoplastic mass and a tumor mass, be it benign or malignant [16]. Although cardiac sarcomas can be a primary site, they have poor prognosis with overall survival < 1 year [17]. Prognosis is generally poor because of the role of chemotherapy may be still ill defined, and complete surgical tumor resection often proves to be challenging [18]. A contributing factor to the negative prognosis is the nature of the heart's unique anatomic and physiologic role which limits complete surgical resection of neoplastic masses. These tumors are rare, and to our knowledge, a metastatic tertiary site to the heart has not been reported.

Our case represents a rare tumor with an unusual course with three different sites involved over the clinical course of many months. It highlights the importance of multimodality imaging, a heart team approach, and oncology support to delineate a successful surgical resection and an optimal clinical result.

References

[1] T. H. Wein and N. M. Bornstein, "Stroke prevention: cardiac and carotid-related stroke," *Neurologic Clinics*, vol. 18, no. 2, pp. 321–341, 2000.

[2] A. Uner, M. Dogan, E. Sal, and E. Peker, "Stroke and recurrent peripheral embolism in left atrial myxoma," *Acta Cardiologica*, vol. 65, no. 1, pp. 101–103, 2010.

[3] Y. D. Kim, J. H. Lee, Y. H. Jung et al., "Safety and outcome after thrombolytic treatment in ischemic stroke patients with high-risk cardioembolic sources and prior subtherapeutic warfarin use," *Journal of the Neurological Sciences*, vol. 298, no. 1-2, pp. 101–105, 2010.

[4] W. J. Powers, A. A. Rabinstein, T. Ackerson et al., "Guidelines for the early management of patients with acute ischemic stroke: 2019 update to the 2018 guidelines for the early management of acute ischemic atroke: a guideline for healthcare professionals from the American Heart Association/American Stroke Association," *Stroke*, vol. 50, no. 12, pp. e344–e418, 2019.

[5] J. L. Dearborn, V. C. Urrutia, and S. R. Zeiler, "Stroke and cancer- a complicated relationship," *Journal of Neurology & Translational Neuroscience*, vol. 2, no. 1, p. 1039, 2014.

[6] M. Mitomi, K. Kimura, Y. Iguchi et al., "A case of stroke due to tumor emboli associated with metastatic cardiac liposarcoma," *Internal Medicine*, vol. 50, no. 14, pp. 1489–1491, 2011.

[7] B. B. Navi, K. Kawaguchi, I. Hriljac, E. Lavi, L. M. DeAngelis, and D. G. Jamieson, "Multifocal stroke from tumor emboli," *Archives of Neurology*, vol. 66, no. 9, pp. 1174-1175, 2009.

[8] G. Serena, J. Gonzalez, J. J. Gaynor, T. Salerno, R. Verzaro, and G. Ciancio, "Pulmonary tumor embolization as early manifestation in patients with renal cell carcinoma and tumor thrombus: perioperative management and outcomes," *Journal of Cardiac Surgery*, vol. 34, no. 10, pp. 1018–1023, 2019.

[9] M. C. Bois, M. D. Eckhardt, V. M. Cracolici et al., "Neoplastic embolization to systemic and pulmonary arteries," *Journal of Vascular Surgery*, vol. 68, no. 204-212, article e207, 2018.

[10] Y. P. Sun, X. Wang, Y. S. Gao, S. Zhao, and Y. Bai, "Primary cardiac sarcoma complicated with cerebral infarction and brain metastasis: a case report and literature review," *Cancer Biomarkers*, vol. 21, no. 1, pp. 247–250, 2017.

[11] D. E. Hallahan, N. J. Vogelzang, K. M. Borow, D. G. Bostwick, and M. A. Simon, "Cardiac metastases from soft-tissue sarcomas," *Journal of Clinical Oncology*, vol. 4, no. 11, pp. 1662–1669, 1986.

[12] N. Mehta, A. Desai, B. Shivdasani et al., "Left atrial spindle cell sarcoma - case report," *Indian Heart Journal*, vol. 64, no. 4, pp. 416–419, 2012.

[13] S. Takenaka, N. Hashimoto, N. Araki et al., "Eleven cases of cardiac metastases from soft-tissue sarcomas," *Japanese Journal of Clinical Oncology*, vol. 41, no. 4, pp. 514–518, 2011.

[14] G. E. Malaret and P. Aliaga, "Metastatic disease to the heart," *Cancer*, vol. 22, no. 2, pp. 457–466, 1968.

[15] M. Alam, F. Gabriel, F. Khaja, and G. Paone, "Transesophageal echocardiographic evaluation of left main coronary artery," *Angiology*, vol. 46, no. 12, pp. 1103–1106, 1995.

[16] K. Randhawa, A. Ganeshan, and E. T. Hoey, "Magnetic resonance imaging of cardiac tumors: part 2, malignant tumors and tumor-like conditions," *Current Problems in Diagnostic Radiology*, vol. 40, no. 4, pp. 169–179, 2011.

[17] N. Kajihara, Y. Tanoue, M. Eto, Y. Tomita, M. Masuda, and S. Morita, "Surgical experience of cardiac tumors: early and late results," *Surgery Today*, vol. 36, no. 7, pp. 602–607, 2006.

[18] Z. Li, T. Hsieh, and A. Salehi, "Recurrent cardiac intimal (spindle cell) sarcoma of the left atrium," *Journal of Cardiothoracic and Vascular Anesthesia*, vol. 27, no. 1, pp. 103–107, 2013.

15

Chronic Type A Aortic Dissection: Rare Presentation of Incidental Pericardial Effusion

Ashraf Abugroun,[1] Ahmed Subahi,[2] Safwan Gaznabi,[1] and Hussein Daoud[1]

[1]*Department of Internal Medicine, Advocate Illinois Masonic Medical Center, 836 W Wellington Avenue, Chicago, IL 60657, USA*
[2]*Department of Internal Medicine, Wayne State University/Detroit Medical Center, Detroit, Michigan, USA*

Correspondence should be addressed to Ashraf Abugroun; ashraf.abugroun@advocatehealth.com

Academic Editor: Man-Hong Jim

Aortic dissection is the most devastating sequelae of aortopathy other than aortic rupture. However, aortic dissection can be asymptomatic in the acute phase with delayed symptomatic presentation or incidental diagnosis upon chest imaging. We report a case of a 63-year-old male who was diagnosed with pericardial effusion upon preoperative workup for elective cholecystectomy. Further investigations confirmed hemorrhagic pericardial effusion secondary to a chronic dissecting ascending aortic aneurysm. The patient condition was successfully managed with open surgical repair with an uneventful postoperative course. This case demonstrates an extremely rare presentation of incidental hemorrhagic pericardial effusion caused by a chronic dissecting ascending aortic aneurysm.

1. Case Report

A 63-year-old male with a history of hypertension, 20 pack-years of smoking, thyroid cancer in remission with partial thyroidectomy, and chronic obstructive lung disease (COPD) presented to the emergency department (ED) with acute abdominal pain. Abdominal ultrasound showed gallstones with no evidence of cholecystitis or biliary obstruction. The patient was diagnosed with biliary colic and discharged home with a plan to perform an elective cholecystectomy. Computed tomography (CT) scan of the abdomen was performed as an outpatient as part of the preoperative workup which showed evidence of gallstones, small bilateral pleural effusions, and moderate pericardial effusion with high density suggestive of hemorrhage (Figure 1). Consequently, the patient was referred to the emergency department for further workup. Upon arrival, the patient was asymptomatic, his vital signs were normal, and his physical examination was unremarkable. An electrocardiogram (EKG) revealed a nonspecific interventricular conduction delay. Chest x-ray showed a mildly enlarged cardiomediastinal silhouette with prominent perihilar opacities suggestive of a prominent vasculature (Figure 2). Complete blood count and basic ?metabolic profile were within normal limits. Further laboratory workup showed normal erythrocyte sedimentation rate, rheumatoid factor, complement level, and procalcitonin with negative serology for antinuclear antibodies and double-stranded DNA antibodies. A transthoracic echocardiogram (TTE) showed a large pericardial effusion without signs of tamponade, moderate aortic regurgitation, and normal left ventricular ejection fraction and size. Given the large volume of pericardial effusion, a pericardial window was attempted. A total of one liter of hemorrhagic fluid was drained. Pericardial tissue biopsy showed acute and chronic inflammatory cells with thickened pericardium, and no malignant cells were detected (Figure 3). Tuberculosis quantiferon assay, acid-fast bacilli staining, and fungal and bacterial cultures of the pericardial tissue were negative. The source of pericardial effusion remained elusive. Given the hemorrhagic nature of the pericardial effusion in the absence of recent use of anticoagulation and the negative workup for infectious or autoimmune etiology, a CT scan of the chest with contrast was obtained to evaluate for possible malignancy. CT showed an ascending aortic aneurysm measuring up to 7.5 cm with

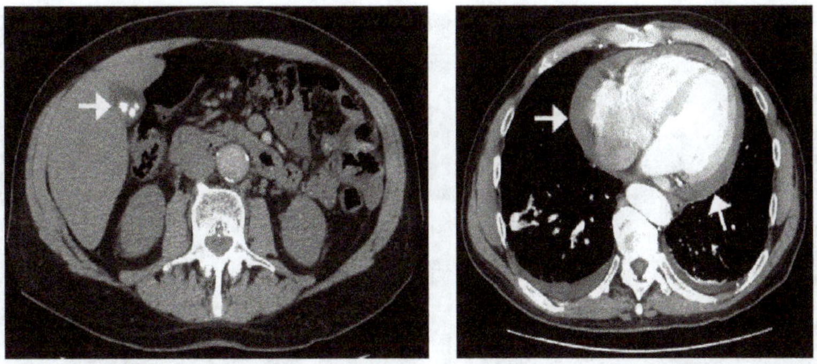

(a) (b)

FIGURE 1: CT scan of the abdomen. (a) Showing gallstones (arrow) with questionable gallbladder wall thickening or pericholecystic fluid. (b) Moderate amount of fluid in the pericardial space appears to be of increased density compared to simple fluid, suggestive of hemorrhage (arrow).

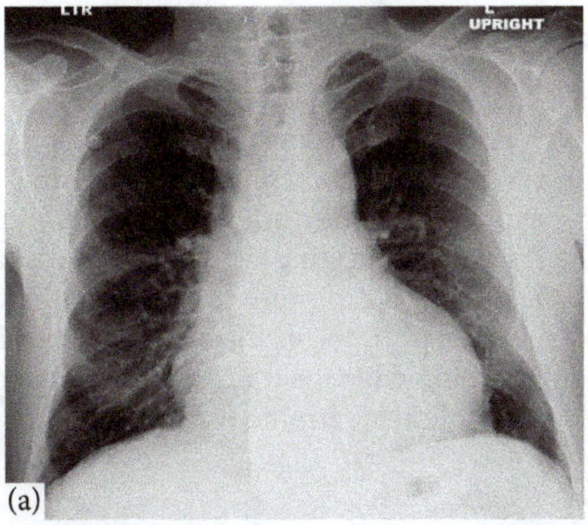

FIGURE 2: CXR of the lungs (posteroanterior view) on admission shows a mildly enlarged cardiomediastinal silhouette that resembles a bottle.

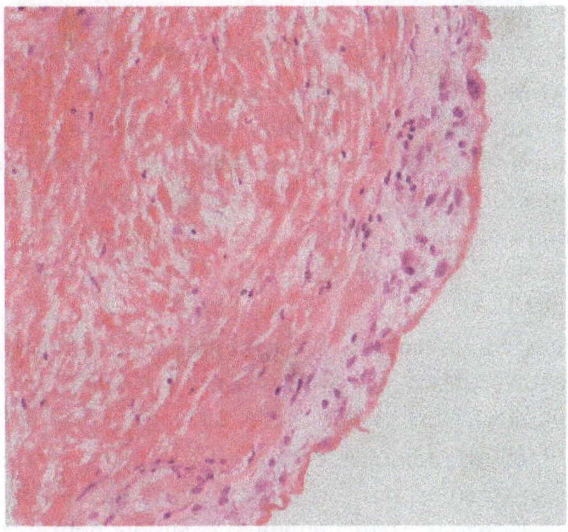

FIGURE 3: H&E stain of biopsy of pericardial tissue showing thickened pericardial tissue with acute and chronic inflammation and reactive mesothelial hyperplasia.

chronic dissection with no involvement of the coronaries or the great vessels (Figure 4). The patient underwent successful open surgical repair of his chronic Stanford type A aortic dissection with an uneventful postoperative course.

2. Discussion

Acute Stanford type A aortic dissection (AD) is a life-threatening condition that serves as an impetus to immediate surgical repair aiming to prevent dissection-associated complications such as acute aortic regurgitation, aortic rupture, myocardial or cerebral ischemia, and pericardial tamponade [1]. However, newly diagnosed chronic type A (CTAD) dissections of a native aorta represent a different subpopulation of patients with atypical or absent symptoms at the time of dissection onset precluding the early diagnosis [2–4]. Patients with de novo chronic AD are usually asymptomatic at the time of diagnosis (like our patient) [2]. Thus, newly diagnosed CTAD is usually discovered incidentally upon chest imaging as a prominent aortic knob or mediastinal widening [2]. Therefore, the accurate timing of dissection is often unfeasible [2]. Careful history is needed to identify previous acute chest pain events (heralding dissection onset). Furthermore, the patient may endorse symptoms related to the enlarging dissection (e.g., hoarseness and persisting or recurrent chest pain), malperfusion (e.g., vision changes, extremity pain, and syncope), or valvular disease (e.g., dyspnea, orthopnea, and lower limb swelling) [1, 2, 5]. Amid any suspicion, CTAD has to be confirmed by further specific imaging modalities including transesophageal echocardiogram (TEE), Computed Tomographic Angiography (CTA), or Magnetic Resonance Angiography (MRA) [1, 2, 5]. Features like thick, immobile intimal flap, aneurysmal dilatation of the thoracic aorta (as in our patient), or the presence of thrombus in the false lumen are suggestive of dissection chronicity [2]. Signs of contained rupture such as pleural effusion or mediastinal hematoma can also be seen in symptomatic patients [2]. Pericardial effusion is a common complication of acute type A AD and usually occurs through two separate mechanisms [5]. The first mechanism is the transudation of fluid across the thin wall of the false lumen into the pericardial cavity which is the most common mechanisms [5]. However, the dissected aorta can rupture directly into the pericardial space with subsequent tamponade [5]. Cardiac tamponade is diagnosed in 8% to 10% of patients presenting with acute type A aortic dissection and is a predictor of poor prognosis, as well as the primary cause of

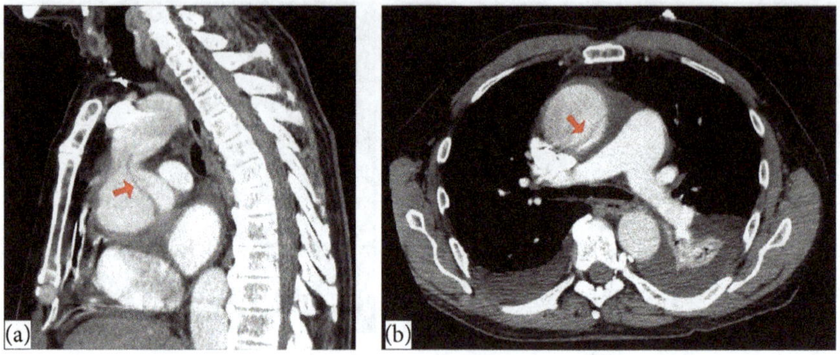

(a) (b)

FIGURE 4: CT scan of the abdomen showing acute ascending thoracic aortic aneurysm measuring up to 7.5 cm with a dissection of the proximal ascending thoracic aorta originates approximately 1.3 cm above the aortic root. (a) Sagittal view of dissection site and (b) coronal view of dissection site. The area of dissection highlighted with an arrow.

mortality in this subgroup of patients mandating urgent aortic repair [5]. In our case, CTAD was asymptomatic and initially was not clinically suspected; thus, pericardial puncture was carried out for the evaluation of the pericardial effusion. Our patient was hemodynamically stable with no contraindications for contrast administration. Given the negative pericardial fluid analysis, the 20 pack-years of smoking, and the thyroid cancer history, hemorrhagic pericardial effusion secondary to metastatic cancer was suspected. Thus, a CT scan of the chest with contrast was obtained and aortic dissection was incidentally discovered.

The first clue for CTAD diagnosis was the detection of high-density pericardial effusion note on abdominal CT scan before elective cholecystectomy. Given the lake of symptoms, transudation of fluid across the wall of the false lumen into the pericardial cavity is the most plausible mechanisms. Also, hemopericardium in our case could be a sign of silent contained rupture.

All patients with aortic dissections will need immediate surgical evaluation independent of location [5]. Patients with type B dissections are typically treated conservatively [6]. On the other hand, those with type A dissection (like in our case) needs immediate surgical intervention. Acute medical management as a bridge to possible surgery consists of initial pain control and anti-impulsive therapy (i.e., heart rate and blood pressure control) to alleviate the shearing forces against the aortic wall and minimize the propagation of the dissection. The systolic blood pressure goal is less than 120 mm Hg. It is imperative that chronotropic medications be used first as vasodilators pose the risk of reflex tachycardia and worsening of the dissection [6].

Our patient had an aorta diameter of 7.5 cm; furthermore, his dissection was complicated by hemorrhagic pericardial effusion and moderate aortic regurgitation. Thus, the open surgical repair was the chosen approach. According to a recent review of a 696 type A patients, following open repair, patients with CTAD had lower in-hospital mortality and longer five- and ten-year survival compared to the acute type A dissection patients [7]. Our patient had successful CTAD repair with an uneventful postoperative course.

3. Conclusion

Chronic type A aortic dissection is a challenging diagnosis with a wide range of clinical presentations including incidental hemorrhagic pericardial effusion. Pericardial puncture in pericarial effusion complicating type A dissection can result in the propagation of the rupture. Accordingly, obtaining a CT scan of the chest prior to any diagnostic pericardial puncture is highly recommended. Surgical repair is the treatment of choice for complicated chronic type A aortic dissection.

References

[1] S. A. Mokashi and L. G. Svensson, "Guidelines for the management of thoracic aortic disease in 2017," *General Thoracic and Cardiovascular Surgery*, vol. 67, no. 1, pp. 59–65, 2019.

[2] R. Erbel, V. Aboyans, C. Boileau et al., "2014 ESC Guidelines on the diagnosis and treatment of aortic diseases: document covering acute and chronic aortic diseases of the thoracic and abdominal aorta of the adult The Task Force for the Diagnosis and Treatment of Aortic Diseases of the European Society of Cardiology (ESC)," *European Heart Journal*, vol. 35, no. 41, pp. 2873–2926, 2014.

[3] C. Hynes, M. Greenberg, S. Sarin, and G. Trachiotis, "Chronic type A aortic dissection: two cases and a review of current management strategies," *Aorta*, vol. 4, no. 1, pp. 16–21, 2016.

[4] G. M. Raffa, M. Pilato, A. Armaro, C. Ruperto, G. Gentile, and F. Follis, "Chronic Stanford type A aortic dissection," *Journal of Cardiovascular Medicine*, vol. 17, Supplement 2, pp. e138–e140, 2016.

[5] L. F. Hiratzka, G. L. Bakris, J. A. Beckman et al., "2010 ACCF/AHA/AATS/ACR/ASA/SCA/SCAI/SIR/STS/SVM Guidelines for the diagnosis and management of patients with thoracic aortic disease. A Report of the American College of Cardiology Foundation/American Heart Association Task Force on Practice Guidelines, American Association for Thoracic Surgery, American College of Radiology,American Stroke Association, Society of Cardiovascular Anesthesiologists, Society for Cardiovascular Angiography and Interventions, Society of Interventional

Radiology, Society of Thoracic Surgeons,and Society for Vascular Medicine," *Journal of the American College of Cardiology*, vol. 55, no. 14, pp. e27–e129, 2010.

[6] R. J. Strayer, P. L. Shearer, and L. K. Hermann, "Screening, evaluation, and early management of acute aortic dissection in the ED," *Current Cardiology Reviews*, vol. 8, no. 2, pp. 152–157, 2012.

[7] B. Rylski, R. K. Milewski, J. E. Bavaria et al., "Outcomes of surgery for chronic type A aortic dissection," *The Annals of Thoracic Surgery*, vol. 99, no. 1, pp. 88–93, 2015.

Retrograde Percutaneous Coronary Intervention in a Case of Takayasu Arteritis with Left Main Coronary Artery Chronic Total Occlusion

Prathap Kumar, Blessvin Jino, Stalin Roy, and Manu Rajendran

Department of Cardiology, Meditrina Hospital, Kollam, Kerala, India

Correspondence should be addressed to Prathap Kumar; prathapndr@gmail.com

Academic Editor: Ertugurul Ercan

Background. Takayasu arteritis (TA) frequently involves the coronary arteries, and restenosis is common after initial percutaneous coronary intervention (PCI). However, PCI remains a good option for patients who develop graft failure after coronary artery bypass graft surgery (CABG). Drug-coated balloons help in repeat revascularization after stent failure in TA. *Case Presentation.* A 31-year-old female with previous history of Takayasu arteritis (TA) and CABG with left internal mammary artery (LIMA) to left anterior descending artery (LAD) grafting in 2012, presented to us with exertional angina of 6-month duration. Her coronary angiogram showed total occlusion of the left main coronary artery (LMCA) ostium and atretic LIMA graft. Since the guiding catheter could not engage the LMCA, a retrograde approach was planned. After lesion crossing, the retrograde guidewire could not be externalized even after multiple attempts. Hence, a repeat antegrade approach was tried, and antegrade wire crossed through the channel created by the retrograde microcatheter. Then, intravascular ultrasound (IVUS) guided LMCA-LAD stenting was done. The patient was started on dual antiplatelets and prednisolone and was on regular follow-up. Three months later, the patient presented to us with non-ST elevation MI. Coronary angiogram showed critical in-stent restenosis of the LMCA stent, and optical coherence tomography (OCT) showed diffuse neointimal hyperplasia. OCT-guided PCI using sirolimus-coated balloon was done. On 8 months of follow-up, the patient remains symptom free. *Conclusion.* Coronary artery disease in TA may require repeated interventions due to stent/graft failure. Drug-coated balloons play a crucial role in repeat revascularization for stent failure in TA. Retrograde approach increases the technical success rate of PCI in LMCA-CTO.

1. Introduction

Coronary arterial lesions are seen in 53.2% of patients with TA on computed tomographic angiography [1]. Immunosuppressive therapies remain the primary treatment of organ ischemia caused by active disease, and interventions are recommended only in progressive organ ischemia [2]. We report an interesting case of left main coronary artery (LMCA) chronic total occlusion (CTO) which was managed by image-guided PCI.

2. Case Report

A 31-year-old female presented to our hospital with exertional angina class III of 6 months duration. She underwent coronary artery bypass grafting (CABG) with left internal mammary artery (LIMA) to left anterior descending artery (LAD) graft in 2012 for critical LMCA disease. She was diagnosed to have TA in 2012 and was on prednisolone 10 mg as maintenance therapy for TA. She had no other risk factors for coronary artery disease. Her electrocardiogram showed T inversion in the anterior leads, and echocardiogram showed left ventricular (LV) anterior wall hypokinesia with an ejection fraction (EF) of 50%. Her CRP level was 2 mg/dl on admission. Coronary angiogram showed LMCA ostial total occlusion and a normal right coronary artery giving collaterals to left system. The left subclavian artery had significant stenosis at the proximal segment, and the LIMA was atretic (Figure 1). The patient was planned for PCI to LMCA using primary retrograde approach through septal

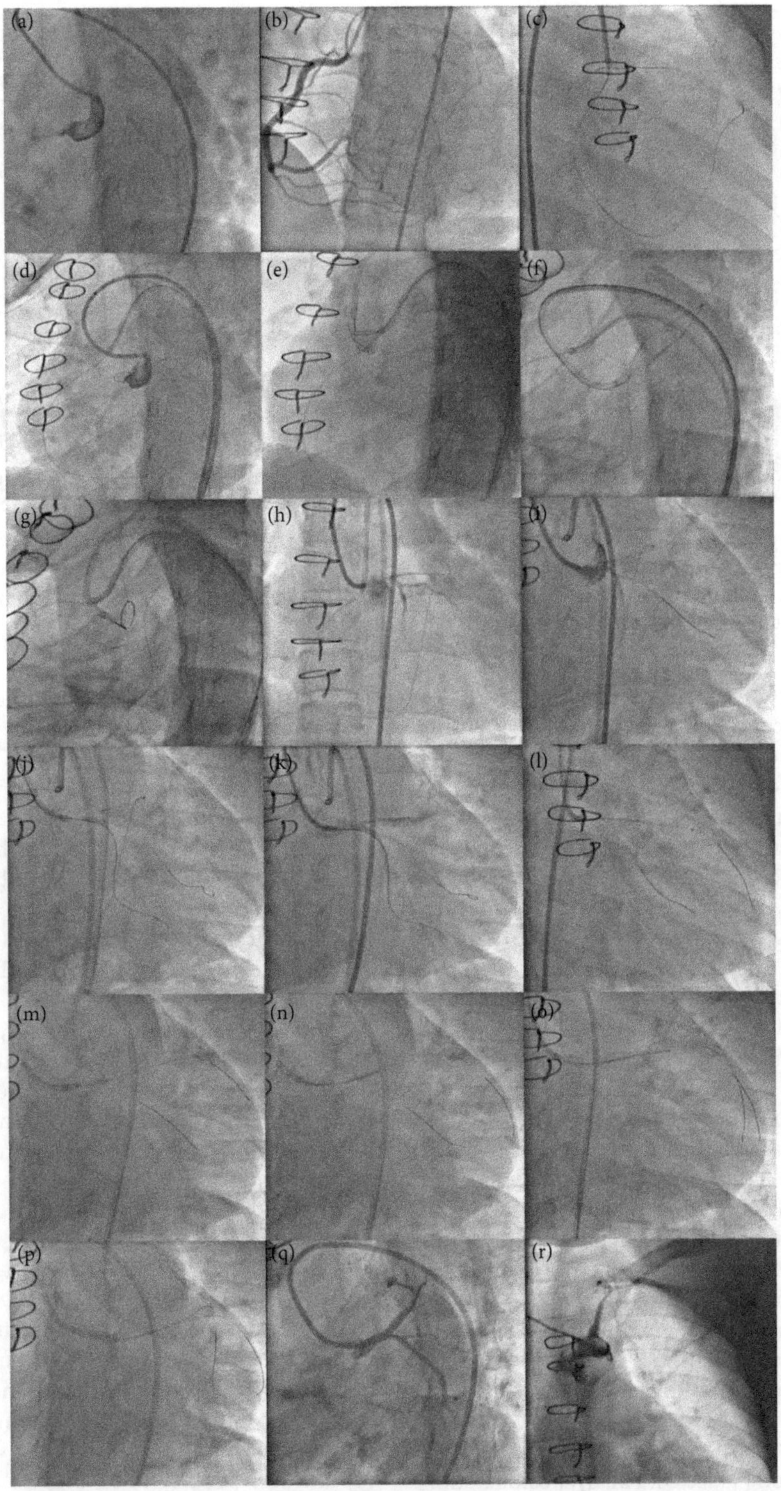

Figure 1: Angiographic images showing initial PCI for LMCA CTO. Left anterior oblique (LAO) caudal view showed LMCA total occlusion (a), and antero posterior (AP) cranial view showed normal RCA giving multiple collaterals to both LAD and LCX (b). LMCA lesion was crossed retrogradely using Fielder FC and caravel through septal collateral from RCA (c), and externalization into 7F EBU 3.5 antegrade guiding catheter was attempted by conventional method (d). After multiple failed attempts to enter antegrade guiding catheter, snaring was attempted using Amplatz goose neck snare (e). After multiple failed attempts of externalization and antegrade wiring (f–h), finally, SION black guidewire crossed LMCA lesion antegradely (i). Then, Fielder XTR guidewire was parked in LCX, and LMCA lesion was dilated with 2.5 × 8 mm NC balloon (j, k). After IVUS analysis (l), LMCA lesion was again dilated with 3 × 10 mm cutting balloon (m). Then, LMCA-LAD stenting was done with 3.5 × 26 mm ZES (n). After stenting, IVUS analysis showed underexpansion (o), and hence, postdilatation was done using 4 × 8 mm NC balloon (p). Final angiogram showed well expanded stent with good distal flow in LAD and LCX (q). Left subclavian artery angiogram showed stenosis at the proximal segment and atretic LIMA (r).

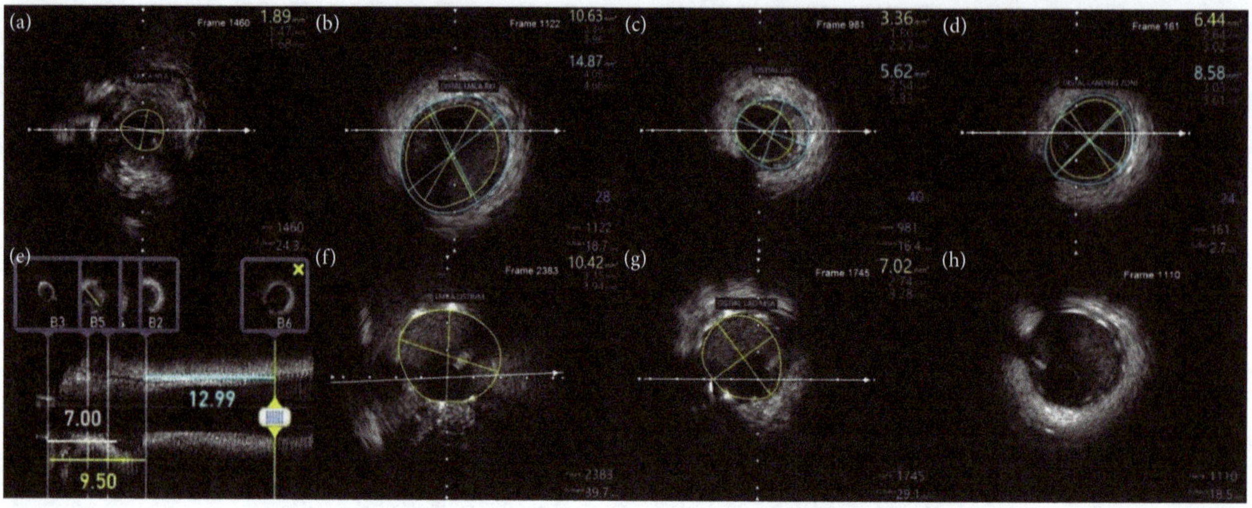

FIGURE 2: IVUS guidance in initial PCI optimization. Initial IVUS run showed LMCA MLA of 1.89 mm^2 (a), and the mean distal LMCA vessel diameter was 4.36 mm (b). MLA of ostial LAD, mean vessel diameter of the distal landing zone, and the total lesion length were 3.36 mm^2, 3.32 mm, and 22.5 mm, respectively (c–e). Post IVUS run showed ostial LMCA MSA of 10.42 mm^2 (f) and ostial LAD MSA of 7.2 mm^2 (g). The distal stent edge was free of edge dissection or malapposition (h).

collaterals from RCA. RCA was engaged using 7F JR 3.5 guiding catheter, and septal collateral was crossed using Fielder FC guidewire and caravel. Since LMCA could not be engaged, 7F JL 3.5 guiding catheter was kept at the aortic root. After lesion crossing, guidewire could not enter the guiding catheter (Video 1), and hence, snaring was attempted using Amplatz goose neck™ snare and KAM snare (Videos 2 and 3). After multiple attempts of snaring, finally, antegrade wiring was tried through the channel created by the guidewire and caravel. SION black was used to cross the lesion antegradely and was parked in the left circumflex (LCX) artery. Then, the LMCA was dilated with a 2.5 × 8 mm noncompliant (NC) balloon, and then, Fielder XTR was parked at LAD. Again, after 3 × 12 mm NC balloon dilatation, intravascular ultrasound (IVUS) run was done. IVUS analysis showed that the disease involved both LMCA and proximal LAD (Video 4), and the minimal luminal area (MLA) of LMCA, mean LMCA vessel diameter, mean proximal LAD vessel diameter, and lesion length were 1.89 mm^2, 4.36 mm, 3.32 mm, and 22.5 mm, respectively (Figure 2). In view of significant fibrotic lesion, another dilatation with 3 × 10 mm cutting balloon was done, and then, ostial LMCA to LAD stenting was done using 3.5 × 26 mm Zotarolimus eluting stent. Poststenting IVUS showed underexpansion at LMCA with stent area at ostial LMCA and ostial LAD were 10.42 mm^2 and 7.02 mm^2, respectively, without distal edge dissection or malapposition (Video 5). Finally, postdilatation was done with a 4 × 8 mm NC balloon, and the final angiogram showed a well expanded stent without any complications (Video 6). The patient was on regular medications including aspirin, ticagrelor, atorvastatin, and prednisolone and was on regular follow-up. Three months later, the patient presented with a non-ST elevation myocardial infarction, and she had COVID-19 vaccination 1 week prior to the chest pain. Her echocardiogram showed LV anterior wall hypokinesia with EF of 45%, and coronary angiogram showed LMCA shaft 95% in-stent restenosis (ISR) with distal TIMI-2 flow (Video 7, Figure 3). Ad hoc PCI was planned, and lesion was crossed with Fielder FC guidewires. After predilatation with a 2.75 × 12 mm NC balloon, optical coherence tomography (OCT) showed diffuse neointimal hyperplasia with LMCA MSA of 1.93 m^2 (Video 8, Figure 4). Lesion was dilated with 3 × 10 mm Flextome™ and 4 × 20 mm sirolimus-coated balloon. Finally, kissing balloon inflation using 4 × 20 mm and 2.75 × 12 mm balloons and proximal optimization (POT) using 4.5 × 8 mm NC balloon were done. Final OCT run showed that stent areas at proximal LMCA, POC, and ostial LAD were 9.9 mm^2, 8.4 mm^2, and 10.01 mm^2, respectively (Video 9). Final angiogram showed no residual stenosis without any complications (Video 10). The patient was discharged without any peri-procedural complications. On 8 months of follow-up, she remains symptom free.

3. Discussion

European League Against Rheumatism (EULAR) recommends vascular intervention in a patient with TA, when a vascular lesion persists despite medical therapy, particularly when it is associated with symptoms or risk of future complications [3]. Vascular interventions should be done preferably after controlling active inflammation, and interventions during active disease are associated with more complications [4] and low patency rates. Studies have shown that PCI is associated with higher risk of ISR and repeat revascularization comparing CABG in TA [5, 6]. In our case, the patient opted for PCI after detailed discussion with our heart team regarding the risks involved in redo CABG and the possibilities of ISR in PCI. LMCA-CTOs are seen mostly in post-CABG patients, and PCI for LMCA-CTO is performed only rarely, around 0.45% of all CTO PCIs in one registry [7]. PCI to an unprotected LMCA-CTO is technically challenging. Subintimal entry and balloon dilatation may compromise the flow in LAD or LCX and may become life-threatening.

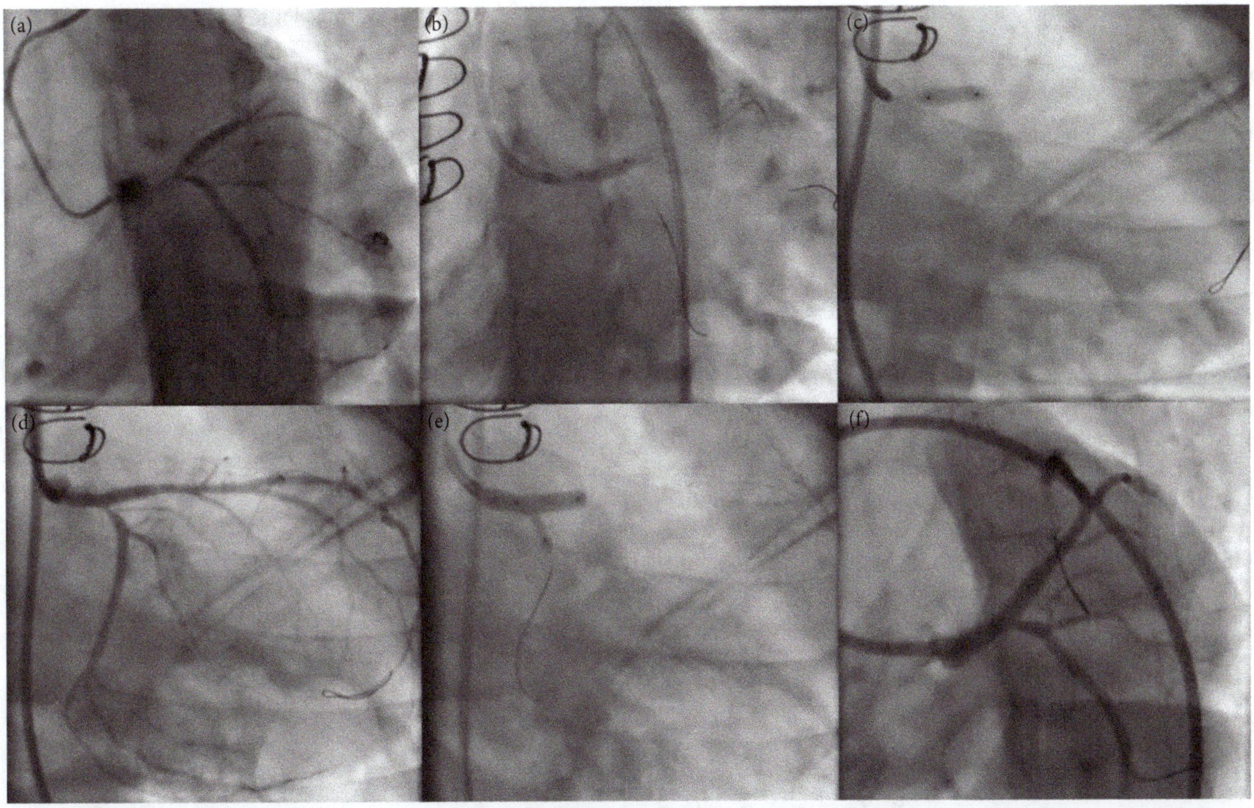

FIGURE 3: Angiographic images of repeat PCI. AP caudal view showed 95% ISR at proximal LMCA (a). Balloon dilatation of the lesion was done using 2.75×12 mm NC balloon and 3×10 mm cutting balloon (b, c). LCX ostium had critical narrowing after balloon dilatation (d), and hence, kissing balloon inflation (e) was done using 4×20 mm sirolimus eluting balloon (LMCA-LAD) and 2.75×12 mm NC balloon (LMCA-LCX). Final angiogram showed well expanded LMCA-LAD stent without residual stenosis (f).

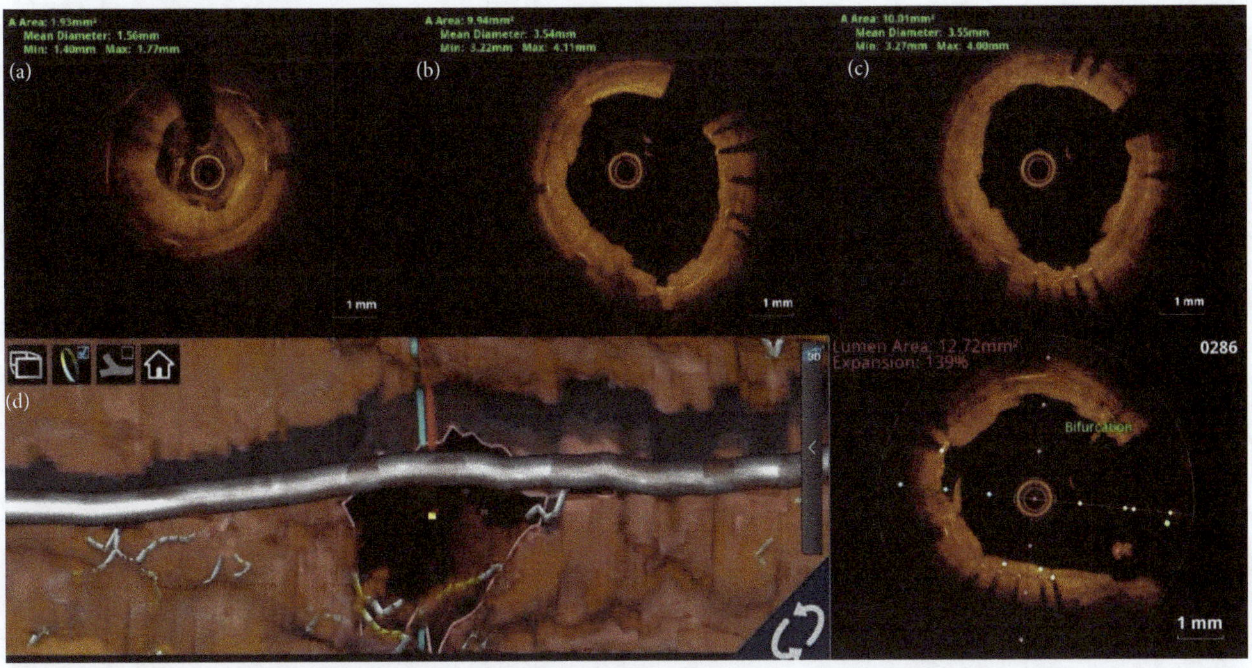

FIGURE 4: OCT images of PCI optimization. Initial OCT run showed diffuse neointimal hyperplasia with LMCA MSA of $1.93\,m^2$ (a). Final OCT run showed MSA at proximal LMCA and ostial LAD as $9.94\,mm^2$ and $10.01\,mm^2$, respectively (b, c). OCT 3D bifurcation mode (ILUMIEN™ Optis™ System—Abbott Vascular) showed adequate LCX ostial area (d).

Hence, dissection reentry techniques are not advisable in an unprotected LMCA-CTO. Though an antegrade approach is possible in distal LMCA-CTOs, a retrograde approach is preferred in ostial LMCA-CTOs due to lack of guide catheter support for an antegrade approach. Externalization of guidewire by pushing the retrograde guidewire into an antegrade guide catheter is technically difficult in ostial LMCA-CTOs, since the guide catheter cannot be engaged, and it has to be floated in the aorta near the LMCA ostium. Hence, snaring may be a better option. PCI with drug-coated balloon (DCB) without stenting is another option in patients with recurrent restenosis, and it has reasonably good outcomes [8]. Intracoronary imaging is essential to delineate the underlying cause for the ISR, because treatment varies according to the underlying etiology [9]. Though both OCT and IVUS can be used in stent failure, OCT is the preferred option because of its excellent resolution to detect the underlying biological causes. Both DCB and drug eluting stents (DES) are recommended for ISR due to biological causes like neointimal hyperplasia and neo-atherosclerosis [10].

4. Conclusion

TA may present with complex coronary artery disease, and its treatment is associated with a high incidence of repeat revascularization. Intracoronary imaging helps in identifying the underlying mechanism for stent failure, which directs the further management. PCI using drug-coated balloons helps to avoid repeated stenting in patients with TA and stent failure. Retrograde approach increases the success rate of PCI in LMCA-CTOs, particularly in ostial LMCA-CTO.

References

[1] E.-J. Kang, S. M. Kim, Y. H. Choe, G. Y. Lee, K.-N. Lee, and D.-K. Kim, "Takayasu arteritis: assessment of coronary arterial abnormalities with 128-section dual-source CT angiography of the coronary arteries and aorta," *Radiology*, vol. 270, no. 1, pp. 74–81, 2014.

[2] M. Maz, S. A. Chung, A. Abril et al., "2021 American College of Rheumatology/Vasculitis Foundation guideline for the management of giant cell arteritis and Takayasu arteritis," *Arthritis & Rhematology*, vol. 73, no. 8, pp. 1349–1365, 2021.

[3] B. Hellmich, A. Agueda, S. Monti et al., "2018 update of the EULAR recommendations for the management of large vessel vasculitis," *Annals of the Rheumatic Diseases*, vol. 79, no. 1, pp. 19–30, 2020.

[4] D. Saadoun, M. Lambert, T. Mirault et al., "Retrospective analysis of surgery versus endovascular intervention in Takayasu arteritis," *Circulation*, vol. 125, no. 6, pp. 813–819, 2012.

[5] H. Wang, Y. Zhang, Z. Shen, L. Fang, Z. Liu, and S. Zhang, "Comparing the effects of different management strategies on long-term outcomes for significant coronary stenosis in patients with Takayasu arteritis," *International Journal of Cardiology*, vol. 306, no. 306, pp. 1–7, 2020.

[6] Y. Yang, T. Tian, K. Yang et al., "Outcomes of percutaneous coronary intervention and coronary artery bypass grafting in patients with Takayasu arteritis," *International Journal of Cardiology*, vol. 241, no. 241, pp. 64–69, 2017.

[7] I. Xenogiannis, D. Karmpaliotis, K. Alaswad et al., "Left main chronic total occlusion percutaneous coronary intervention: a case series," *The Journal of Invasive Cardiology*, vol. 31, no. 7, pp. E220–E225, 2019.

[8] K. L. X. Chiew and P. O. Lim, "Three-year outcome with drug-coated balloon percutaneous coronary intervention in coronary Takayasu arteritis: a case review," *Catheterization and Cardiovascular Interventions*, vol. 97, no. 5, pp. 841–846, 2021.

[9] L. Raber, G. S. Mintz, K. C. Koskinas et al., "Clinical use of intracoronary imaging. Part 1: guidance and optimization of coronary interventions. An expert consensus document of the European Association of Percutaneous Cardiovascular Interventions," *European Heart Journal*, vol. 39, no. 35, pp. 3281–3300, 2018.

[10] E. Shlofmitz, M. Iantorno, and R. Waksman, "Restenosis of drug-eluting stents. A new classification system based on disease mechanism to guide treatment and state-of-the-art review," *Circulation. Cardiovascular Interventions*, vol. 12, no. 8, article e007023, 2019.

17

Achieving Hemostasis Post transcatheter Aortic Valve Replacement in a Patient with Aortobifemoral Bypass Graft using Perclose Device: A Novel Technique

Ebubechukwu Ezeh,[1] **Mohammad Amro**,[2] **Esiemoghie Akhigbe**,[1] **Mackenzie Hamilton**,[1] **and Mehrette Maru**[3]

[1]*Internal Medicine Department, Marshall University, Huntington WV, USA*
[2]*Internal Medicine Residency, The Palestinian Ministry of Health and Higher Education, State of Palestine*
[3]*Department of Cardiology, St. Mary's Medical Center, Huntington WV, USA*

Correspondence should be addressed to Ebubechukwu Ezeh; eoezeh18@gmail.com

Academic Editor: Ertugurul Ercan

The presence of aortobifemoral bypass graft can complicate vascular access during percutaneous intervention. Choosing an access route for transcatheter aortic valve replacement (TAVR) in this patient population can be challenging. Access options are further limited by the presence of coexisting vascular comorbidities such as extensive peripheral artery diseases in these patients. Adequate preoperative planning to determine the suitability of different access sites is, therefore, very crucial. Our case report shows that the use of Perclose can be a viable option for achieving hemostasis after a direct puncture of an aortobifemoral bypass graft during transfemoral TAVR.

1. Introduction

Transcatheter aortic valve replacement (TAVR) has become a common treatment option for patients with severe symptomatic aortic valve stenosis, and a transfemoral (TF) arterial approach is the most common approach [1]. Thus, whenever feasible, the TF should be employed for TAVR because it is more effective than alternative approaches, including transapical, transsubclavian, and direct aortic procedures [2]. Distorted anatomy of the femoral arteries as seen in patients with aortobifemoral bypass graft can, however, make TF access challenging. In this, we present a case where we used successfully used Perclose to close an aortobifemoral graft bypass puncture site during percutaneous transfemoral TAVR.

2. Case Presentation

Patient is an 81-year-old male with a history of nonrheumatic aortic stenosis who was admitted for a planned TAVR after complaining of a 6-month history of progressive dyspnea that had markedly impacted his quality of life. He denied palpitation, chest pain, or syncope. Notably, he had past medical history of peripheral artery disease status post-aortobifemoral bypass grafting, abdominal aortic aneurysm repair, and lung cancer status postradiotherapy. He also had a history of coronary artery disease status postright coronary artery (RCA) stent. Coronary angiography performed one month prior to admission showed patent RCA stent and stable left coronary disease.

Upon admission, his vital signs were blood pressure 145/49 millimeter of mercury (mmHg), pulse 68 beats/minute, and oxygen saturation of 96%. Cardiac auscultation revealed a systolic, grade 4 murmur maximally heard at the second right intercostal space and that radiated towards the carotid. Transthoracic echocardiogram confirmed severe aortic stenosis (maximal velocity > 4.0 m/s, and mean gradient > 40 mmHg and aortic valve area 0.8 squared centimeter). Ejection fraction (EF) was 60% with mild left atrial

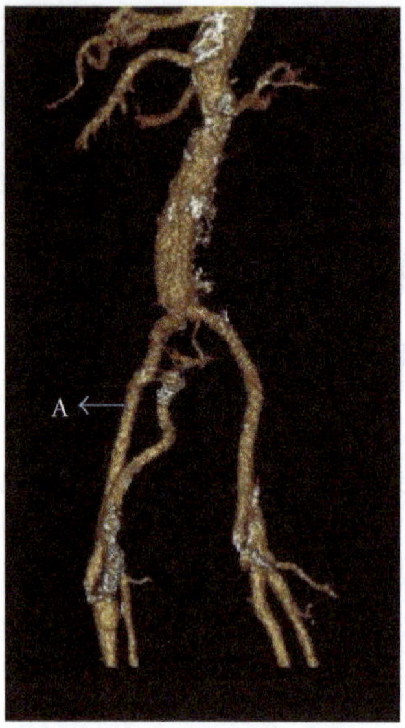

Figure 1: Showing graft (A) and stenosed, native femoral artery.

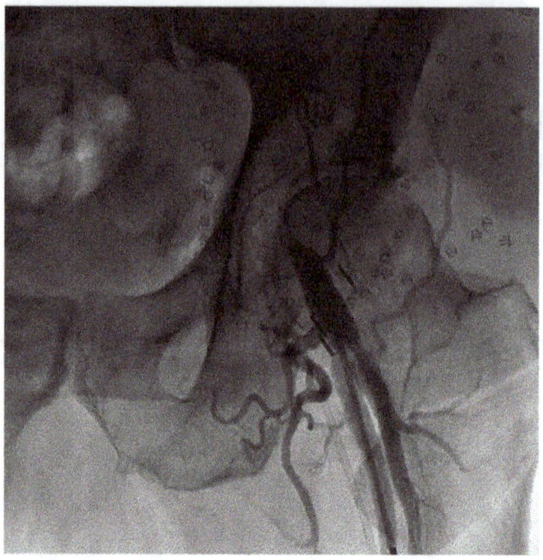

Figure 3: Angiogram showing graft puncture site without complications.

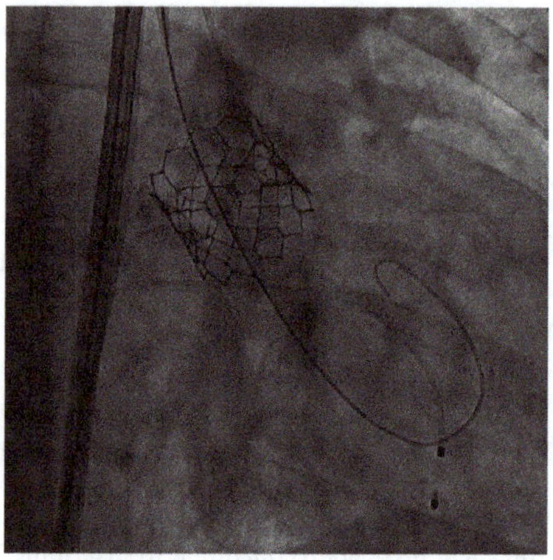

Figure 2: Showing deployed Sapien 3 valve.

enlargement. His Society of Thoracic Surgeons Predicted Risk of Mortality (STS-PROM) score was calculated to be 19%; he was, therefore, admitted for transcatheter aortic valve replacement (TAVR). Pre-TAVR work up with computed tomography angiogram (CTA) showed subclavian artery stenosis. CTA abdomen and pelvis showed widely patent graft aortobifemoral graft and widely patent femoral bifurcation bilaterally with moderate atheromatous calcification. These are shown in Figure 1.

Considering his comorbidities, the decision was made to utilize the TF approach in accessing the graft using adequate cutaneous anesthesia. TAVR was performed, and Perclose was successfully used to secure the puncture site with no complication. Patient's symptom improved afterwards. He had an uneventful recovery and was discharged.

3. Discussion

There have been few cases of TAVR in patients with previous aortobifemoral bypass grafting. Two previous case reports demonstrated the importance of thorough pre-TAVR planning including angiography to identify optimal access [3]. This is especially true in patients with previous aortobifemoral bypass grafting like our patient. Defining the most optimal strategy—as well as bail-out options—for access and closure of the large-bore arteriotomy is an absolute necessity in cases of previous aortobifemoral bypass grafts [3]. Also, peripheral artery disease, which is a major comorbidity in patients referred for TAVR, provides challenge in completing the TF-TAVR procedure in patients with comorbidities associated with femoral access routes such as iliofemoral arteries with severe narrowing, or an artificial bypass graft [4]. In these situations, other access routes like subclavian access are more typically utilized [5]. Our patient had stenosed subclavian artery; thus, we elected to use the TF route despite his history of aortobifemoral bypass graft.

During the procedure, the left common femoral artery was accessed with a needle under ultrasound guidance. A guidewire was introduced followed by a 6-French sheath using a modified Seldinger technique. A transvenous pacing wire was introduced into the right ventricle through the common femoral vein; it was interrogated and was confirmed to be functioning well. Using a guidewire, an angle pigtail catheter was introduced into the ascending aorta through the left common femoral artery. At the root of the aorta, an angiogram was performed to obtain the optimal angle for valve deployment. At this time, the right common femoral artery was accessed with a needle under ultrasound guidance. With a modified Seldinger technique, a guidewire followed by a 6-French sheath was introduced. Then, two Perclose devices, to be deployed at the end of the procedure, were placed at the access sites with the help of a guidewire. After obtaining adequate systemic heparinization, an 8-French sheath followed by a stiff Amplatz guidewire was introduced into the arch of the aorta. Dilators were used after which a 14-French Edwards Sapien sheath was introduced into the thoracic aorta. Then, with the help of a catheter, the guidewire was passed across the aortic valve. After that, a pigtail catheter was introduced into the left ventricle.

Subsequently, a 29-millimeter Sapien ultra 3 bioprosthetic valve, which was mounted on delivery system was then introduced with the help of Amplatz guidewire across the aortic valve (Figure 2). The bioprosthetic valve was deployed under fluoroscopy, under rapid pacing when the blood pressure was low. TTE was obtained and confirmed proper positioning of valve with no paravalvular leak. Then, the Perclose devices were completely deployed, and heparin was reversed with protamine. Sterile dressing was applied after the left common artery was closed with angio-seal. Angiogram showed no complication (Figure 3). Immediate postprocedure period was unremarkable.

4. Conclusion

Closure of distorted anatomies such as aortobifemoral graft can present a great challenge during TAVR. This case report demonstrates that TF-TAVR with Perclose closure of the femoral access in a patient with vascular endograft is feasible approach—after careful preprocedural imaging, assessment, and planning. As a result, the transfemoral TAVR approach can reasonably be expanded to patients with previous aorto-bifemoral bypass graft surgery who have contraindications to general anesthesia and/or alternative access routes.

References

[1] G. C. M. Siontis, F. Praz, T. Pilgrim et al., "Transcatheter aortic valve implantation vs. surgical aortic valve replacement for treatment of severe aortic stenosis: a meta-analysis of randomized trials," *European Heart Journal*, vol. 37, no. 47, pp. 3503–3512, 2016.

[2] G. M. Fröhlich, P. D. Baxter, C. J. Malkin et al., "Comparative Survival After Transapical, Direct Aortic, and Subclavian Transcatheter Aortic Valve Implantation (Data from the UK TAVI Registry)," *The American Journal of Cardiology*, vol. 116, no. 10, pp. 1555–1559, 2015.

[3] L. Rosseel, I. Degrieck, B. de Bruyne, L. Søndergaard, and O. de Backer, "Percutaneous transfemoral TAVR with direct puncture and successful closure of aortobifemoral bypass graft," *CJC Open*, vol. 2, no. 1, pp. 34–37, 2020.

[4] I. Ben-Dor, R. Waksman, N. N. Hanna et al., "Utility of radiologic review for noncardiac findings on multislice computed tomography in patients with severe aortic stenosis evaluated for transcatheter aortic valve implantation," *The American Journal of Cardiology*, vol. 105, no. 10, pp. 1461–1464, 2010.

[5] D. A. Raptis, M. A. Beal, D. C. Kraft, H. S. Maniar, and A. J. Bierhals, "Transcatheter aortic valve replacement: alternative access beyond the femoral arterial approach," *Radiographics*, vol. 39, no. 1, pp. 30–43, 2019.

18

Surgical Management of Right Atrial Mass Associated with a Vascular Access Catheter

David Ferreira,[1,2] **Anthony Le**,[3] **John Khoo**,[1] **Paul Nguyen**,[1] **Manish Jain**,[3] **Timothy Spicer**,[2,4] **and Craig Juergens**[1,2]

[1]*Department of Cardiology, Liverpool Hospital, NSW, 2170 Sydney, Australia*
[2]*Department of Medicine, University of New South Wales, NSW, 2052 Sydney, Australia*
[3]*Department of Cardiothoracic Surgery, Liverpool Hospital, NSW, 2170 Sydney, Australia*
[4]*Department of Nephrology, Liverpool Hospital, NSW, 2170 Sydney, Australia*

Correspondence should be addressed to David Ferreira; dave_7@live.com.au

Academic Editor: Assad Movahed

Atrial masses are an uncommon but serious clinical problem. The authors report a case of an atrial mass associated with a tunnelled vascular access catheter in an immunosuppressed haemodialysis patient. In the setting of immunosuppression with fevers, a broad differential for the atrial mass was considered. Multidisciplinary team review was pursued to guide management decisions. Ultimately, surgical excision of the mass was pursued with an excellent result. The causes and management of this complex clinical scenario are discussed.

1. Introduction

Atrial masses pose an infrequent diagnostic and management dilemma. The differential diagnoses are broad and include primary and secondary malignancy, benign neoplasms, thrombi, and infective foci [1, 2]. Assessment and management require integration of clinical, laboratory, and imaging investigations and may necessitate involvement from multiple specialty teams. In this report, the authors describe a case of a right atrial mass complicating immunosuppression for lupus nephritis and haemodialysis via a tunnelled vascular access catheter. Ultimately, a diagnosis of atrial thrombus was confirmed on histology. The considered differential diagnoses and management strategy will be described. The management of atrial thrombus associated with vascular access catheters will then be discussed.

2. Case Presentation

An 18-year-old female with lupus nephritis, treated with tacrolimus and rituximab, was referred for admission to hospital. She had, until recently, required haemodialysis via a tunnelled permanent vascular access catheter which was still in situ. Complicating her immunosuppression, *Cryptococcus neoformans* meningitis was diagnosed through lumbar puncture seven months earlier. She was initially treated with intravenous amphotericin and flucytosine and was subsequently placed on therapeutic oral fluconazole.

Outpatient transthoracic echocardiography demonstrated a large echogenic mass in the right atrium at the tip of the vascular access catheter. Transoesophageal echocardiography confirmed an echogenic mass in the right atrium measuring 23 mm × 26 mm (see Figure 1) and a patent foramen ovale (PFO) with left to right shunt (see Clip 1). The differential diagnoses considered were that of atrial thrombus complicating vascular access, as well as an infective focus. A primary tumour was unlikely given a normal transthoracic echocardiogram four months before.

Inflammatory markers and septic screening with blood cultures were performed. C-reactive protein was 0.9 mg/L, and the neutrophil count was 9.5×10^9. Three blood cultures were negative for bloodstream infection. Ventilation perfusion scanning revealed segmental pulmonary emboli. After multidisciplinary discussion, standard percutaneous catheter

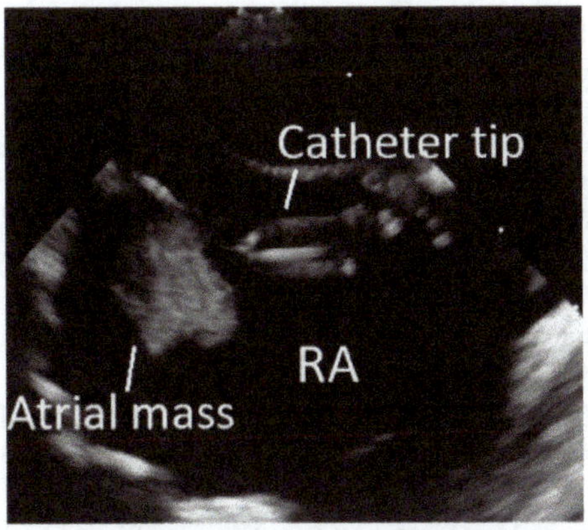

FIGURE 1: Transoesophageal echocardiography demonstrating vascular catheter tip abutting a right atrial mass.

removal was deemed high risk due to potential embolisation. Anticoagulation with Apixaban was initiated for suspected atrial thrombus, and serial cardiac imaging was organised. Removal of the vascular access catheter was to be planned after thrombus resolution, and the patient was discharged [3].

Four weeks later, she represented with lethargy and fevers to 39.4 degrees Celsius. Inflammatory markers were elevated with a C-reactive protein of 157 mg/L and neutrophils of 10.2×10^9. A repeat infective panel was performed, and empiric therapy with intravenous gentamicin and vancomycin was provided due to skin colonisation with methicillin-resistant *Staphylococcus aureus*. Blood cultures, including vascular catheter cultures, were positive for *Stenotrophomonas maltophilia*, and a diagnosis of line-associated bacteraemia was made. Infectious diseases input was sought, and broad-spectrum antimicrobials with intravenous trimethoprim-sulfamethoxazole and cefepime were administered. Regular therapeutic oral fluconazole was continued. Rapid clinical response to antimicrobial therapy was seen with defervescence within 24 hours.

Repeat transthoracic echocardiogram showed no interval change in the right atrial mass despite anticoagulation. This placed the diagnosis of thrombus in doubt, and in the setting of bacteraemia, complicating infection could not be excluded. After multidisciplinary review by infectious diseases, cardiology, cardiothoracic surgery, nephrology, and interventional radiology, definitive management of the atrial mass was deemed appropriate. This decision was made considering the diagnosis of thrombus was in doubt after anticoagulation failed to reduce its size, and in the setting of bacteraemia, complicating infection could not be excluded. Endovascular removal and thrombolysis were deemed high risk due to potential for embolisation. The decision was made to pursue open surgical thrombectomy, PFO closure, and vascular catheter removal. Brain magnetic resonance imaging (MRI) was negative for ischaemic stroke prior to on-pump cardiothoracic surgery.

Surgery was performed (see Figure 2) with no postoperative complications, and she was discharged seven days later. Histology demonstrated organised thrombus with no evidence of abscess, granuloma, endocarditis, or myxoma (see Figure 3).

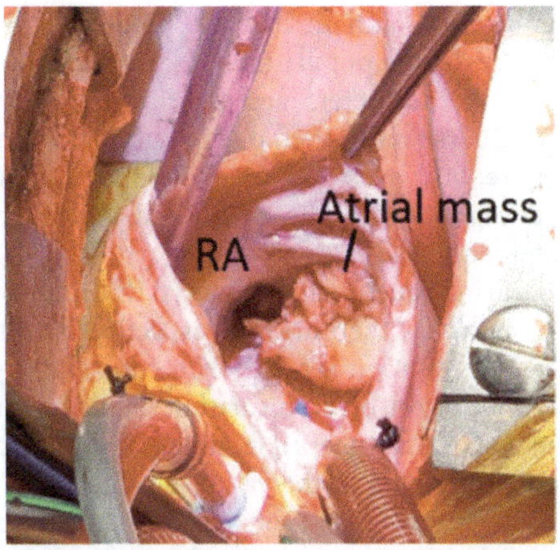

FIGURE 2: Intraoperative image of open right atrium with right atrial mass.

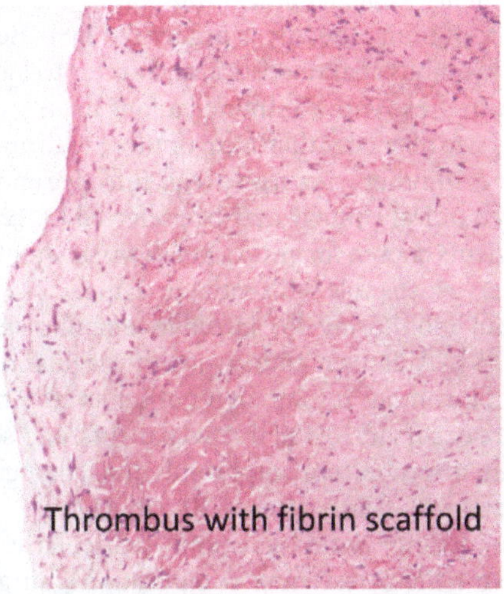

FIGURE 3: Histology of the atrial mass demonstrating organised thrombus with fibrin scaffold.

3. Discussion

Though infrequent, atrial masses can pose a significant diagnostic and management challenge. The differential diagnosis is broad and includes primary and secondary cardiac tumours, infective processes, and thrombi. Primary tumours are rare and have an incidence of 0.02% based on large autopsy series [4]. Secondary cardiac metastases occur 20 times more often, the most common primaries being mesothelioma, lung cancer, and melanoma [4]. Primary atrial mural endocarditis is rare with reported organisms including staphylococcus species, streptococci species, aspergillus, and candida [2, 5–7]. Secondary infection complicating myxoma has also been reported with similar bacterial pathogens [8].

In this case, the atrial mass was histologically confirmed as organised thrombus without an infective component. While atrial thrombi are rare, they can complicate 5-18% of vascular access catheters for haemodialysis patients [9, 10]. This is related to factors including the intra-atrial prothrombotic foreign body, frequent complicating infections in the immunosuppressed, and thrombotic predisposition in the chronic kidney disease population [11]. Atrial thrombi complicating vascular catheters are associated with mortality rates of 18.3-20.6%, most often due to pulmonary embolism, cardiac failure, and overwhelming sepsis [3, 12]. Mortality rates appear high (44%) in those managed without thrombus specific intervention [3].

Due to the infrequent nature of atrial thrombi complicating vascular catheters, there are no prospective data informing management. Prevention is better than cure, and in the haemodialysis population, fistula formation should be considered over vascular access catheters if feasible [12]. When a thrombus is present, removal of the vascular catheter is ideal [3]. Percutaneous removal may not be possible due to risk of thrombus dislodgement and life-threatening pulmonary embolism. Current retrospective reviews have shown that in 50% of cases, therapeutic anticoagulation was the initial treatment of choice. Primary surgical thrombectomy is pursued in 25% of patients while first line thrombolysis occurs in 7-17%. The choice of initial therapy is influenced by patient comorbidities, thrombus characteristics, and access to local surgical expertise. In those with contraindications to anticoagulation, thrombus size of greater than 6 cm or those with another indication for cardiothoracic surgery (e.g., infective endocarditis), a primary surgical strategy may be preferred [3, 12].

In patients chosen for anticoagulation, six months of therapy appears reasonable with serial imaging, close follow-up, and careful monitoring for infective, embolic, and cardiac sequelae [9]. A longer course of anticoagulation may be required if thrombus resolution is not achieved. Anticoagulation failure occurs in 30% of treated patients, and second-line options are thrombectomy or thrombolysis, though the latter is associated with failure rates of 30-75% [12].

When failing anticoagulation, particularly with the potential for life-threatening complications, surgical intervention for vascular access catheter associated atrial thrombus is a potential management option in complex patients [13, 14].

Consent

Informed written consent has been provided by the patient.

References

[1] R. Mankad and J. Herrmann, "Cardiac tumors: echo assessment," *Echo Research and Practice*, vol. 3, no. 4, pp. R65–R77, 2017.

[2] S. O. Soman, G. Vijayaraghavan, N. P. Padmaja, A. R. Warrier, and M. Unni, "Aspergilloma of the heart," *Indian Heart Journal*, vol. 66, no. 2, pp. 238–240, 2014.

[3] A. Stavroulopoulos, V. Aresti, and C. Zounis, "Right atrial thrombi complicating haemodialysis catheters. A meta-analysis of reported cases and a proposal of a management algorithm," *Nephrology, Dialysis, Transplantation*, vol. 27, no. 7, pp. 2936–2944, 2012.

[4] F. Silvestri, R. Bussani, N. Pavletic, and T. Mannone, "Metastases of the heart and pericardium," *Giornale Italiano di Cardiologia*, vol. 27, no. 12, pp. 1252–1255, 1997.

[5] S. Hosokawa, H. Okayama, G. Hiasa et al., "Isolated left atrial infective mural endocarditis," *Internal Medicine*, vol. 57, no. 7, pp. 957–960, 2018.

[6] Y. Agrawal, R. Dada, J. Dada, and M. Degregorio, "Primary mural infective endocarditis with associated central line infection," *BMJ Case Reports*, vol. 11, no. 1, 2018.

[7] W. Chowdhury, M. U. Lodhi, I. A. Syed, U. Rahim, M. Miller, and M. Rahim, "Catheter-related Candida endocarditis on the right atrial septum - a case report," *Cureus*, vol. 10, no. 2, article e2158, 2018.

[8] S.-M. Yuan, "Infected cardiac myxoma: an updated review," *Brazilian Journal of Cardiovascular Surgery*, vol. 30, no. 5, pp. 571–578, 2015.

[9] A. Shah, M. Murray, and C. Nzerue, "Right atrial thrombi complicating use of central venous catheters in hemodialysis," *The Journal of Vascular Access*, vol. 6, no. 1, pp. 18–24, 2018.

[10] M. Dilek, C. Kaya, A. Karatas, I. Ozer, N. Arik, and O. Gulel, "Catheter-related atrial thrombus: tip of the iceberg?," *Renal Failure*, vol. 37, no. 4, pp. 567–571, 2015.

[11] K. Wattanakit and M. Cushman, "Chronic kidney disease and venous thromboembolism: epidemiology and mechanisms," *Current Opinion in Pulmonary Medicine*, vol. 15, no. 5, pp. 408–412, 2009.

[12] M.-H. Tran, T. Wilcox, and P. N. Tran, "Cather-related right atrial thrombosis," *The Journal of Vascular Access*, vol. 21, no. 3, article 1129729819873851, 2020.

[13] N. Hussain, P. E. Shattuck, M. H. Senussi et al., "Large right atrial thrombus associated with central venous catheter requiring open heart surgery," *Case Reports in Medicine*, vol. 2012, Article ID 501303, 4 pages, 2012.

[14] M. Akçay, S. B. Deşer, Ö. Gedikli, S. Yüksel, and O. Gülel, "Successful management of complications after inappropriate positioning of a hemodialysis catheter," *Anatolian Journal of Cardiology*, vol. 18, no. 4, pp. E7–E8, 2017.

19

Impact of Percutaneous Coronary Intervention and Implantation of Intra-Aortic Balloon Pump on the Outcome of an Acute Total Obstruction of the Left Main Coronary Artery

Hamza Hamayel,[1] Yahya Ismail,[2,3] Sajed Majadla,[2,3] Yousef Hamshari,[1] and Yunis Daralammouri[2,3]

[1]*Department of Internal Medicine, An-Najah National University Hospital, Nablus, State of Palestine*
[2]*Department of Cardiology, An-Najah National University Hospital, Nablus, State of Palestine*
[3]*Department of Medicine, Faculty of Medicine and Health Sciences, An-Najah National University, Nablus, State of Palestine*

Correspondence should be addressed to Yahya Ismail; hartdocyahya@yahoo.com

Academic Editor: Antonio de Padua Mansur

Background. Acute total occlusion of the left main coronary artery (LMCA) is a fatal event; most patients die before reaching hospitals. Few of them reach the hospital alive. Revascularization of the LMCA can be achieved by surgical intervention or percutaneous coronary intervention with unknown optimal modality. However, mortality of those patients is very high even with either; few cases reported successful management of acute total occlusion of the LMCA including our patient. *Case Presentation.* A 56-year-old male patient who is a smoker presented with typical chest pain worsened 2 hours prior to admission. He was hemodynamically stable, but he had respiratory failure due to pulmonary edema. An electrocardiogram showed anterior ST-elevation myocardial infarction. He was given loading doses of dual antiplatelet agents, in addition to respiratory support, then transferred immediately to the cardiac catheterization laboratory. Urgent cardiac catheterization showed total occlusion of the LMCA. Recanalization was done successfully, and a stent was inserted in the LMCA and left anterior descending artery. The patient developed cardiogenic shock during the procedure. An intra-aortic balloon pump (IABP) was applied which improved his hemodynamic status and enhanced his coronary flow. He is clinically improved, there was resolution of ST elevation, and cardiogenic shock gradually resolved. IABP was removed, and the patient was discharged in good general condition. *Conclusions.* Survival after acute total occlusion of the LMCA is very rare. The good outcome in this patient is attributed to early recognition and timely successful intervention, with good respiratory and hemodynamic support. The surgical and anaesthesia team should be on stand-by until complete revascularization and stabilization of the patient are achieved.

1. Background

Acute total occlusion of the left main coronary artery (LMCA) is an emergency condition and a catastrophic event. It is a very rare presentation of acute coronary syndrome [1]. Sudden death due to cardiogenic shock or arrhythmia is usually the outcome which occurred before any intervention can be done [2, 3]. The remaining patients mostly presented with cardiogenic shock and critical condition with a very high mortality rate even with revascularization [4].

Literature case reports revealed successful management of acute total occlusion of the LMCA with coronary artery bypass graft (CABG) and percutaneous coronary intervention (PCI). However, optimal modality is unknown yet [5]. There is limited data about the presentation with ST-elevation myocardial infarction (STEMI) and cardiogenic shock.

Our report describes a 56-year-old man with acute total occlusion of the LMCA presenting as ST-elevation myocardial infarction (STEMI) that developed cardiogenic shock during the procedure and treated with emergency primary PCI and simultaneous implantation of IABP.

2. Case Presentation

In December 2018, a 56-year-old male patient who is a heavy smoker without other comorbidities was referred to our hospital as a case of acute coronary syndrome for cardiac catheterization. The history of the patient revealed that he had typical retrosternal chest pain for 8 hours increased in intensity 2 hours prior to hospital admission. He received his first medical assessment 40 minutes before presentation to our hospital where he was given 300 mg chewable aspirin, 300 mg clopidogrel, and 5000 international unit (IU) of heparin for a diagnosis of STEMI by electrocardiogram (ECG). Upon arrival to our hospital, he was conscious but in severe respiratory distress in terms of tachypnea and hypoxemia, in addition to anginal chest pain. Blood pressure was 135/90 mmHg, and heart rate was 50 beats/min with regular pulse, SpO_2 75% on room air. Physical examination showed elevated jugular venous pressure (JVP), bilateral chest crepitation up to mid-chest-zones, and unremarkable cardiac auscultation findings. Pulmonary edema was diagnosed, and oxygen was started by nonrebreather mask (NRM) along with intravenous (IV) furosemide and nitroglycerine infusion, to relieve chest pain and improve respiratory condition. ECG showed left axis deviation, and STEMI in the anterior chest leads with premature ventricular complexes (PVCs) in bigeminy pattern (Figure 1). The patient was transferred to the cardiac catheterization laboratory for primary PCI.

The door to balloon time was eighty minutes. During preparation for cardiac catheterization, his symptoms from pulmonary edema did not improve. So, we put the patient on noninvasive ventilation which resulted in significant improvement of his respiratory symptoms. We proceeded with cardiac catheterization using the left Judkins guide catheter through femoral access; the 1st injection of contrast material revealed total occlusion of the left main coronary artery (LMCA) with thrombolysis in myocardial infarction (TIMI) flow "0" (Figure 2). Meanwhile, the cardiac surgery and anaesthesia team was called and remained on standby in case CABG surgery become necessary. Successful Recanalization of the Left Coronary Circulation LCS using 0.014 × 180 cm floppy guide wire, subsequently predilation with 2.00 × 20 mm balloon was done followed by deployment of 4.00 × 28 mm everolimus drug-eluting stent (Figure 3). During intervention, he developed hypotension which required starting norepinephrine infusion, dose titrated up to 0.15 mcg/kg/min to keep mean arterial BP over 65 mmHg. Also, he developed two attacks of ventricular tachycardia with hypotension terminated with defibrillation. He was started on amiodarone infusion. Lidocaine infusion was added after the second attack of ventricular tachycardia. As soon as the procedure on the left coronary artery was completed, the right coronary artery was examined which showed a dominant artery with significant proximal stenosis, and moderate diffuse stenosis from mid to distal segment (Figure 4). On the following 24 hours, the patient maintained on heparin infusion at a rate of 1000 unit/hour titrated on the basis of activated thromboplastin time (aPTT) to achieve twice the normal value, and tirofiban with initial of bolus of 25 microgram/kg over 3 minutes followed by continuous infusion at a rate of 0.15 mcg/kg/min.

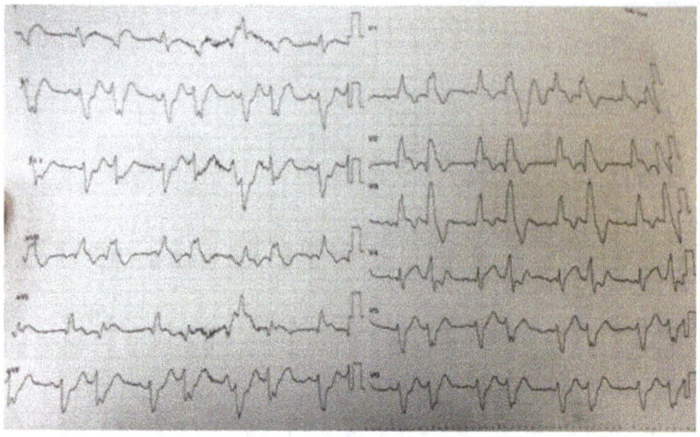

FIGURE 1: Electrocardiogram at presentation: sinus rhythm, STEMI in anterior chest leads, left axis deviation, PVCs in bigeminy pattern.

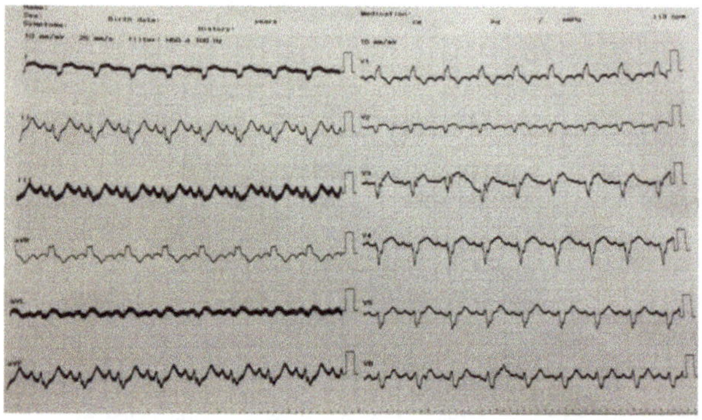

FIGURE 2: Electrocardiogram after primary PCI: it showed resolution of STEMI.

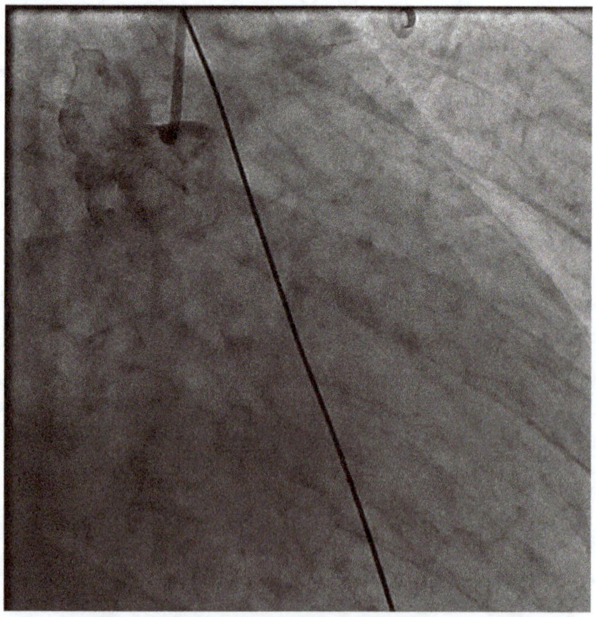

FIGURE 3: Cardiac catheterization showed total occlusion of LMCA.

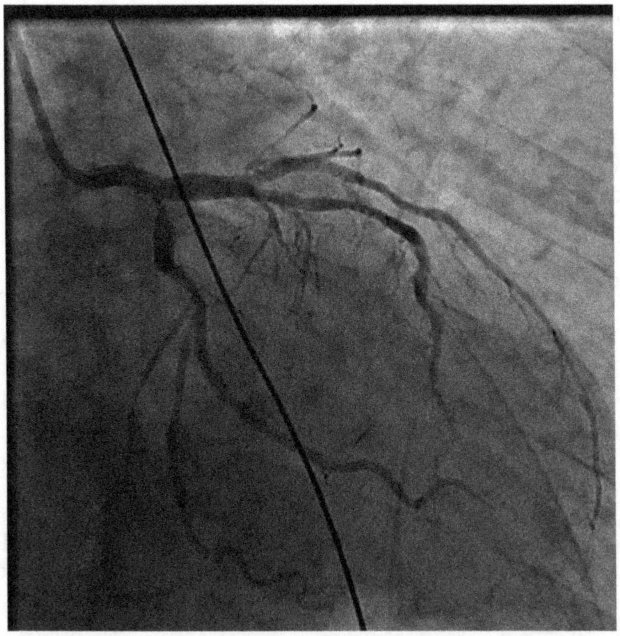

FIGURE 4: Left coronary artery after stenting LMCA with restoration of blood flow.

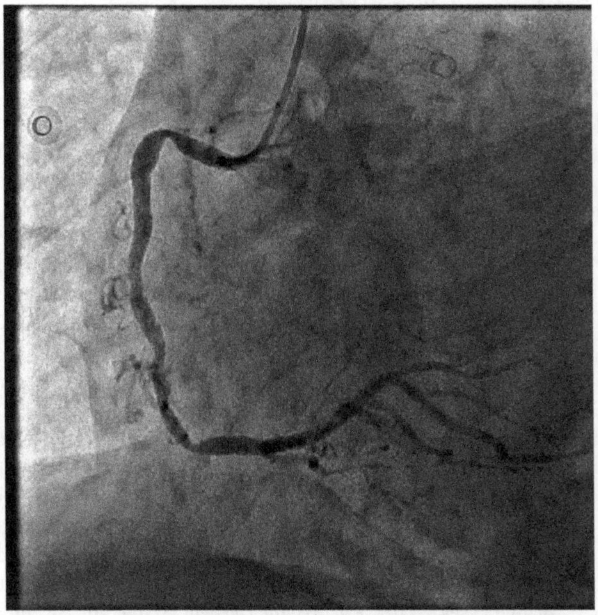

FIGURE 5: Cardiac catheterization for right coronary artery, dominant artery and showed proximal significant stenosis, and moderate diffuse stenosis from mid to distal segment.

At the end of the procedure, the patient remained hypotensive with slow coronary flow. An intra-aortic balloon pump (IABP) was positioned under fluoroscopy via femoral access, and 1 : 1 augmentation was started. On admission, troponin was normal. Six hours after the procedure, troponin was 1028 ng/ml, reference range (0.1-0.4). ECG showed resolving of ST-elevation and PVCs with a bigeminy pattern (Figure 5). After the PCI, blood pressure started to improve. Two days after intervention, he was weaned from IABP, and norepinephrine infusion was tapered down gradually till we stopped it on day four; troponin continued to decrease gradually till it became negative, and Transthoracic Echocardiography (TTE) after removal of IABP showed ejection fraction (EF) 40%. The patient was discharged after 8 days of hospitalization in good general condition with stable vital signs on the following medications: aspirin 100 mg once daily, clopidogrel 75 mg twice daily for the first 2 weeks then once daily, atorvastatin 80 mg once daily, furosemide 40 mg once daily, bisoprolol 2.5 mg once daily, and enalapril 5 mg once daily.

3. Discussion

Total occlusion of the LMCA is a rare and fatal event. It is reported in less than 0.6% of acute coronary syndrome who were admitted for primary PCI. Most of them die before arriving to the hospital. While mortality for those patients is very high even with appropriate management, only half of the patients survived and discharged alive from the hospital [1].

As the LMCA supplies most of the left ventricular mass, acute occlusion will lead to catastrophic massive myocardial infarction and arrhythmia. This explain differences in the outcome and mortality when it is compared with occlusion of distal coronary bed especially in the absence of collateral circulation [1].

It is still unknown what is the best management of such cases, either to proceed with PCI or CABG [5]. Successful revascularization by angioplasty and stenting of the LMCA was reported with a good final result [6–9]. Emergency CABG is also effective in restoring blood flow, but it is time consuming and may carry risk of irreversible damage by ischemia [9]. There are reported cases where PCI failed and the patient underwent emergency CABG to restore blood flow [10]. However, this could be different right now with the improvement of intervention technique and stent technology. In our case, ECG for the patient was confusing and its changes did not give any hint for total occlusion of the LMCA. So, when the first injection of contrast material revealed total occlusion of the left main coronary artery, it was obvious that PCI is the appropriate approach for time interest. Meanwhile, the cardiac surgery and anaesthesia team was called to be on standby for any need for urgent CABG surgery. Fortunately, our hospital is a tertiary hospital, well-staffed, and with equipment for primary PCI. Opening of the occlusion and restoration of blood flow was successfully done within 80 minutes.

Periprocedure cardiogenic shock, no flow after intervention, and late presentation were reported as a poor prognostic factor and carry a high mortality rate [1]. Our case survived because of early recognition, timely preparation of cardiac catheterization laboratory, and successful revascularization. This was a result of good and proper communication between emergency room doctors, cardiologist on call, and cardiac catheterization laboratory team. Moreover, early supportive management of respiratory failure with noninvasive ventilation and early treatment of pulmonary edema in addition to hemodynamic support using norepinephrine and IABP kept the patient stable until reperfusion was achieved.

Hypotension during the procedure as a result of reperfusion injury was suspected before revascularization. For which, femoral access was selected instead of radial access, and vasopressor and IAPB were prepared before reperfusion. Hemodynamic support with norepinephrine was the initial vasopressor according to guidelines [11]. It was started during intervention once his blood pressure started to drop before any hypotension episode; then, it was titrated according to mean arterial pressure reading keeping it more than 65 mmHg. After reperfusion was done and due to slow flow (TIMI 1 flow), IABP was applied as stabilizing measure and to enhance coronary perfusion. There is conflicting result about the benefit of IABP in cardiogenic shock [12]. In the IABP-SHOCK II trial, there was no difference in the outcome between patients that underwent IABP insertion and those who did not [13]. However, this cannot be generalized to LMCA disease which constitutes 9% of cases in that trial. Moreover, it is usually inserted when other devices like the left ventricular assistance device (LVAD) are not available.

In conclusion, this report describes a 56-year-old male patient who survived acute LMCA occlusion treated with primary PCI. Early recognition and timely intervention with appropriate management resulted in good outcome. The patient survived until discharge from the hospital. At 2-year follow-up, he remained in good general condition.

Abbreviations

LMCA: Left main coronary artery
ECG: Electrocardiogram
STEMI: ST-elevation myocardial infarction
CABG: Coronary artery bypass graft
PCI: Percutaneous coronary intervention
IABP: An intra-aortic balloon pumps (IABP)
PVC: Premature ventricular complex.

Consent

This is a case report with no identifiable content; despite this, written consent form was taken from the patient himself for participation and publication. There are no images or other personal data that might compromise the anonymity of the patients.

Authors' Contributions

Authors YI, YA, and SM have contributed to the diagnosis and management of this patient. YI did cardiac catheterization and stent insertion. HH and YH participated in the drafting of the manuscript. All authors read and approved the final manuscript.

Acknowledgments

The authors thank the Clinical Research Centre of An-Najah National University Hospital for their wise pieces of advice. Moreover, we are very thankful to the cardiac catheterization and cardiology team at our hospital for providing support for completing this report.

References

[1] N. Patel, G. L. de Maria, G. Kassimis et al., "Outcomes after emergency percutaneous coronary intervention in patients with unprotected left main stem occlusion: the BCIS national audit of percutaneous coronary intervention 6-year experience," *JACC. Cardiovascular Interventions*, vol. 7, no. 9, pp. 969–980, 2014.

[2] G. de Luca, H. Suryapranata, K. Thomas et al., "Outcome in patients treated with primary angioplasty for acute myocardial infarction due to left main coronary artery occlusion," *The American Journal of Cardiology*, vol. 91, no. 2, pp. 235–238, 2003.

[3] J. Takahashi, T. Sugiki, J. Okude et al., "Emergency surgical treatment for acute occlusion of the left main coronary artery-report of a case," *Annals of Thoracic and Cardiovascular Surgery*, vol. 9, no. 1, pp. 73–78, 2003.

[4] I. F. Édes, Z. Ruzsa, L. Gellér et al., "Acute, total occlusion of the left main stem: coronary intervention options, outcomes, and recommendations," *Advances in Interventional Cardiology*, vol. 14, no. 3, pp. 233–239, 2018.

[5] G. Saeed, "Survival after acute and total occlusion of the left main coronary artery," *Asian Cardiovascular & Thoracic Annals*, vol. 18, no. 6, p. 599, 2010.

[6] M. Yamane, S. Inoue, A. Yamane, O. Kinebuchi, and H. Yokozuka, "Primary stenting for left-main shock syndrome," *EuroIntervention: journal of EuroPCR in collaboration with the Working Group on Interventional Cardiology of the European Society of Cardiology*, vol. 1, no. 2, pp. 198–203, 2005.

[7] M. S. Lee, C.-H. Tseng, C. M. Barker et al., "Outcome after surgery and percutaneous intervention for cardiogenic shock and left main disease," *The Annals of Thoracic Surgery*, vol. 86, no. 1, pp. 29–34, 2008.

[8] N. Aygül, M. U. Aygül, K. Özdemir, and B. B. Altunkeser, "Emergency revascularization procedures in patients with acute ST-elevation myocardial infarction due to acute total occlusion of unprotected left main coronary artery: a report of five cases," *Türk Kardiyoloji Derneği Arşivi*, vol. 38, no. 2, pp. 131–134, 2010.

[9] M. M. Abuzahra, A. Mesa, and B. Treistman, "Unprotected left main coronary artery intervention for acute myocardial infarction and cardiogenic shock," *Texas Heart Institute Journal*, vol. 34, no. 4, pp. 479–484, 2007.

[10] R.-B. Hsu, C.-Y. Chien, S.-S. Wang, and S.-H. Chu, "Surgical revascularization for acute total occlusion of left main coronary artery," *Texas Heart Institute Journal*, vol. 27, no. 3, pp. 299–301, 2000.

[11] E. M. Antman, D. T. Anbe, P. W. Armstrong et al., "ACC/AHA guidelines for the management of patients with ST-elevation myocardial infarction: a report of the American College of Cardiology/American Heart Association task force on practice guidelines (committee to revise the 1999 guidelines

for the management of patients with acute myocardial infarction)," *Journal of the American College of Cardiology*, vol. 44, no. 3, pp. E1–E211, 2004.

[12] Authors/Task Force Members, P. G. Steg, S. K. James et al., "ESC guidelines for the management of acute myocardial infarction in patients presenting with ST-segment elevation," *European Heart Journal*, vol. 33, no. 20, pp. 2569–2619, 2012.

[13] H. Thiele, U. Zeymer, F.-J. Neumann et al., "Intraaortic balloon support for myocardial infarction with cardiogenic shock," *The New England Journal of Medicine*, vol. 367, no. 14, pp. 1287–1296, 2012.

20

Rare Association between Giant Right Ventricular Myxoma and Right Coronary Artery Tumour Blush with Complicating Pulmonary Tumour Embolism

Robin Yeong Hong Goh,[1] **Shreeja Mehrotra**,[2] **Stefan Buchholz**,[1] **Deepak Mehrotra**,[2] **and Allison Morton**[1]

[1]*Heart Care, Western Australia, Suite 21, St. John of God Bunbury Hospital, 700 Robertson Dr, College Grove, Western Australia, Australia*
[2]*Department of Cardiothoracic Surgery, Heart and Lung Centre, Mount Hospital, 150 Mounts Bay Rd, Perth, Western Australia, Australia*

Correspondence should be addressed to Robin Yeong Hong Goh; wwwrgrobin@gmail.com

Academic Editor: Gianluca Di Bella

Cardiac myxoma is a benign primary cardiac tumour which can present with nonspecific symptoms of right heart failure, syncope, exertional dyspnea, and pulmonary embolism. We describe a case of a right ventricular myxoma complicated with bilateral pulmonary embolism, with an incidental right coronary artery fistula but otherwise normal coronary anatomy on coronary angiogram. This case report emphasizes the importance of performing a transesophageal echo in the setting of pulmonary embolism to search for the origin of thrombus/tumour, and performing a comprehensive assessment is also necessary to rule out coronary artery disease, coronary artery fistula that may also represent a tumour blush.

1. Background

Cardiac myxoma is the most prevalent (50%) benign primary cardiac tumour [1], with 85% arising from the left atrium, 10% from the right atrium, and 5% from the ventricles [2]. Patients can present with constitutional symptoms (fever, lethargy, and weight loss), infection (endocarditis), or nonspecific symptoms of right heart failure, syncope, exertional dyspnea, and pulmonary embolism [3, 4].

2. Case Summary

A 60-year-old man presented with pleuritic chest pain and shortness of breath on a background of exertional dyspnea associated with self-limiting central chest pain over the past eight years increasing over the past three weeks. Apart from having symptoms suggestive of obstructive sleep apnea, he is a nonsmoker and is in the low-risk group for developing thromboembolism with a Wells' score of zero on initial assessment. The patient also had no history of familial or recurrent myxoma or stigmata associated with Carney's complex [5]. In the work-up process, he was found to have no deep venous thrombosis (DVT), but computed tomography pulmonary angiogram (CTPA) showed large pulmonary embolism more on the left side (Figures 1 and 2). Transthoracic and transesophageal echo confirmed right ventricular filling defect (Figure 2), which initially was thought to be a right ventricular thrombus and was placed on intravenous heparin therapy. An angiogram revealed incidental distal right coronary artery fistula (Figure 3), without haemodynamic compromise, likely also represents "tumour blush." During surgery on cardiopulmonary bypass (CPB), a myxoma arising from the right ventricular septum beneath the septal leaflet of the tricuspid valve, approximately 5 cm × 4 cm in size was identified (Figure 4) and removed without spilling and further fragmentation (Figure 5). The tumour

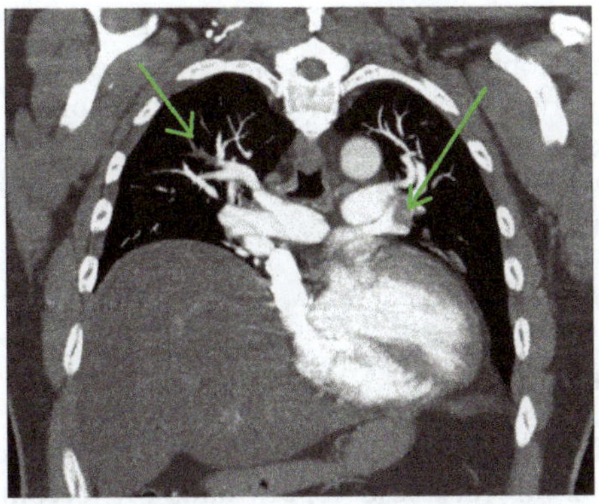

FIGURE 1: Computed tomography pulmonary angiogram revealed bilateral pulmonary emboli (green arrows).

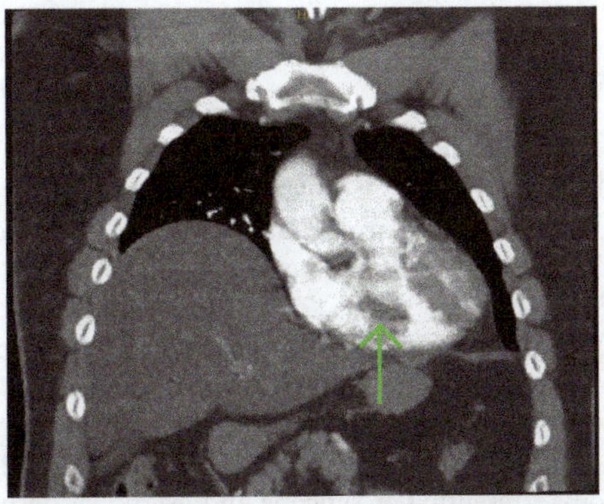

FIGURE 2: Computed tomography pulmonary angiogram revealed a broad-based filling defect in the right ventricle (green arrow), with incidental finding of preoperative raised right hemidiaphragm.

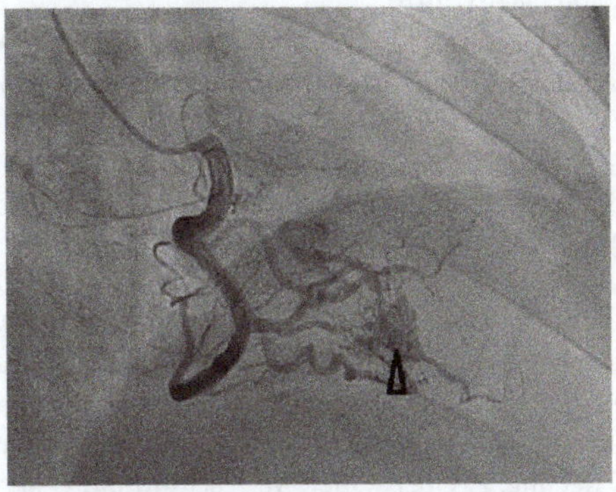

FIGURE 3: Coronary angiogram revealed no evidence of coronary artery disease, right coronary artery fistula, or tumour blush demonstrating blood supply to the base of tumour in the ventricular septum.

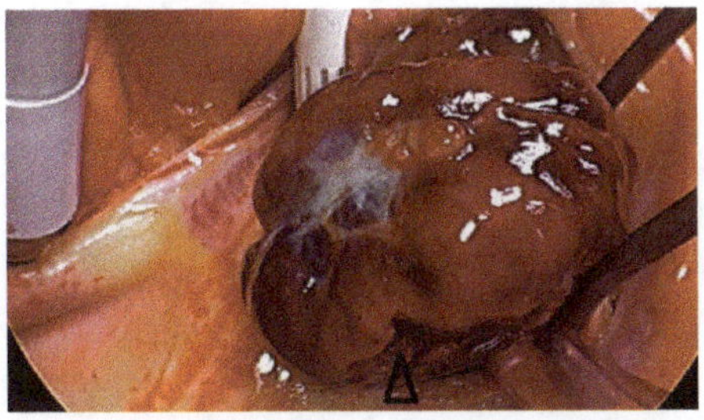

FIGURE 4: Intraoperative photograph of histologically proven large 5 cm × 4 cm right ventricular myxoma beneath the septal leaflet of the tricuspid valve. Area where part of myxoma have fragmented and embolized (arrowhead).

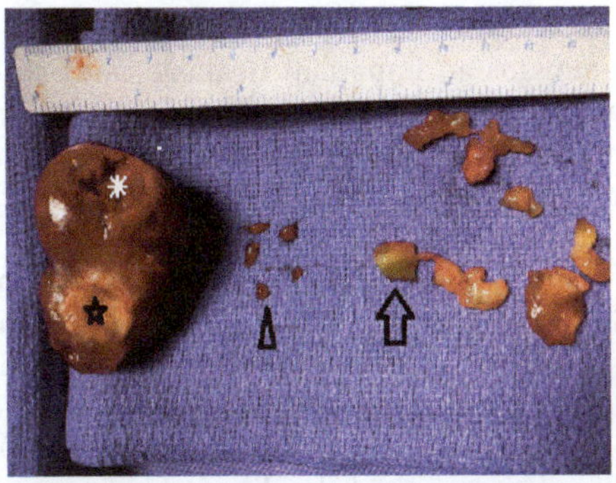

FIGURE 5: Pathology specimen of large 55 mm × 30 mm × 30 mm smooth right ventricular myxoma with attachment site to ventricular septum (star), part of myxoma that fragmented and embolized (asterisk), blood clot removed (arrowhead), and myxoma accessories (arrow).

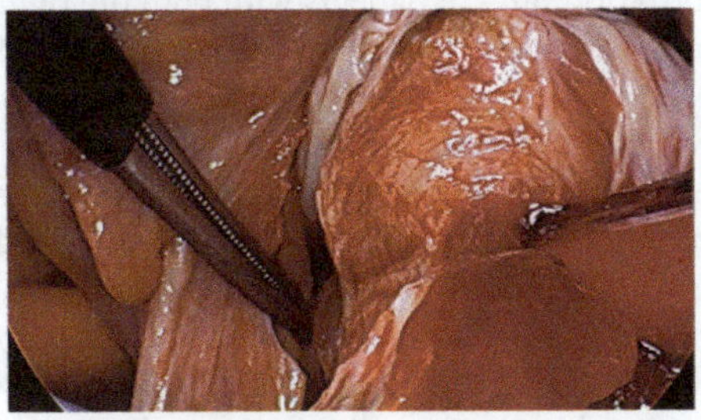

FIGURE 6: Right ventricular myxoma being excised and shaved off from ventricular septum. Note the origin of tumour beneath the septal and anterior leaflets of the tricuspid valve.

was shaved from the septum without creating any ventricular septal defect (VSD) and protecting the tricuspid valve leaflets (Figure 6). A patent foramen ovale (PFO) was enlarged to create an atrial septal defect (ASD) to inspect the left-sided chambers of the heart, which was subsequently closed. The main pulmonary artery was opened to perform extensive tumour embolectomy, and tumour was retrieved in piecemeal. Histology of tumour and emboli both confirmed to be myxomatous in origin (Figure 7). The patient's postoperative recovery was uneventful. Postoperatively, he was anticoagulated with Clexane for 4 days and discharged with warfarin with a recommended therapeutic INR between 2 and 2.5 for his pulmonary embolism for a total of six months before reviewing in the follow-up consultation.

3. Discussion

Cardiac myxoma is associated with embolic phenomena in 30-40% of all cases [6]. Unlike in the left atrial myxoma where systemic arterial embolism is of concern, right-sided

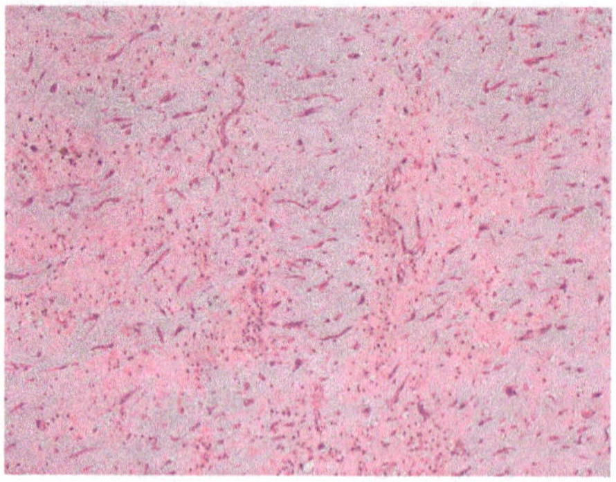

FIGURE 7: Histology of ventricular myxoma.

myxoma remains an important treatable cause to be ruled out in patients with idiopathic pulmonary embolism [6, 7]. Embolism is likely due to exposed nature and constant agitation of tumour which results in detachment of fragment either of the tumour or of the overlying thrombus.

High degree of suspicion of pulmonary embolism is necessary with consequent diagnosis. Missing the diagnosis can have fatal outcome. CTPA is gold standard for diagnosis and then search for thrombus/emboli origin. In current case, Doppler ultrasound of leg veins was negative for DVT, but echocardiogram confirmed the diagnosis of tumour in the right ventricle. These tumours have a tendency to prolapse into atrium and ventricle with each heartbeat. In this process, they can embolize or even obstruct the major atrioventricular valves with fatal outcome. Urgent surgery is mandatory for good outcome.

Embolization rates of patients with both the right and left cardiac myxomas vary between 25.3% [8] and 43% [9]. Studies have shown that morphology of cardiac myxoma is the most predictive factor of embolic events. Villous or papillary myxomas have multiple fine surface extensions that are more fragile and hence more easily embolized than round-shaped myxomas with a smooth surface [10, 11]. Other variables that were associated with embolic events include atrial fibrillation and small tumour size. Tumour size has been shown to be inversely related to the embolic event rate but related to the size of emboli. Friable myxomas tend to fragment and cannot grow large [6]. Conversely, even though it is rare for large cardiac myxomas to undergo total detachment, they still serve as a source for large embolic fragments [12]. Recurrence amongst nonfamilial cardiac myxomas is rare (Up to 3% after surgical resection), and time to recurrence for right-sided cardiac myxomas was reported between 36 and 72 months as compared to recurrence for left-sided cardiac myxomas which can recur earlier between 5 and 60 months [13].

In summary, this case report illustrates and supports early diagnosis to search for the cause of pulmonary embolism to reemphasize the importance of transesophageal echocardiogram in the diagnosis of origin of thrombus/tumour and early referral to surgery for good outcome as demonstrated in this case. Furthermore, long-term follow-up is essential to rule out the recurrence of such tumours. A high degree of suspicion is required to include tumour as an important entity in differential diagnosis of pulmonary embolism. Comprehensive assessment is necessary to rule out coronary artery disease, which is common in patients with cardiac myxomas [14], and other rare anomalies like coronary artery fistula [15]. In certain cases like this, it may represent tumour blush.

Consent

Written informed consent was obtained from the patient for publication of this case report and any accompanying images. A copy of the written consent is available for review by the Editor-in-Chief of this journal.

References

[1] L. S. Canale, A. S. Colafranceschi, E. S. Leal Botelho, and A. J. de Oliveira Monteiro, "Surgical treatment of right atrial myxoma complicated with pulmonary embolism," *Interactive CardioVascular and Thoracic Surgery*, vol. 9, no. 3, pp. 535-536, 2009.

[2] M. Demir, O. Akpinar, and E. Acarturk, "Atrial myxoma: an unusual cause of myocardial infarction," *Texas Heart Institute Journal*, vol. 32, no. 3, pp. 445–447, 2005.

[3] O. Azevedo, J. Almeida, T. Nolasco et al., "Massive right atrial myxoma presenting as syncope and exertional dyspnea: case report," *Cardiovascular Ultrasound*, vol. 8, no. 1, p. 23, 2010.

[4] H. J. Cho, S. H. Seol, B. J. Choi et al., "A case of a right atrial and inferior vena caval thrombus resembling a right atrial myxoma," *Journal of Cardiovascular Ultrasound*, vol. 18, no. 2, pp. 58–61, 2010.

[5] S. A. Boikos and C. A. Stratakis, "Carney complex: the first 20 years," *Current Opinion in Oncology*, vol. 19, no. 1, pp. 24–29, 2007.

[6] M. G. St John Sutton, L. A. Mercier, E. R. Giuliani, and J. T. Lie, "Atrial myxomas: a review of clinical experience in 40 patients," *Mayo Clinic Proceedings*, vol. 55, no. 6, pp. 371–376, 1980.

[7] A. Ikeda, T. Tsukada, T. Konishi, K. Matsuzaki, T. Jikuya, and Y. Hiramatsu, "Right atrial myxoma with a large tumor embolus in the left pulmonary artery," *Journal of Surgical Case Reports*, vol. 2014, no. 10, article rju115, 2014.

[8] I. M. Keeling, P. Oberwalder, M. Anelli-Monti et al., "Cardiac myxomas: 24 years of experience in 49 patients," *European Journal of Cardio-Thoracic Surgery*, vol. 22, no. 6, pp. 971–977, 2002.

[9] K. Boyacıoğlu, M. Kalender, A. A. Dönmez, B. Çayhan, and M. A. Tuncer, "Outcomes following embolization in patients with cardiac myxoma," *Journal of Cardiac Surgery*, vol. 32, no. 10, pp. 621–626, 2017.

[10] K. Reynen, "Cardiac myxomas," *New England Journal of Medicine*, vol. 333, no. 24, pp. 1610–1617, 1995.

[11] A. Grimaldi, A. Fumero, M. Taramasso et al., "Polypoid atrial myxoma," *Journal of Cardiovascular Medicine*, vol. 13, no. 8, pp. 529-530, 2012.

[12] B. R. Fang, C. P. Chang, C. W. Cheng, N. I. Yang, M. C. Shieh, and N. Lee, "Total detachment of cardiac myxoma causing

saddle embolization and mimicking aortic dissection," *Japanese Heart Journal*, vol. 45, no. 2, pp. 359–363, 2004.

[13] C. Mendoza, E. Bernstein, and A. Ferreira, "Multiple recurrences of nonfamilial cardiac myxomas: a report of two cases," *Texas Heart Institute Journal*, vol. 34, no. 2, pp. 236–239, 2007.

[14] N. Erdil, S. Ates, L. Cetin, U. Demirkilic, E. Sener, and H. Tatar, "Frequency of left atrial myxoma with concomitant coronary artery disease," *Surgery Today*, vol. 33, no. 5, pp. 328–331, 2003.

[15] T. Murakawa, H. Takeuchi, Y. Oda, K. Taki, T. Takaoka, and K. Yagyu, "Coronary artery fistula with left atrial myxoma: report of a case," *Kyobu Geka. The Japanese Journal of Thoracic Surgery*, vol. 51, no. 12, pp. 1035–1038, 1998.

21

Percutaneous Coronary Intervention (PCI) Strategies under Hemodynamic Support for Cardiogenic Shock: A Single-Center Experience with Two Patients

Talha Ahmed,[1] **Diljon Chahal**,[2] **Ronson J. Madathil**,[2] **David Kaczorowski**,[2] **and Anuj Gupta**[2]

[1]*University of Maryland Medical Center Midtown Campus, USA*
[2]*University of Maryland Medical Center, School of Medicine, USA*

Correspondence should be addressed to Talha Ahmed; atalha858@yahoo.com

Academic Editor: Antonio de Padua Mansur

We describe two cases of profound cardiogenic shock complicating acute myocardial infarction (CSAMI) requiring mechanical circulatory support (MCS) with venoarterial extracorporeal membrane oxygenation (VA-ECMO) allowing complex, high-risk, and staged percutaneous interventions with successful decannulation but with unfortunate outcomes.

1. Introduction

Mechanical circulatory support (MCS) is utilized for refractory cardiogenic shock (CS) that does not respond to inotropes and vasopressors. However, evidence for use of this treatment strategy to improve mortality outcomes is limited. In light of current guidelines, MCS with some preference based on availability, institutional experience, presence of hypoxia, and right ventricle (RV) dysfunction should be considered in refractory CS [1, 2]. We describe two cases of refractory cardiogenic shock complicating acute myocardial infarction (CSAMI) requiring venoarterial extracorporeal membrane oxygenation (VA-ECMO) support and left ventricle (LV) venting that allowed for complex and staged percutaneous coronary interventions (PCI). Both patients were eventually weaned off the ECMO but died during the hospitalization.

2. Case 1

A 52-year-old male with past history of hypertension, diabetes, stroke, and seizure disorder presented to an outside facility with chest pain, dyspnea, and syncope. His electrocardiogram (EKG) showed anterior ST elevation MI (STEMI). Chest X-ray (CXR) revealed pulmonary edema. Emergent coronary angiography "*first stage*" was performed revealing severe triple vessel disease for which he underwent stenting of the left anterior descending (LAD) artery with a drug-eluting stent (DES). An intra-aortic balloon pump (IABP) was placed due to elevated left ventricle end-diastolic pressure (LVEDP). The patient became progressively hypoxic and was intubated with high requirements for fraction of inspired oxygen (FiO_2) of 100% and positive end-expiratory pressure (PEEP) of 20 cmH_2O. He was referred to our hospital for consideration for ECMO support.

On presentation to our hospital, he was on hemodynamic support with inotropes (epinephrine at 0.21 mcg/kg/min) and vasopressors (norepinephrine at 0.38 mcg/kg/min) along with IABP. His troponin I peaked at 444 ng/ml with lactate of 11 mmol/l. Echocardiogram revealed severely decreased left ventricle ejection fraction (LVEF) of 20% with wall motion abnormalities involving LAD territory and normal RV size and function. Due to severe hypoxic respiratory failure and refractory cardiogenic shock, he was cannulated for VA-ECMO at bedside followed by an Impella CP (Abiomed) placement using a right femoral artery approach for LV

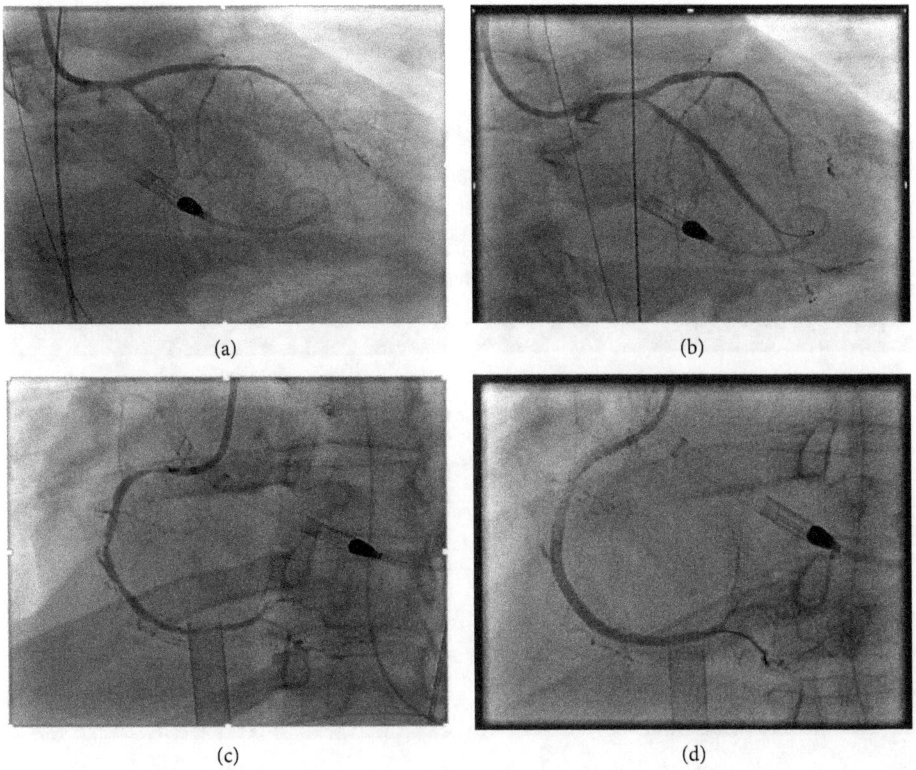

FIGURE 1: (a) Coronary angiogram showing left coronary artery disease with chronic total occlusion (CTO) of the obtuse marginal 1 (OM1) branch of the left circumflex (LCx) artery. (b) Postcoronary intervention with restoration of TIMI 3 flow in the OM1 branch. (c) Coronary angiogram showing severe diffuse right coronary artery (RCA) disease. (d) Postcoronary intervention with restoration of TIMI 3 flow in RCA.

venting and the IABP was removed. The ECMO inflow cannula (19 French/Fr) was at the left femoral artery while the outflow cannula (25 Fr) at the right common femoral vein with blood flow of 3.16 liters per min.

In the "*second stage*" of PCI, the proximal and distal RCA lesions were predilated and then stented with three DES followed by aggressive postdilation. CTO of mid left circumflex (LCx) extending into the distal obtuse marginal 1 (OM1) was predilated followed by placement of DES. TIMI-3 flow was demonstrated with no evidence of dissection or perforation (Figures 1(a)–1(d)).

The patient's clinical status started to improve and was weaned off inotropic and vasopressor support. He was decannulated from ECMO, and Impella device was removed on the 7th day of admission. He however developed severe pneumonia and had a cardiac arrest for which he was placed back on ECMO with Impella CP (Abiomed) insertion via the left femoral artery approach due to severe hypoxic respiratory failure from pulmonary edema. His lactate trended down to 1.7 mmol/l on day 3 of the first ECMO cannulation and stayed normal after decannulation from ECMO but again trended up to 6.1 mmol/l after the second arrest. He was found to have multiple new strokes on brain imaging, and considering worsening clinical status and poor outcomes, the family decided to withdraw care. The patient died a few hours later as the discussion regarding continuation versus withdrawal of hemodynamic support including ECMO and Impella was being discussed with the family.

3. Case 2

A 79-year-old African American male with past history of hypertension, hyperlipidemia, and insulin-dependent diabetes mellitus presented with exertional chest pain and dyspnea that got progressively worse to the point that he presented to an outside hospital. Examination revealed trace pedal edema, and auscultation of chest revealed mild crackles but no murmurs. His EKG and initial troponin I were normal which later peaked at 1.50 ng/ml and trended down. CXR revealed cardiomegaly and mild pulmonary edema. Echocardiogram revealed dilated LV with global hypokinesia (LVEF of 15%) and normal RV size and function. Coronary angiography revealed severe three vessel disease, and he was referred to our facility for coronary artery bypass grafting (CABG) evaluation. On presentation to our hospital, he suffered a pulseless electrical activity (PEA) arrest on day 1 complicated by refractory CS and was cannulated for VA-ECMO. The ECMO inflow cannula (19 Fr) was at the right femoral artery while the outflow cannula (25 Fr) at the left common femoral vein with blood flow of 3.1 liters per min. After initial stabilization, he underwent staged high-risk and complex PCI on days 2 and 10 of presentation.

During the "*first stage*," 100% occlusion of ostial to distal LAD was managed by successful rotational atherectomy with the deployment of four DES. LCx had severe proximal to mid calcific disease managed by rotational atherectomy and one DES. Large OM2 had CTO treated with an antegrade wire

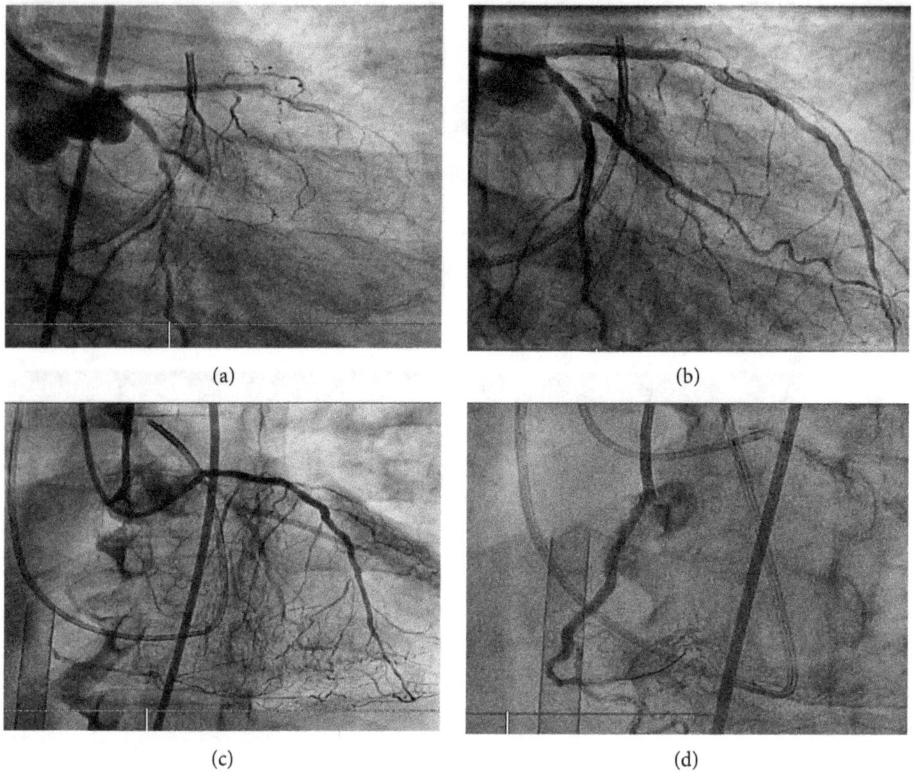

FIGURE 2: (a) Coronary angiogram showing severe disease in the left anterior descending (LAD) and left circumflex (LCx) arteries. (b) Postfirst stage of coronary intervention with restoration of TIMI 3 flow in the LAD and LCx. (c) Coronary angiogram showing severe diffuse right coronary artery (RCA) disease with CTO. (d) Postsecond stage of coronary intervention with restoration of TIMI 3 flow in RCA.

escalation technique and placement of a DES using modified T and small protrusion strategy with final bifurcation kissing balloon inflation (Figures 2(a) and 2(b)). CTO of RCA was seen with retrograde filling via LAD septals to the right posterior descending artery septals. For this reason and also to limit the complications from contrast use, RCA intervention was not performed in the first stage. Given significant pulmonary edema with an elevated LVEDP, an Impella CP (Abiomed) device was placed via the left femoral artery at the completion of the case for LV unloading. Post PCI, stress testing showed viable RCA territory and matched metabolic-perfusion defect in LAD and LCx territory. In the "*second stage*," CTO at the ostial RCA was managed by successful deployment of two overlapping DES via an antegrade approach guided by intravascular ultrasound (IVUS) (Figures 2(c) and 2(d)). Impella was replaced with left axillary Impella 5.0 (Abiomed) due to anticipated long-term need, with a goal to decannulate from VA-ECMO.

The patient was decannulated from VA-ECMO to axillary Impella on day 14 due to improvement in hemodynamic status. His echocardiogram on day 1 (at time of PEA arrest) showed dilated LV with diffuse hypokinesia (EF of 10%) and nondilated RV with moderately decreased function. A follow-up echocardiogram almost 1 month later showed slightly improved LVEF of 25% with global hypokinesia and normal right RV size and function. The patient however continued to require axillary Impella 5.0 support as well as vasopressor (norepinephrine at 0.14 mcg/kg/min, vasopressin at 0.03 units/min) and inotropic support (epinephrine at 0.05 mcg/kg/min). He developed severe pneumonia and suffered a cardiac arrest after 54 days of admission from which he could not be resuscitated.

4. Discussion

Cardiogenic shock (CS) is a state of low tissue perfusion, inadequate to meet the needs of the body that results from primary cardiac dysfunction [1]. The clinical presentation of CS is varied from hemodynamic abnormalities of preshock to mild shock, progressing to more profound shock and finally refractory shock, which is associated with high mortality rates. Acute coronary syndrome continues to be the most common cause of CS, and mortality from CSAMI remains high despite early revascularization and advents in medical therapy [2].

First-line treatment for cardiogenic shock involves hemodynamic support with inotropes and vasopressors [3]. Percutaneous MCS for refractory CS have been in practice for some years now. These include but are not limited to IABP, Impella device, tandom heart, and VA-ECMO [3]. VA-ECMO is most commonly considered for patients with biventricular failure and profound hypoxemia refractory to other medical or device-based intervention [4].

Risk factors associated with worse long-term outcomes after VA-ECMO include increasing age; comorbidities like ischemic heart disease, diabetes mellitus, renal failure, and chronic obstructive lung disease; degree of acid base disturbance; liver/kidney dysfunction; and inadequate unloading at the time of ECMO initiation. Risk scores including ENCOURAGE score, SAVE (survival after VA-EMCO), and the simple cardiac ECMO scores can assess likelihood of survival to hospital discharge with modest discrimination [5–7]. In our cases, patient 1 had a ENCOURAGE score of 28 (with 30-day and 6-month survival post ECMO initiation of 17% and 7%, respectively) and SAVE score of -12/Class V (18% in-hospital mortality) while patient 2 had ENCOURAGE score of 19 (30-day and 6-month survival post ECMO initiation were 35% and 25%, respectively) and SAVE score of -18/Class V (18% in-hospital mortality).

In patients with signs of LV distension and worsening pulmonary edema, some form of LV unloading or venting strategy needs to be introduced. A number of LV venting strategies have been used historically each with its own limitations and advantage. The use of Impella device as LV venting has demonstrated reduction in LV end-diastolic dimension and pulmonary edema while axillary Impella allows for patients' mobility while being on support [8].

According to the 2014 American Heart Association/-American College of Cardiology (AHA/ACC) NSTEMI guidelines, a revascularization strategy with multivessel PCI in contrast to culprit lesion-only PCI may be reasonable in patients undergoing coronary revascularization as part of treatment for NSTEMI [9]. This however does not account for patients in cardiogenic shock since results from the CULPRIT-SHOCK trial reveal that in patients with cardiogenic shock complicating myocardial infarction, culprit lesion-only PCI improves outcomes including 30-day mortality and time to renal revascularization therapy as compared to the multivessel approach [10]. The 2018 European guidelines recommend using the revascularization strategy based on clinical status, comorbidities, and disease severity of patients. Similarly in patients with STEMI, current data favors complete revascularization before hospital discharge; however, optimal timing (single stage vs. multiple staged) of procedures should be determined by clinical status of the patient [11].

In a single-center study, Shaukat et al. described high-risk PCI using VA-ECMO support in five patients who presented with either LV systolic dysfunction or NSTEMI [12]. In an interesting observational study involving almost 287 patients from a large registry, Basir et al. concluded that early initiation of MCS even before initiation of inotropes or vasopressors was associated with increased survival in patients presenting with CSAMI. In their study, Impella device was used as MCS [13]. Whether or not these results will hold true for VA-ECMO support has not been evaluated thus far.

5. Conclusion

These cases highlighted that MCS can support staged PCI, but we need more data before this can become routine practice. However, great emphasis should be placed on patient selection in order to gain maximal benefit out of these invasive devices while limiting their inherent side effects. This particularly is true for elderly frail patients and those with multiple comorbidities leading to poor prognosis as determined by various risk predictors.

Abbreviations

MCS: Mechanical circulatory support
CS: Cardiogenic shock
VA-ECMO: Venoarterial extracorporeal membrane oxygenation
RV: Right ventricle
LV: Left ventricle
IABP: Intra-aortic balloon pump
CSAMI: Cardiogenic shock complicating acute myocardial infarction
PCI: Percutaneous coronary intervention
STEMI: ST elevation MI
CXR: Chest X-ray
LAD: Left anterior descending
DES: Drug-eluting stent
LVEDP: Left ventricle end-diastolic pressure
LVEF: Left ventricle ejection fraction
CTO: Chronic total occlusion
LCx: Left circumflex
OM: Obtuse marginal
LHC: Left heart catheterization
CABG: Coronary artery bypass grafting
PEA: Pulseless electrical activity
TAP: T and small protrusion
rPDA: Right posterior descending artery
IVUS: Intravascular ultrasound
SAVE: Survival after VA-ECMO
AHA/ACC: American Heart Association/American College of Cardiology.

Additional Points

Learning Points. (1) The use of MCS in patients with CS has not shown mortality benefit so far but does prove to be substantial in refractory cardiogenic shock. (2) In patients undergoing urgent or emergent VA-ECMO cannulation, various risk predictors can determine in-hospital mortality. (3) Early initiation of VA-ECMO either simultaneously or even prior to inotropes or vasopressors has not been evaluated so far. (4) However, needed evidence and studies are underway to determine the effects of the MCS on both short-term and long-term outcomes as well as their cost-effectiveness in patients with CS (ANCHOR trial and EURO SHOCK trial) [14, 15].

Authors' Contributions

Diljon Chahal and Anuj Gupta (Department of Cardiovascular Medicine, UMMC) and Ronson J. Madathil and David Kaczorowski (Department of Cardiothoracic Surgery, UMMC) are coauthors.

References

[1] H. R. Reynolds and J. S. Hochman, "Cardiogenic shock," *Circulation*, vol. 117, no. 5, pp. 686–697, 2008.

[2] D. Kolte, S. Khera, W. S. Aronow et al., "Trends in incidence, management, and outcomes of cardiogenic shock complicating ST-elevation myocardial infarction in the United States," *Journal of the American Heart Association*, vol. 3, no. 1, 2014.

[3] H. Thiele, E. M. Ohman, S. Desch, I. Eitel, and S. De Waha, "Management of cardiogenic shock," *European Heart Journal*, vol. 36, no. 20, pp. 1223–1230, 2015.

[4] R. Jimenez-Espinosa, I. Galvan, D. Roldan-Morales et al., "Six-year results of consecutive patients treated with extracorporeal membrane oxygenation for refractory postoperative cardiogenic shock," *European Journal of Heart Failure*, vol. 19, 2017.

[5] M. Schmidt, A. Burrell, L. Roberts et al., "Predicting survival after ECMO for refractory cardiogenic shock: the survival after veno-arterial-ECMO (SAVE)-score," *European Heart Journal*, vol. 36, no. 33, pp. 2246–2256, 2015.

[6] G. Peigh, N. Cavarocchi, S. W. Keith, and H. Hirose, "Simple new risk score model for adult cardiac extracorporeal membrane oxygenation: simple cardiac ECMO score," *The Journal of Surgical Research*, vol. 198, no. 2, pp. 273–279, 2015.

[7] G. Muller, E. Flecher, G. Lebreton et al., "The ENCOURAGE mortality risk score and analysis of long-term outcomes after VA-ECMO for acute myocardial infarction with cardiogenic shock," *Intensive Care Medicine*, vol. 42, no. 3, pp. 370–378, 2016.

[8] S. Chocron, A. Perrotti, C. Durst, and B. Aupècle, "Left ventricular venting through the right subclavian artery access during peripheral extracorporeal life support," *Interactive CardioVascular and Thoracic Surgery*, vol. 17, no. 1, pp. 187–189, 2013.

[9] J. L. Anderson, C. D. Adams, E. M. Antman et al., "ACC/AHA 2007 guidelines for the management of patients with unstable angina/non–ST-elevation myocardial infarction: executive summary," *Circulation*, vol. 116, no. 7, pp. 803–877, 2007.

[10] P. T. O'Gara, F. G. Kushner, D. D. Ascheim et al., "2013 ACCF/AHA Guideline for the Management of ST-Elevation Myocardial Infarction: Executive Summary: A Report of the American College of Cardiology Foundation/American Heart Association Task Force on Practice Guidelines," *Journal of the American College of Cardiology*, vol. 61, no. 4, pp. 485–510, 2013.

[11] B. Ibanez, S. James, S. Agewall et al., "2017 ESC guidelines for the management of acute myocardial infarction in patients presenting with ST-segment elevation," *European Heart Journal*, vol. 39, no. 2, pp. 119–177, 2018.

[12] A. Shaukat, K. Hryniewicz-Czeneszew, B. Sun et al., "Outcomes of extracorporeal membrane oxygenation support for complex high-risk elective percutaneous coronary interventions: a single-center experience and review of the literature," *The Journal of Invasive Cardiology*, vol. 30, no. 12, pp. 456–460, 2018.

[13] M. B. Basir, T. L. Schreiber, C. L. Grines et al., "Effect of early initiation of mechanical circulatory support on survival in cardiogenic shock," *The American Journal of Cardiology*, vol. 119, no. 6, pp. 845–851, 2017.

[14] A. Combes, "Assessment of ECMO in acute myocardial infarction with non-reversible cardiogenic shock to halt organ failure and reduce mortality," https://clinicaltrials.gov/ct2/show/NCT04184635?term=ANCHOR+TRIAL&cond=Cardiogenic+Shock&draw=2&rank=1.

[15] H. A. Gershlick et al., "EURO SHOCK testing the value of novel strategy and its cost efficacy in order to improve the poor outcomes in cardiogenic shock," https://clinicaltrials.gov/ct2/show/NCT03813134?term=EUROSHOCK&cond=Cardiogenic+Shock&draw=2&rank=1.

22

Use of Idarucizumab to Revert the Anticoagulant Effect of Dabigatran in Heart Transplant Surgery: An Institutional Experience

Álvaro Herrera-Escandón,[1,2,3] Orlando Castaño-Cifuentes,[2] and Carlos A. Plata-Mosquera[2,3]

[1]*Internal Medicine Department, Universidad del Valle, Cali, Colombia*
[2]*Cardiology Department, DIME Clínica Neurocardiovascular, Cali, Colombia*
[3]*Heart Failure and Cardiac Transplant Unit, DIME Clínica Neurocardiovascular, Cali, Colombia*

Correspondence should be addressed to Álvaro Herrera-Escandón; alvaro.escandon@correounivalle.edu.co

Academic Editor: Christian Machado

Heart transplant is a surgical procedure with a high risk of perioperative bleeding in patients with a previous history of sternotomy, congestive liver disease, and/or use of oral anticoagulants. Anticoagulation is usually done with coumarin agents (warfarin, acenocoumarol), while on the waiting list, vitamin K is available allowing for partial reversal of the anticoagulant effect, although with variable INR and risk of uncontrolled bleeding. Direct oral anticoagulants have emerged as an alternative to the use of coumarins in patients with nonvalvular atrial fibrillation (NVAF). The main disadvantage of this group of drugs is that there was no specific reversal agent available that would allow an urgent reversal of the anticoagulant effect. The recent commercialization of idarucizumab (specific reversal agent) has allowed patients with NVAF on the waiting list for heart transplant to be treated with dabigatran. We present the case of a patient with advanced chronic heart failure and NVAF anticoagulated with dabigatran, who underwent urgent heart transplant after administration of idarucizumab, without complications derived from its use or from anticoagulation.

1. Introduction

New oral anticoagulants have emerged as an alternative to warfarin in the treatment of venous thromboembolic disease and as prevention of thromboembolic events in nonvalvular atrial fibrillation (NVAF). Dabigatran inhibits coagulation-activated factor II while apixaban and rivaroxaban inhibit factor Xa [1]. These anticoagulants are classified as direct-acting anticoagulants and are as effective as warfarin in ischemic event prevention with a better security profile [2, 3]; however, there was no available antidote that allowed for urgent reversal of the anticoagulant effect to realize urgent invasive procedures, mainly surgery.

Idarucizumab is a reversal agent specific for dabigatran. It is a fragment of immunized monoclonal antibody (Fab) that attaches to dabigatran and its metabolites with high affinity. It is approximately 350 times more potent than the affinity of dabigatran for thrombin. Compounded idarucizumab-dabigatran is characterized by a fast association constant and an extremely slow dissociation constant, giving way to a very stable compound. Idarucizumab attaches to dabigatran and its metabolites in a potent and specific manner, neutralizing its anticoagulant effect. It is indicated in adult patients treated with dabigatran etexilate when a fast reversal of its anticoagulant effects is needed (emergency surgical interventions or in the case of potentially deadly or uncontrolled hemorrhaging) with good clinical results and equal bleeding rates as patients not anticoagulated.

Patients with chronic heart failure (CHF) present with atrial fibrillation rhythm in as much as 30% of cases [4, 5].

The benefits offered by NOAC by not requiring monitorization of therapeutic effects, and having less variability between subjects and having a more predictable effect compared to warfarin make them an option in NVAF treatment.

We present a case of a patient with advanced chronic heart failure and NVAF anticoagulated with dabigatran who was subjected to an emergency heart transplant after idarucizumab administration.

2. Clinical Case Description

A 60-year-old, group A Rh-negative male had been waitlisted for heart transplant due to dilated cardiomyopathy of nonischemic origin, stage D with INTERMACS 5 profile with an ejection fraction of 20%.

Disease debut in the year 2012 with embolic ischemic cerebrovascular event with intracavitary apical thrombus causes the event, with small sequela in left upper extremity (monoparesis). Patient received medical treatment in accordance to clinical practice guidelines, including resynchronization therapy (150 msec QRS) and defibrillation for primary prevention. The patient had advanced heart failure, with NYHA IIIA class of symptoms and VO2 peak less than 10 ml/kg/min in cardiopulmonary exercise test.

Evolution of the latest years shows multiple hospitalizations due to congestion, hypoperfusion, renal dysfunction, and arrhythmic storm with discharges appropriate to defibrillator treated with amiodarone.

Of note in the first follow-up is the development of atrial fibrillation with ischemic risk calculated CHADS2 VASC of 4 (heart failure, AHT, ischemic stroke) and risk of bleeding HASBLED of 1 in anticoagulation treatment with dabigatran 150 mg every 12 hours since 2015. We did not use any type of heparin prior to the procedure.

After 6 months on the waiting list, an effective and compatible donation alert was activated at 22:00 hours. Patient takes the last dose of dabigatran at 09:00 hours (13 hours) and administration of reversal agent determined previous to heart transplant surgery.

Upon arrival, the first laboratory exams are taken noting a creatinine elevation compared to basal state as single additional finding.

Reversal with bolus of total dose of 5.0 g from 2 vials (2.5 g) of idarucizumab at 23:57 and 00:15, respectively, was passed in the surgical room.

After 3:46 hours of ischemic time of the graft, with subjectively considered normal bleeding by the surgical team, the patient is transferred to the intensive care unit (ICU). We had standard bleeding during perioperative state, and the patient needed 3 more units of erythrocyte concentrate after immediate surgery, without additional transfusion requirements after 24 hours in ICU. Our group uses intraoperative hemostatic factors as a surgical adhesive, careful hemostasis prior to sternal closure.

Patient is required with inotropic infusion in accordance with transplant protocol with 0.03 mcg/kg/min of isoproterenol and 7.5 mcg/kg/min of dobutamine. Immunosuppression induction performed with 20 mg of basiliximab on days 0 and 4 and extubation was programmed upon 24 hours of surgical procedure. At 48 hours of ICU arrival, mediastinal drains were removed with a total bleed of 295 ml in the first 6 hours, 835 ml at 30 hours, and finally 1045 ml at 48 hours, thereby completing security protocol for retrieval. Coagulation times, platelet count, hemoglobin, and creatinine behavior were adequate (Supplement 1).

The total ICU stay time was 7 days and protocol prophylaxis was started with valganciclovir, trimethoprim sulfamethoxazole, and nistatin.

On the tenth day, herpes zoster is evidenced and successfully treated on T8 dermatome; this is a single finding during hospital stay.

The 15th day endomyocardial biopsy was negative for cellular and humoral rejection, with adequate biventricular function of graft. Patient was released 17 days after transplant and until now lives free of further clinical findings. We used the usual thromboprophylaxis with enoxaparin during the hospital stay.

3. Discussion

The idarucizumab effectively reversed the anticoagulant effect of dabigatran in patient taken to heart transplant, obtaining good hemostasis during surgery and without presenting bleeding requiring transfusion support post operation. Normal coagulation tests and an adequately functioning coagulation system are key to contributing to a favorable outcome in patient subject to mayor surgery.

The dabigatran reaches its peak plasma anticoagulant activity upon 2 hours of ingestion, having a bioavailability of between 3 and 7% and attaching 35% to plasma proteins, with up to 80% of renal elimination, with a half-life of between 12 and 17 hours if renal function is normal [6]. Different control studies and meta-analyses have demonstrated its efficacy as an anticoagulant and its security profile [1]. Current international guides recommend it as thromboembolic prevention in patients with atrial fibrillation [7]. Until recent years, the main limitation in the use of these medicines was the lack of a reversal agent and the inability to monitor its anticoagulant effect through conventional exams measuring coagulation and those that approximate the measurement of its activity are not available in our region.

As opposed to warfarin, the lack of an effective reversal agent in restoring hemostasis in the case of severe hemorrhaging or emergency or urgent surgery was seen for many years as a limitation in the use of dabigatran and other direct anticoagulants. The arrival of idarucizumab supported in RE-VERSE AD [8] study opened the field for those patients with mayor hemorrhage who require urgent surgery to establish hemostasis within minutes of its administration.

Our case is the first reported in Colombia and in Latin America on the use of idarucizumab in heart transplant. Two similar cases to ours were found in the literature [9, 10] in which the successful use in patients with mayor surgery is documented; however, although in the REVERSE-AD study, there were no patients with heart transplant; these 3 reported cases in the medical literature suggest that this medication is equally as effective and safe in this population [11], which has high prevalence of atrial fibrillation [12].

In conclusion, idarucizumab is an effective and safe specific reversal agent in patients anticoagulated with dabigatran including those who have been subjected to mayor surgery such as heart transplant. The fact of having a reversal agent makes dabigatran a medication of choice in these patients with advanced heart failure who require anticoagulation and need emergency surgery.

References

[1] S. J. Connolly, M. D. Ezekowitz, S. Yusuf et al., "Dabigatran versus warfarin in patients with atrial fibrillation," *The New England Journal of Medicine*, vol. 361, no. 12, pp. 1139–1151, 2009.

[2] T. van der Hulle, J. Kooiman, P. L. den Exter, O. M. Dekkers, F. A. Klok, and M. V. Huisman, "Effectiveness and safety of novel oral anticoagulants as compared with vitamin K antagonists in the treatment of acute symptomatic venous thromboembolism: a systematic review and meta-analysis," *Journal of Thrombosis and Haemostasis*, vol. 12, no. 3, pp. 320–328, 2014.

[3] C. T. Ruff, R. P. Giugliano, E. Braunwald et al., "Comparison of the efficacy and safety of new oral anticoagulants with warfarin in patients with atrial fibrillation: a meta-analysis of randomised trials," *Lancet*, vol. 383, no. 9921, pp. 955–962, 2014.

[4] H. H. van der Wal, V. M. van Deursen, P. van der Meer, and A. A. Voors, "Comorbidities in heart failure," in *Heart Failure*, Handbook of Experimental Pharmacology, pp. 35–66, Springer, 2017.

[5] D. Mozaffarian, E. J. Benjamin, A. S. Go et al., "Heart disease and stroke statistics–2015 update: a report from the American Heart Association," *Circulation*, vol. 131, no. 4, pp. e29–322, 2015.

[6] J. Stangier, "Clinical pharmacokinetics and pharmacodynamics of the oral direct thrombin inhibitor dabigatran etexilate," *Clinical Pharmacokinetics*, vol. 47, no. 5, pp. 285–295, 2008.

[7] P. Kirchhof, S. Benussi, D. Kotecha et al., "2016 ESC guidelines for the management of atrial fibrillation developed in collaboration with EACTS," *European Journal of Cardio-Thoracic Surgery*, vol. 50, no. 5, pp. e1–e88, 2016.

[8] C. V. Pollack Jr., P. A. Reilly, J. Eikelboom et al., "Idarucizumab for dabigatran reversal," *The New England Journal of Medicine*, vol. 373, no. 6, pp. 511–520, 2015.

[9] J. Rimsans, M. Rhoten, K. Sylvester, S. K. Singh, and J. M. Connors, "Idarucizumab for urgent reversal of dabigatran for heart transplant: A case report," *American Journal of Hematology*, vol. 92, no. 3, pp. E34–E35, 2017.

[10] A. Tralhao, C. Aguiar, J. Ferreira et al., "Dabigatran reversal with idarucizumab in a patient undergoing heart transplantation: first European report," *Thrombosis Journal*, vol. 5, no. 15, p. 23, 2017.

[11] F. Schiele, J. van Ryn, K. Canada et al., "A specific antidote for dabigatran: functional and structural characterization," *Blood*, vol. 121, no. 18, pp. 3554–3562, 2013.

[12] S. A. Batul and R. Gopinathannair, "Atrial fibrillation in heart failure: a therapeutic challenge of our times," *Korean Circulation Journal*, vol. 47, no. 5, pp. 644–662, 2017.

Suspected Brugada Phenocopy Secondary to Coronary Slow Flow

Alicia Shim,[1] Rajeev Seecheran,[2] Valmiki Seecheran,[2] Sangeeta Persad,[2] Shiva Sreenivasan,[3] Ronald Henry,[1] and Naveen Anand Seecheran[4]

[1]*Cardiology Unit, Advanced Cardiovascular Institute, Port of Spain, Trinidad and Tobago*
[2]*Department of Medicine, North Central Regional Health Authority, Mt. Hope, Trinidad and Tobago*
[3]*School of Medicine, Dentistry, and Biomedical Sciences, Queen's University, Belfast, UK*
[4]*Department of Clinical Medical Sciences, University of the West Indies, St. Augustine, Trinidad and Tobago*

Correspondence should be addressed to Naveen Anand Seecheran; nseecheran@gmail.com

Academic Editor: Man-Hong Jim

Brugada syndrome (BrS) is a genetic condition that accentuates the risk of potentially lethal ventricular arrhythmias and sudden cardiac death (SCD) in a structurally normal heart. The Brugada electrocardiographic pattern may manifest separately from the syndrome—this clinical scenario has been described as Brugada phenocopy (BrP). Many etiologies of BrP have been reported, but it has not yet been reported as a result of coronary slow flow (CSF) phenomenon. This case report highlights a suspected coronary slow flow-associated Brugada type 1 electrocardiographic pattern, which subsequently normalized following the institution of guideline-directed medical therapy for acute coronary syndrome.

1. Introduction

Brugada syndrome (BrS), initially described in 1992, is a genetic condition with a characteristic electrocardiographic (ECG) pattern and is associated with an elevated risk of life-threatening ventricular arrhythmia (VA) and sudden cardiac death (SCD) [1]. It is typically considered a primary electrical condition without structural heart disease [2]. The ECG pattern comprises ST-segment elevation > 2 mm in one or more leads from V_1 to V_3 with "coved-type" descending to inverted T wave or "saddleback" morphology consistent with Brugada type 1 and type 2 patterns, respectively [3, 4]. The prevalence varies internationally and genealogically, typically with a male predilection. Appropriate risk stratification and management of these patients remain a topic of considerable debate [2].

The Brugada type 1 electrocardiographic pattern can manifest separately from the definite syndrome, and this clinical scenario has been called Brugada phenocopy (BrP) [2]. Diagnostic maneuvers (e.g., cardiac sodium channel blockade provocation testing) are often performed to differentiate true BrS from BrP, which can be encountered in a multitude of clinical scenarios and, ultimately, can result potentially in life-saving interventions [5, 6].

Currently, there are no cases reported on BrP observed in patients with coronary slow flow, although it has been recognized in ischemia [7–9]. This report describes a patient with coronary slow flow who presented with a Brugada type 1 ECG pattern, which subsequently normalized following resolution of the endothelial dysfunction.

2. Case Report

A fifty-nine-year-old lady of mixed Caribbean-Black and Asian descent with a history of essential hypertension, dyslipidemia, obesity, generalized anxiety disorder, and pharmacological nonadherence presented with chest pain which followed an emotionally stressful encounter (abrupt marital separation). There was no prior history of syncope, presyncope, or palpitation; however, there was a paternal history of sudden cardiac death. Physical examination revealed hypertension but was otherwise normal. Initial routine laboratory results, including cardiac biomarkers, were normal.

The admission electrocardiogram displayed coved ST-segment elevation in V_1 and V_2 suggestive of a Brugada type 1 pattern (Figure 1(a)). She was treated with aspirin, ticagrelor, intravenous heparin and nitroglycerin infusions,

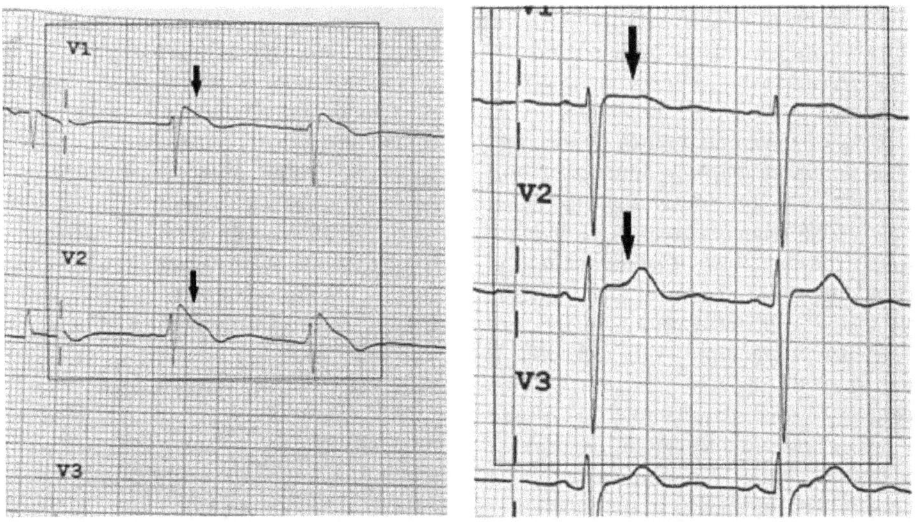

(a) (b)

Figure 1: There is the characteristic ST-segment elevation ≥ 2 mm in ≥1 right precordial leads (V_1 to V_3), following an r'-wave and a straight ST-segment. Additionally, the descending ST-segment crosses the isoelectric line and is followed by a negative and symmetric T wave. At 40 ms of high takeoff, the decrease in amplitude of ST is ≤4 mm and the duration of QRS is longer than that in a right bundle branch block [3]. No high-pass filters were applied to attenuate low-frequency noise [15, 16]. (a) Admission ECG leads V_1 and V_2 upon presentation, showing coved ST-segment elevation (black arrows) with elevated J points, suggestive of a Brugada type 1 pattern. (b) Subsequent ECG showing resolution of the Brugada type 1 pattern (black arrows).

high-intensity statin, beta-adrenergic and calcium channel blockade, angiotensin-converting enzyme inhibition, and mineralocorticoid receptor antagonist pharmacotherapy. A chest radiograph was unremarkable, with transthoracic echocardiography showing preserved left ventricular function, with no regional wall abnormalities, and grade 1 diastolic dysfunction. Tentative diagnoses for ST-segment elevation at this juncture included aneurysm formation, dissection, hyperkalemia, and pulmonary embolism, which were all effectively excluded with requisite investigations [10].

Coronary angiography revealed mild luminal irregularities with Thrombolysis In Myocardial Infarction (TIMI) 2 antegrade flow suggestive of endothelial dysfunction in the right coronary artery (Supplemental Video Files, 2a, 2b, and 2c). Subsequent ECGs done when pain-free revealed normalization of the Brugada pattern (Figure 1(b)).

Serial measurements of cardiac biomarkers remained normal throughout her inpatient stay, and she was discharged on guideline-directed medical therapy with scheduled outpatient follow-up. The patient subsequently declined further cardiac sodium channel blockade provocation testing and genetic testing for *SCN5A* [11–13]. The patient and her family were counseled with respect to accessing online resources such as the Brugada phenocopy international registry and online educational portal for further insight into her suspected condition [14].

3. Discussion

Coronary slow flow (CSF) phenomenon, initially described by Tambe et al. in 1972, is an angiographic entity characterized by delayed progression of the injected contrast medium through the coronary vasculature, typically encountered in patients presenting with clinical features of acute coronary syndrome [17]. It is reported to have an incidence of approximately 7% in patients undergoing coronary angiography. The pathophysiology has not been fully elucidated; however, several structural and mechanistic effects with a resultant maladaptive milieu have been proposed [18, 19]. It has been implicated with life-threatening arrhythmias and sudden cardiac death; however, the most common clinical presentation is that of unstable angina [20, 21]. It is defined by the presence of angiographically normal or near-normal coronary arteries and Thrombolysis In Myocardial Infarction (TIMI) 2 flow (i.e., requiring ≥3 beats to opacify prespecified branch points in the distal vasculature of at least one of the three major epicardial coronary vessels) [22, 23].

The endothelium plays a pivotal role in vasomotor regulation and platelet reactivity and is intimately involved in atherogenesis [18]. Patients with CSF have diffuse intimal thickening and microcalcification along the vessel wall [24] and also tend to have elevated endogenous inflammatory markers such as C-reactive protein and interleukin-6 [25]. Additionally, impaired laminar flow occurs in arterial segments with tortuosity and bifurcations [26]. Clinically, CSF tends to appear in patients with metabolic syndrome—high total cholesterol and low-density lipoprotein cholesterol, elevated fasting glucose, and raised body mass index, all of which were present in our patient [27, 28].

Statin therapy appears beneficial for patients with CSF and is likely to be as a result of their anti-inflammatory properties [29, 30]. Beta-adrenergic blockade can also improve endothelial function and attenuate symptoms by increased nitric oxide release [31]. Our patient's symptoms and ECG appearances quickly resolved after administration of these therapies.

BrP may occur in relation to cardiac sodium (Na) and potassium (K) channel blocking effects or cardiac structural abnormalities, particularly those affecting the right ventricle, such as right ventricular outflow tract ischemia (RVOT) [32]. Occlusion or spasm of the conus branch of the right coronary artery and ischemia of the right ventricular outflow tract and BrP have been previously reported. This has also been replicated in experiments involving acetylcholine, giving credence to the hypothesis that ischemia and vagal influences act additively or synergistically with the substrate responsible for ST-segment elevation in BrS and precipitation of ventricular fibrillation (VF) [33, 34]. It has been postulated that ST-segment elevation occurs maybe due to a decrease in ionized calcium (iCa) caused by acetylcholine or an increase in the adenosine triphosphate- (ATP-) sensitive K channels caused by ischemia resulting in voltage gradients contributing to the manifestation of the Brugada ECG pattern [8, 35]. Furthermore, it has recently been demonstrated that reduced Na channel availability in the ventricular epicardium may contribute to electrical depression and thus may contribute to the ST-segment changes in acute myocardial ischemia [36]. Additionally, in 2015, Agrawal et al. reported BrP during stent implantation distal to the conus branch, which resolved after deployment. They postulated that ischemia of the Purkinje system of the right ventricle might have slowed conduction to the RVOT. Resolution of ischemia restored normal conduction and resolved the ECG pattern. Repolarization abnormalities are less likely to be attributed to this finding because flow reduction was not confined to the conus branch and would have therefore not directly impacted on the RVOT [37]. This case is similar to the one previously described by Peter and further highlights the possible association between RVOT ischemia and BrP [38].

It is difficult to estimate the impact of BrS due to its uncertain prevalence; however, the incidence of the BrS electrocardiographic pattern remains less than 1% in several studies while accounting for approximately 10% of sudden deaths [39]. Implantable cardioverter-defibrillator device therapy is considered the gold standard; however, radiofrequency catheter ablation is rapidly gaining traction as an emerging strategy [2].

Clinical conditions separate from BrS, which electrocardiographically mimic the BrS type 1 ECG pattern, which then resolves with appropriate treatment, have been referred to as Brugada phenocopies [40]. Differentiation between these two entities is critical, as BrP usually represents a more benign prognosticator [14]. The BrP ECG pattern is indistinguishable from that of BrS, and misdiagnosis can have devastating sequelae [41–43]

Our patient's initial ECG was consistent with a Brugada "coved type 1" phenocopy for several reasons, although the presence of a negative P wave component in V_2 could suggest electrode malposition [2, 4]. There is the characteristic ST-segment elevation ≥ 2 mm in ≥ 1 right precordial leads (V_1 to V_3), following an r'-wave and a straight ST-segment. Additionally, the descending ST-segment crosses the isoelectric line and is followed by a negative and symmetric T wave. At 40 ms of high takeoff, the decrease in amplitude of ST is ≤ 4 mm and the duration of QRS is longer than that in a right bundle branch block [3]. No high-pass filters were applied to attenuate low-frequency noise [15, 16].

Our patient's pretest probability of BrS was determined to be intermediate, as there was no previous history of syncope, palpitations, or witnessed nocturnal agonal respiration; however, there was a positive family history of sudden cardiac death. She declined provocative testing as well as genetic testing for the *SCN5A* gene mutation. Genetic testing, however, is not considered mandatory, as the *SCN5A* mutation is identifiable in only 20% to 30% of probands affected by true BrS [44].

As per the BrP morphologic classification criteria, our patient would potentially be classified as a type 1B BrP (as drug challenge was not performed), which resolved with administration of the acute coronary syndrome and neurohormonal therapies [45].

Differentiating between BrS and BrP is critical because patients with BrS are susceptible to SCD and may require an implantable cardioverter-defibrillator (ICD) with its attendant complications.

4. Conclusion

We report the first case of a patient with a suspected Brugada phenocopy thought to be as a result of coronary slow flow and whose ECG reverted to normal following institution of guideline-directed medical therapy.

Additional Points

Key Clinical Message. Be cognizant that coronary slow flow may induce a transient, reversible Brugada-type electrocardiographic pattern (phenocopy), which normalizes upon resolution of the underlying endothelial dysfunction.

Consent

The patient has provided written informed consent to have the details of her case published.

Authors' Contributions

AS, RS, VS, SP, SS, RH, and NS all contributed equally to writing the manuscript. All authors read and approved the final manuscript.

References

[1] P. Brugada and J. Brugada, "Right bundle branch block, persistent ST segment elevation and sudden cardiac death: A distinct clinical and electrocardiographic syndrome: A multicenter report," *Journal of the American College of Cardiology*, vol. 20, no. 6, pp. 1391–1396, 1992.

[2] J. Brugada, O. Campuzano, E. Arbelo, G. Sarquella-Brugada, and R. Brugada, "Present Status of Brugada Syndrome:," *Journal of the American College of Cardiology*, vol. 72, no. 9, pp. 1046–1059, 2018.

[3] A. Bayés de Luna, J. Brugada, A. Baranchuk et al., "Current electrocardiographic criteria for diagnosis of Brugada pattern: a consensus report," *Journal of Electrocardiology*, vol. 45, no. 5, pp. 433–442, 2012.

[4] A. B. de Luna, J. Garcia-Niebla, and A. Baranchuk, "New electrocardiographic features in Brugada syndrome," *Current Cardiology Reviews*, vol. 10, no. 3, pp. 175–180, 2014.

[5] Y. G. Yap, E. R. Behr, and A. J. Camm, "Drug-induced Brugada syndrome," *Europace*, vol. 11, no. 8, pp. 989–994, 2009.

[6] W. Shimizu, "Acquired forms of the Brugada syndrome," *Journal of Electrocardiology*, vol. 38, 4 Supplement, pp. 22–25, 2005.

[7] H. Kataoka, "Electrocardiographic patterns of the Brugada syndrome in right ventricular infarction/ischemia," *The American Journal of Cardiology*, vol. 86, no. 9, p. 1056, 2000.

[8] M. Yamaki, N. Sato, T. Myojo et al., "Possible contribution of ischemia of the conus branch to induction or augmentation of Brugada type electrocardiographic changes in patients with coronary artery disease," *International Heart Journal*, vol. 51, no. 1, pp. 68–71, 2010.

[9] F. Ferrando-Castagnetto, A. Garibaldi-Remuñan, G. Vignolo, R. Ricca-Mallada, and A. Baranchuk, "Brugada phenocopy as a dynamic electrocardiographic pattern during acute anterior myocardial infarction," *Annals of Noninvasive Electrocardiology*, vol. 21, no. 4, pp. 425–428, 2016.

[10] K. Wang, R. W. Asinger, and H. J. L. Marriott, "ST-segment elevation in conditions other than acute myocardial infarction," *New England Journal of Medicine*, vol. 349, no. 22, pp. 2128–2135, 2003.

[11] A. Ueoka, H. Morita, A. Watanabe et al., "Prognostic significance of the sodium channel blocker test in patients with Brugada syndrome," *Journal of the American Heart Association*, vol. 7, no. 10, 2018.

[12] G. Sarquella-Brugada, O. Campuzano, E. Arbelo, J. Brugada, and R. Brugada, "Brugada syndrome: clinical and genetic findings," *Genetics in Medicine*, vol. 18, no. 1, pp. 3–12, 2016.

[13] C. Antzelevitch and B. Patocskai, "Brugada syndrome: clinical, genetic, molecular, cellular, and ionic aspects," *Current Problems in Cardiology*, vol. 41, no. 1, pp. 7–57, 2016.

[14] B. H. Gottschalk, D. D. Anselm, and A. Baranchuk, "Brugada phenocopy international registry and online educational portal," 2014, http://www.brugadaphenocopy.com.

[15] J. García-Niebla, P. Llontop-García, J. I. Valle-Racero, G. Serra-Autonell, V. N. Batchvarov, and A. B. de Luna, "Technical mistakes during the acquisition of the electrocardiogram," *Annals of Noninvasive Electrocardiology*, vol. 14, no. 4, pp. 389–403, 2009.

[16] B. P. Knight, F. Pelosi, G. F. Michaud, S. A. Strickberger, and F. Morady, "Clinical consequences of electrocardiographic artifact mimicking ventricular tachycardia," *The New England Journal of Medicine*, vol. 341, no. 17, pp. 1270–1274, 1999.

[17] A. A. Tambe, M. A. Demany, H. A. Zimmerman, and E. Mascarenhas, "Angina pectoris and slow flow velocity of dye in coronary arteries–A new angiographic finding," *American Heart Journal*, vol. 84, no. 1, pp. 66–71, 1972.

[18] X. Wang and S.-P. Nie, "The coronary slow flow phenomenon: characteristics, mechanisms and implications," *Cardiovascular Diagnosis & Therapy*, vol. 1, no. 1, pp. 37–43, 2011.

[19] P. K. Goel, S. K. Gupta, A. Agarwal, and A. Kapoor, "Slow coronary flow: a distinct angiographic subgroup in syndrome X," *Angiology*, vol. 52, no. 8, pp. 507–514, 2001.

[20] S. Saya, T. A. Hennebry, P. Lozano, R. Lazzara, and E. Schechter, "Coronary slow flow phenomenon and risk for sudden cardiac death due to ventricular arrhythmias: a case report and review of literature," *Clinical Cardiology*, vol. 31, no. 8, pp. 352–355, 2008.

[21] S. M. Victor, A. Gnanaraj, V. Subban, and A. s. Mullasari, "AS-274: Coronary slow flow phenomenon: risk profile," *The American Journal of Cardiology*, vol. 109, 7 Supplement, pp. S132–S133, 2012.

[22] J. H. Chesebro, G. Knatterud, R. Roberts et al., "Thrombolysis in Myocardial Infarction (TIMI) trial, phase I: a comparison between intravenous tissue plasminogen activator and intravenous streptokinase. Clinical findings through hospital discharge," *Circulation*, vol. 76, no. 1, pp. 142–154, 1987.

[23] C. M. Gibson, C. P. Cannon, W. L. Daley et al., "TIMI frame count," *Circulation*, vol. 93, no. 5, pp. 879–888, 1996.

[24] V. G. Cin, H. Pekdemir, A. Çamsar et al., "Diffuse intimal thickening of coronary arteries in slow coronary flow," *Japanese Heart Journal*, vol. 44, no. 6, pp. 907–919, 2003.

[25] J.-J. Li, X.-W. Qin, Z.-C. Li et al., "Increased plasma C-reactive protein and interleukin-6 concentrations in patients with slow coronary flow," *Clinica Chimica Acta*, vol. 385, no. 1-2, pp. 43–47, 2007.

[26] Y. S. Chatzizisis, A. U. Coskun, M. Jonas, E. R. Edelman, C. L. Feldman, and P. H. Stone, "Role of endothelial shear stress in the natural history of coronary atherosclerosis and vascular remodeling: molecular, cellular, and vascular behavior," *Journal of the American College of Cardiology*, vol. 49, no. 25, pp. 2379–2393, 2007.

[27] H. Yilmaz, I. Demir, and Z. Uyar, "Clinical and coronary angiographic characteristics of patients with coronary slow flow," *Acta Cardiologica*, vol. 63, no. 5, pp. 579–584, 2008.

[28] H. Sanati, R. Kiani, F. Shakerian et al., "Coronary slow flow phenomenon clinical findings and predictors," *Research in Cardiovascular Medicine*, vol. 5, no. 1, article e30296, 2016.

[29] M. Cakmak, H. Tanriverdi, N. Cakmak, H. Evrengul, S. Cetemen, and O. Kuru, "Simvastatin may improve myocardial perfusion abnormality in slow coronary flow," *Cardiology*, vol. 110, no. 1, pp. 39–44, 2008.

[30] M. Caliskan, D. Erdogan, H. Gullu et al., "Effects of atorvastatin on coronary flow reserve in patients with slow coronary flow," *Clinical Cardiology*, vol. 30, no. 9, pp. 475–479, 2007.

[31] S. Albayrak, S. Ordu, H. Yuksel, H. Ozhan, O. Yazgan, and M. Yazici, "Efficacy of nebivolol on flow-mediated dilation in patients with slow coronary flow," *International Heart Journal*, vol. 50, no. 5, pp. 545–553, 2009.

[32] A. Baranchuk, *Brugada Phenocopy: The Art of Recognizing the Brugada ECG Pattern*, Academic Press, 2018.

[33] J. Sieira, G. Dendramis, and P. Brugada, "Pathogenesis and management of Brugada syndrome," *Nature Reviews Cardiology*, vol. 13, no. 12, pp. 744–756, 2016.

[34] T. Noda, W. Shimizu, A. Taguchi et al., "ST-segment elevation and ventricular fibrillation without coronary spasm by intracoronary injection of acetylcholine and/or ergonovine maleate in patients with Brugada syndrome," *Journal of the American College of Cardiology*, vol. 40, no. 10, pp. 1841–1847, 2002.

[35] T. Miyazaki, H. Mitamura, S. Miyoshi, K. Soejima, Y. Aizawa, and S. Ogawa, "Autonomic and antiarrhythmic drug modulation of ST segment elevation in patients with Brugada syndrome," *Journal of the American College of Cardiology*, vol. 27, no. 5, pp. 1061–1070, 1996.

[36] J. M. Cordeiro, M. Mazza, R. Goodrow, N. Ulahannan, C. Antzelevitch, and J. M. Di Diego, "Functionally distinct sodium channels in ventricular epicardial and endocardial cells contribute to a greater sensitivity of the epicardium to electrical depression," *American Journal of Physiology-Heart and Circulatory Physiology*, vol. 295, no. 1, pp. H154–H162, 2008.

[37] S. Agrawal, S. Stevens, J. Shirani, J. Garg, and S. Nanda, "Ischemia-induced Brugada phenocopy," *Journal of Electrocardiology*, vol. 48, no. 5, pp. 815–817, 2015.

[38] S. Peters, "Brugada phenocopy in percutaneous coronary intervention of the right coronary artery," *International Journal of Cardiology*, vol. 203, p. 675, 2016.

[39] X.-Q. Quan, S. Li, R. Liu, K. Zheng, X.-F. Wu, and Q. Tang, "A meta-analytic review of prevalence for Brugada ECG patterns and the risk for death," *Medicine*, vol. 95, no. 50, article e5643, 2016.

[40] A. Baranchuk, T. Nguyen, M. H. Ryu et al., "Brugada phenocopy: new terminology and proposed classification," *Annals of Noninvasive Electrocardiology*, vol. 17, no. 4, pp. 299–314, 2012.

[41] B. H. Gottschalk, D. D. Anselm, J. Brugada et al., "Expert cardiologists cannot distinguish between Brugada phenocopy and Brugada syndrome electrocardiogram patterns," *Europace*, vol. 18, no. 7, pp. 1095–1100, 2016.

[42] B. H. Gottschalk and A. Baranchuk, "Differentiation between brugada syndrome and brugada phenocopy ECG patterns: is it possible?," *Brugada Phenocopy*, vol. 1, pp. 119–124, 2018.

[43] S. M. Al-Khatib, W. G. Stevenson, M. J. Ackerman et al., "2017 AHA/ACC/HRS guideline for management of patients with ventricular arrhythmias and the prevention of sudden cardiac death: executive summary: a report of the American College of Cardiology/American Heart Association Task Force on Clinical Practice Guidelines and the Heart Rhythm Society," *Heart Rhythm*, vol. 15, no. 10, pp. e190–e252, 2018.

[44] V. Probst, A. A. M. Wilde, J. Barc et al., "SCN5A mutations and the role of genetic background in the pathophysiology of Brugada syndrome," *Circulation. Cardiovascular Genetics*, vol. 2, no. 6, pp. 552–557, 2009.

[45] D. D. Anselm, B. H. Gottschalk, and A. Baranchuk, "Brugada phenocopies: consideration of morphologic criteria and early findings from an international registry," *The Canadian Journal of Cardiology*, vol. 30, no. 12, pp. 1511–1515, 2014.

24

Systemic Inflammation-Related Bradycardia in COVID-19

Aswin Srinivasan ,[1] Tusharkumar Pansuriya,[1] Branden Wilson,[1] Siva T. Sarva,[2] Turuvekere Jayaram,[1,2] Salman Alim,[2] Ramesh Kesavan,[2] and Syed Raza[3]

[1]*Department of Internal Medicine, HCA Houston Kingwood/University of Houston College of Medicine, USA*
[2]*Department of Pulmonology/Critical Care, HCA Houston Kingwood/University of Houston College of Medicine, USA*
[3]*Department of Cardiology, HCA Houston Kingwood/University of Houston College of Medicine, USA*

Correspondence should be addressed to Aswin Srinivasan; aswin.srinivasan@hcahealthcare.com

Academic Editor: Celestino Sardu

Systemic inflammation-related sinus bradycardia in COVID-19 infection has not been well described yet. This six-patient case series excludes common causes of bradycardia. As bradycardia may be a sequela of COVID-19 infection, we recommend closely monitoring hemodynamics and stopping medications that can exacerbate bradycardia in these patients.

1. Introduction

Coronavirus disease 2019 (COVID-19), caused by the pathogen SARS-CoV-2, is primarily a respiratory illness with secondary systemic and cardiovascular involvement reported [1]. Acute myocardial injury is the most commonly reported cardiac manifestation, with elevations in serum troponin reported in 8-10% of patients and troponin elevations associated with increased mortality [2]. Additionally, it has been reported that COVID-19 patients with hyperglycemia, even without known diabetes, have higher risk of severe disease than those with normoglycemia [3]. This issue in COVID-19 patients is important as tight glycemic control has been described as affecting cardiovascular outcome [4]. Arrhythmias have also been noted, with a recent report from Wuhan, China, noting that 16.4% of hospitalized patients and 44% of ICU patients developed arrhythmias [1]. This phenomenon was also reported in a global survey of electrophysiologists conducted by the Heart Rhythm Society, which reported that bradyarrhythmias occurred in conjunction with COVID-19 [2]. In this case series, we report a new arrhythmic phenomenon of sinus bradycardia without underlying myocardial injury in six patients with COVID-19. We recommend close monitoring of hemodynamic stability and stopping medications that can further exacerbate bradycardia in these patients.

2. Case Description

Patient 1 presented with weakness, dyspnea, and dizziness since testing positive for SARS-CoV-2 five days before admission. His admission electrocardiogram (EKG) and laboratory studies were unremarkable (Table 1). He required high-flow nasal cannula (HFNC). Chest X-ray (CXR) showed pulmonary infiltrates consistent with bilateral pneumonia. Given his worsening respiratory status, convalescent plasma, dexamethasone, and full-dose enoxaparin were started. He experienced persistent bradycardia for five days, starting on day six of his hospitalization (Figures 1, 2). His oxygen requirements progressively increased, with a CXR on hospital day eleven showing worsening moderate bilateral pneumothorax, for which a thoracostomy was performed. Despite treatment, the patient became hypothermic, tachypneic, hypotensive, and eventually passed away from pulseless electrical activity.

Patient 2 presented with worsening shortness of breath (SOB) after testing positive for SARS-CoV-2 five days before admission. Her admission EKG and laboratory results were unremarkable (Table 1). She required a nonrebreather and BiPAP. CXR revealed extensive bilateral pulmonary infiltrates. Dexamethasone, ceftriaxone, azithromycin, and full-dose enoxaparin were initiated. Remdesivir and convalescent plasma initiated when her respiratory status worsened. She

Table 1: Patient characteristics and data.

Patient	Age (year)	Sex	Relevant past medical history	Initial clinical presentation	Relevant laboratory results on admission	Findings on admission EKG	Days between COVID-19 diagnosis and onset of persistent bradycardia	Findings on EKG(s) after onset of persistent bradycardia
1	45	Male	Hypertension	Weakness, shortness of breath, and dizziness	Troponin: <0.012 Potassium: 3.6 Creatinine: 0.7 TSH: 0.205	Sinus tachycardia; intervals within normal limits; no conduction system blocks	10 days	Hospital day 4: Sinus bradycardia; intervals within normal limits; no conduction system blocks
2	34	Female	Type II diabetes mellitus	Shortness of breath	Troponin: <0.012 Potassium: 4.0 Creatinine: 0.8 TSH: 0.515	Sinus tachycardia; intervals within normal limits; no conduction system blocks	9 days	Hospital day 8: Sinus bradycardia; intervals within normal limits; no conduction system blocks
3	60	Female	Hypertension, hypothyroidism, type II diabetes mellitus	Shortness of breath, cough, fever, myalgias	Troponin: <0.012 Potassium: 4.2 Creatinine: 0.7 TSH: 0.667	Normal sinus rhythm; intervals within normal limits; no conduction system blocks	6 days	Hospital days 3, 4, & 6: Sinus bradycardia; intervals within normal limits; no conduction system blocks
4	67	Female	Hypertension, hypothyroidism, deep vein thrombosis, anxiety disorder	Shortness of breath, cough, fever	Troponin: <0.012 Potassium: 4.1 Creatinine: 0.5 TSH: 0.139	Normal sinus rhythm; intervals within normal limits; no conduction system blocks	12 days	Hospital day 6: Sinus bradycardia; intervals within normal limits; no conduction system blocks
5	54	Male	Hypertension, obstructive sleep apnea	Shortness of breath	Troponin: <0.012 Potassium: 4.1 Creatinine: 0.5 TSH: 0.508	Normal sinus rhythm; intervals within normal limits; no conduction system blocks	8 days	Hospital day 10: Sinus bradycardia; intervals within normal limits; no conduction system blocks Hospital day 15: Sinus bradycardia; prolonged QT/QTc interval (482/477 milliseconds); no conduction system blocks
6	41	Male	Hypertension, obesity	Shortness of breath	Troponin: <0.012 Potassium: 4.9 Creatinine: 0.6 TSH: NA	Normal sinus rhythm; intervals within normal limits; no conduction system blocks	9 days	Hospital day 4: Sinus bradycardia; intervals within normal limits; right bundle branch block, left posterior fascicular block Hospital day 8 (discharge day): Sinus bradycardia; intervals within normal limits; no conduction system blocks

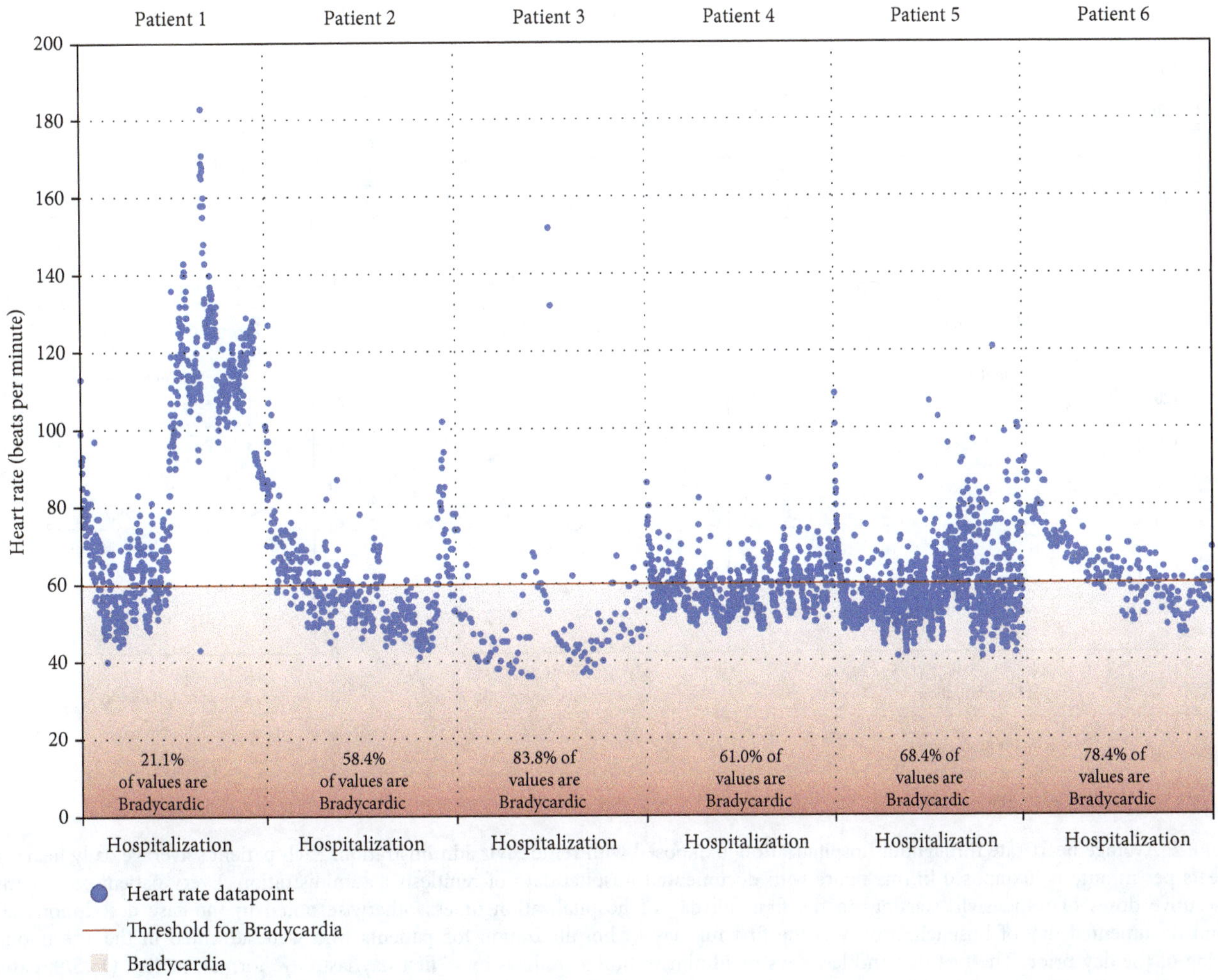

FIGURE 1: Heart rate throughout hospitalization for each patient. Every discrete heart rate datapoint as recorded in the electronic medical record throughout each patient's hospital stay, with patients' data shown adjacent to one another using a uniform *y*-axis, but individually labeled *x*-axes. The proportion of recorded values found to be bradycardic is noted at the bottom of each patient's dataset. HR: heart rate; %: percentage; *x*-axis: duration of hospitalization (continuous measure of time, no discrete intervals used); *y*-axis: heart rate in beats per minute.

developed bradycardia on hospital day four, which resolved on day 9 (Figures 1 and 2). Once her respiratory status improved and oxygen requirements decreased, she was discharged home with dexamethasone.

Patient 3 presented with ten days of worsening SOB, dry cough, fever, and generalized body pain. She tested positive for SARS-CoV-2 four days before admission. CXR revealed extensive bilateral pulmonary infiltrates. Though she required HFNC, her admission EKG and laboratory studies were unremarkable. Dexamethasone, remdesivir, convalescent plasma, and azithromycin were initiated. On hospital day three, she developed eight days of persistent bradycardia (Figures 1 and 2). Once her respiratory status improved, oxygen requirement decreased, and heart rate improved, she was discharged with prednisone.

Patient 4 presented with SOB and cough after testing positive for SARS-CoV-2 nine days before admission. CXR revealed bilateral pneumonia. Though she required HFNC, her admission EKG and laboratory studies were unremarkable. Remdesivir, convalescent plasma, azithromycin, dexamethasone, and full-dose anticoagulation were started on admission. She started experiencing persistent bradycardia lasting eight days on hospital day four (Figures 1 and 2). Once her respiratory status and heart rate improved, she was discharged.

Patient 5 presented with SOB after testing positive for SARS-CoV-2 seven days before admission and being discharged from the ED on steroids. His admission EKG and laboratory studies were only remarkable for elevated liver function tests; he now required HFNC (Table 1). CT of the chest showed ground glass opacities. He received convalescent plasma, dexamethasone, and full-dose enoxaparin, with remdesivir initiation on hospital day three after improvement in kidney and liver function (Tables 1 and 2). He developed sinus bradycardia on the same day. Once his respiratory status improved, he was discharged on albuterol and dexamethasone.

Patient 6 presented with SOB after testing positive for COVID-19 infection seven days before admission. His admission EKG and laboratory studies were unremarkable,

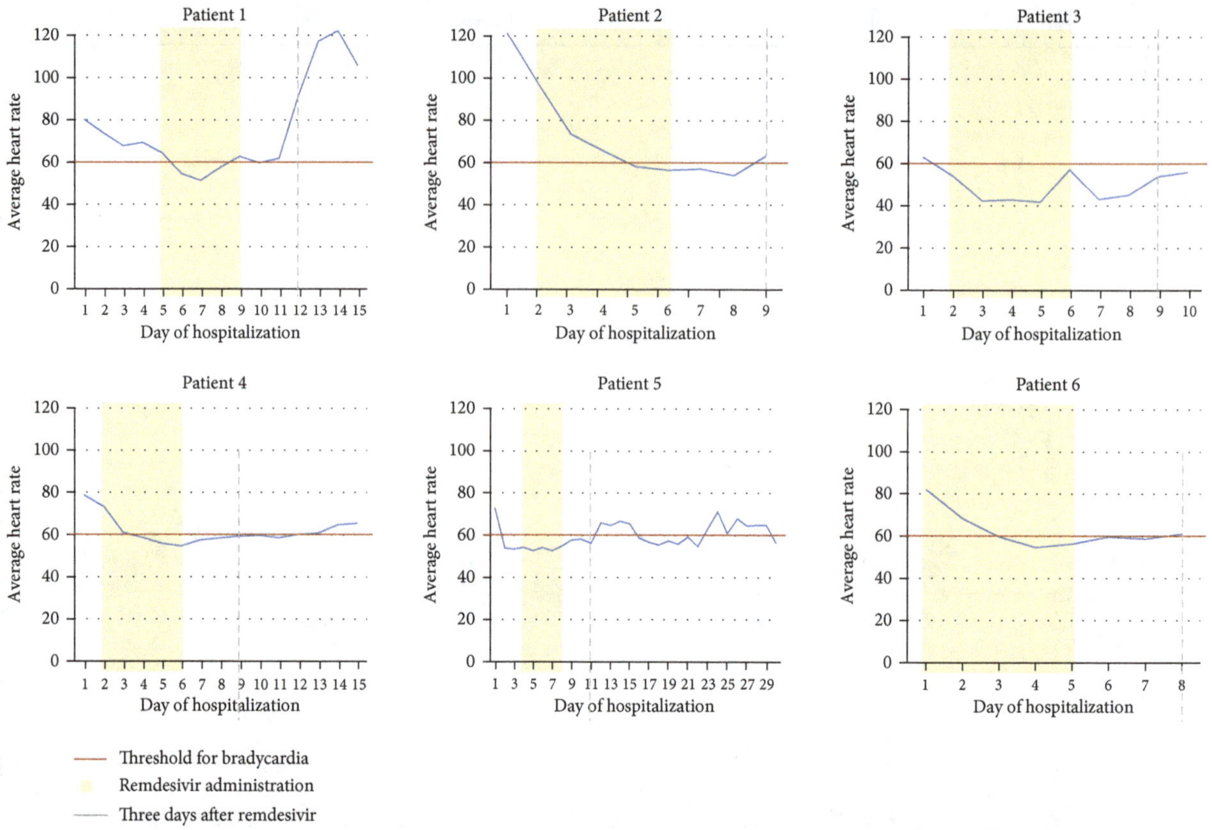

Figure 2: Average heart rate throughout hospitalization juxtaposed with remdesivir administration. Each patient's average daily heart rate in beats per minute is juxtaposed in this figure with documented hospital days of remdesivir administration. Every patient received five consecutive doses of remdesivir, starting on the first full day of hospitalization unless otherwise noted in the case descriptions. The second documented day of hospitalization was the first full day of hospitalization for patients who were admitted in the afternoon or evening of the day prior. The first day and last days of administration as follows in a "first day/last day" format: patient (1) 5/9, patient (2) 2/6, patient (3) 2/6, patient (4) 2/6, patient (5) 4/8, patient (6) 1/5. The threshold for bradycardia is noted, and the third day after the last dose of Remdesivir is noted. Recovery from bradycardia was expected at this point should remdesivir be causative.

Table 2: Additional patient data.

Patient	Lowest HR between 8 AM and 5 PM (bpm)	Peak D-dimer (ng/mL)	Peak CRP (normal range: 0-12.4 mg/L)	IL-6 (normal range: 0-14.6 pg/mL)
1	46	1843	181.4	20.0
2	43	294	167.7	108.9
3	36	831	67.4	NA
4	48	1240	48.1	NA
5	42	41352	201.2	93.6
6	35	878	179.8	125.7

bpm: beats per minute; CRP: C-reactive protein; HR: heart rate; IL-6: interleukin 6; L: liter; mL: milliliter; mg: milligrams; NA: not available; ng: nanograms; pg: picograms.

although he required HFNC and subsequently BiPAP (Table 1). CXR showed bilateral pneumonia. He received convalescent plasma, remdesivir, dexamethasone, cefepime, and full-dose enoxaparin. On hospital day three, he developed persistent bradycardia lasting five days (Figures 1 and 2). Once his respiratory status and oxygen requirement improved, he was discharged with dexamethasone and amlodipine.

3. Discussion

Cardiac phenomena associated with COVID-19 include direct myocardial injury, myocarditis, heart failure, and cardiogenic shock [1]. However, COVID-19-associated arrhythmias are not well described in the literature. In this case series, we present several patients with sinus bradycardia associated with COVID-19 in the absence of myocardial injury.

Our case series includes six patients—three male and three female. None had any reported history of coronary artery disease. Five patients had a prior history of hypertension. Echocardiography was unremarkable except a mildly reduced ejection fraction of 45-50% in patient 5. On admission, every patient exhibited normal sinus rhythm on EKG, with patients developing sinus bradycardia while hospitalized despite their generally healthy baseline cardiac status (Table 1). The lowest daytime heart rates for every patient were 46, 43, 36, 48, 42, and 35 beats/min, respectively. Severity of bradycardia that each patient exhibits does not appear to be related to their cardiovascular morbidity.

On admission, EKG on all patients revealed normal sinus rhythm. A retrospective cohort study from Wuhan, China, showed an increase in cardiac troponin I in fatal cases that started around 16 days into their illness [2]. All the six patients in this series had serial troponin enzymes of less than 0.012 during bradycardia episodes, which indicates that sinus bradycardia was not associated with myocardial injury. Thyroid function was within normal limits for all patients. In patients 3 and 4, home thyroid medications were resumed on admission and thyroid function was normal during hospitalization. All patients had a normal range of potassium levels during the bradycardia period. All patients did not receive any AV nodal blocking agents or sedatives prior to or during the period of bradycardia. The patients were not given any AV nodal blocking agents or sedatives prior or during their periods of bradycardia (Table 1).

Recent literature shows remdesivir to be a potential cause of sinus bradycardia [5]. But patient 5 developed bradycardia prior to administration of remdesivir. The half-life of remdesivir is approximately one hour, and the half-life of its active metabolite is approximately 27 hours. However, patients 2, 3, and 4 did not recover to normal sinus rhythm even after three to four days of the last dose of remdesivir administration (Figure 2). This finding indicates remdesivir likely is not the sole cause of bradycardia.

Another virus in the same family, severe acute respiratory syndrome coronavirus (SARS-CoV), has been found to resemble closely with SARS-CoV-2 [6]. Interestingly, sinus bradycardia has been previously reported in 18 patients (14.1%) with SARS-CoV [6]. It is possible that the SARS-CoV-2 and related viruses may be associated with bradycardia secondary to structural interactions at a molecular level between these pathogens and their biological hosts.

Possible mechanisms for bradycardia such as direct myocardial injury, hypoxia, enhanced inflammatory stages, and drug toxicity have been postulated in recent reports [1]. In a multicenter autopsy study performed on 21 patients with SARS-CoV-2, 18 cases showed macrophage interstitial infiltration in the myocardium, while the other 3 cases showed lymphocytic myocarditis [7]. These high levels of myocardial macrophages in COVID-19 patients may largely result from systemic elevations of proinflammatory cytokines such as interleukin-6 (IL-6). Four of the patients in this case series had elevated IL-6 levels (Table 2) at the onset of bradycardia. All six patients exhibited elevated CRP at the onset of bradycardia. The inflammatory cytokines including IL-6 released during the host inflammatory response phase could act on sinoatrial (SA) node. This finding suggests a possible association between bradycardia and host inflammatory response. Finally, the age range of the six patients in this series was 41 and 67 years. The age range of nearly 30 years makes this observation limited to potential bias. Therefore, more studies are needed to investigate and establish the correlation between bradycardia and COVID-19 infection.

4. Conclusion

As per our knowledge and published data, association of sinus bradycardia in COVID-19 patients has not been well described yet. In this case series, we excluded all major causes of bradycardia. We recommend closely monitoring these patients for hemodynamic stability, especially the patients with underlying cardiovascular conditions. As described, arrhythmia gets better along with improvement in clinical condition in most cases. We also believe it is important to exclude other main causes of bradycardia and to know that sinus bradycardia is a potential sequela of COVID-19 infection. We recommend to be prudent about not taking any medications that can exacerbate the severe bradycardia further. More studies need to be done in survivors for long-term cardiac sequelae.

Abbreviations

COVID-19:	Coronavirus disease 2019
EKG:	Electrocardiogram
HFNC:	High-flow nasal cannula
CXR:	Chest X-ray
SOB:	Shortness of breath
SARS-CoV:	Severe acute respiratory syndrome coronavirus
IL-6:	Interleukin-6
CRP:	C-reactive protein
SA:	Sinoatrial node.

Additional Points

Learning Objectives. (i) To recognize bradycardia as a sequela of COVID-19 infection. (ii) Needs close monitoring of these patients for hemodynamic instability.

Consent

No written consent has been obtained from the patients as there is no patient identifiable data included in this case series.

References

[1] R. Gopinathannair, F. Merchant, D. Lakkireddy et al., "COVID-19 and cardiac arrhythmias: a global perspective on arrhythmia characteristics and management strategies," *Journal of Interventional Cardiac Electrophysiology*, vol. 59, no. 2, pp. 329–336, 2020.

[2] T. Guo, Y. Fan, M. Chen et al., "Cardiovascular implications of fatal outcomes of patients with coronavirus disease 2019 (COVID-19)," *JAMA Cardiology*, vol. 5, no. 7, pp. 811–818, 2020.

[3] C. Sardu, N. D'Onofrio, M. L. Balestrieri et al., "Outcomes in patients with hyperglycemia affected by COVID-19: can we do more on glycemic control?," *Diabetes Care*, vol. 43, no. 7, pp. 1408–1415, 2020.

[4] R. Marfella, F. C. Sasso, F. Cacciapuoti et al., "Tight glycemic control may increase regenerative potential of myocardium during acute infarction," *The Journal of Clinical Endocrinology and Metabolism*, vol. 97, no. 3, pp. 933–942, 2012.

[5] A. K. Gupta, B. M. Parker, V. Priyadarshi, and J. Parker, "Cardiac adverse events with remdesivir in COVID-19 infection," *Cureus*, vol. 12, no. 10, 2020.

[6] C. Yu, R. S. Wong, E. B. Wu et al., "Cardiovascular complications of severe acute respiratory syndrome," *Postgraduate Medical Journal*, vol. 82, no. 964, pp. 140–144, 2006.

[7] C. Basso, O. Leone, S. Rizzo et al., "Pathological features of COVID-19-associated myocardial injury: a multicentre cardiovascular pathology study," *European Heart Journal*, vol. 41, no. 39, pp. 3827–3835, 2020.

25

High Risk Features of an Anomalous Origin of the Right Coronary Artery

Dre Eleonore Campiche[1] **Jean-Paul Vallée**[2] **and David Carballo**[1]

[1]*Cardiology Department, University Hospitals of Geneva, 1205 Geneva, Switzerland*
[2]*Radiology Department, University Hospitals of Geneva, 1205 Geneva, Switzerland*

Correspondence should be addressed to Dre Eleonore Campiche; eleonore.campiche@hcuge.ch

Academic Editor: Assad Movahed

Anomalous aortic origin of the coronary arteries (AAOCA) is a rare congenital abnormality. It is usually asymptomatic and often found incidentally during coronary angiography. However, it can also be discovered during the autopsy of young healthy adults who have suffered from sudden cardiac death (SCD). AAOCA represents the second most common cause of SCD in young athletes. Herein, we report a case of a 39-year-old patient with left-sided right coronary anomaly with multiple high-risk features who presented with life-threatening symptoms for SCD but normal electrocardiography, echocardiography, and cardiac markers. The coronary computed tomography revealed an anomalous coronary artery from the left sinus of Valsalva with a hypoplasic origin and a high-risk path between the aorta and the pulmonary artery with a short intramural path. He was surgically managed with a coronary artery bypass with an uneventful follow-up.

1. Background

Anomalous aortic origin of the coronary arteries (AAOCA) is a rare congenital abnormality. It can be asymptomatic but usually found during diagnostic angiography for workup of symptoms or during acute myocardial infarctions making the management options very complicated. However, it can also be discovered during autopsy of young healthy adults who suffered from sudden cardiac death (SCD) [1]. AAOCA represent the second most common cause of SCD in young athletes [2].

Herein, we report a case of a patient with left-sided right coronary anomaly with multiple high-risk features who presented with life-threatening symptoms for SCD.

2. Case Presentation

A 39-year-old nonsmoking male native from Cameroun without any significant personal medical history or family history of cardiovascular disease presented to the emergency department with sudden loss of consciousness. At the end of a two-hour run ending on an uphill path, the patient felt unwell with blurred vision. This was followed by chest pain, palpitations, shortness of breath, and eventually a brief loss of consciousness.

The patient was brought to the emergency department by ambulance. On admission, the electrocardiogram showed no signs of ischemia, and the troponin T levels were slightly elevated but remained stable (15 ng/l at admission, 29 ng/l after one hour, and 15 ng/l after two hours). An acute coronary syndrome was ruled out. An echocardiography performed by the specialist revealed a preserved left ventricular systolic function with an estimated ejection fraction of 60-65% and normal left ventricular parietal kinesis. The patient was admitted for further investigations.

A coronary computed tomography (CT) (Figures 1 and 2) showed a congenital anomaly of the right coronary artery (RCA) originating from the contralateral sinus of Valsalva, 18 millimetres above the left coronary leaflet. The right and left coronary arteries were located close to each other, but separate from the ostia; this was corroborated on the coronary angiogram (CA) which furthermore did not show any

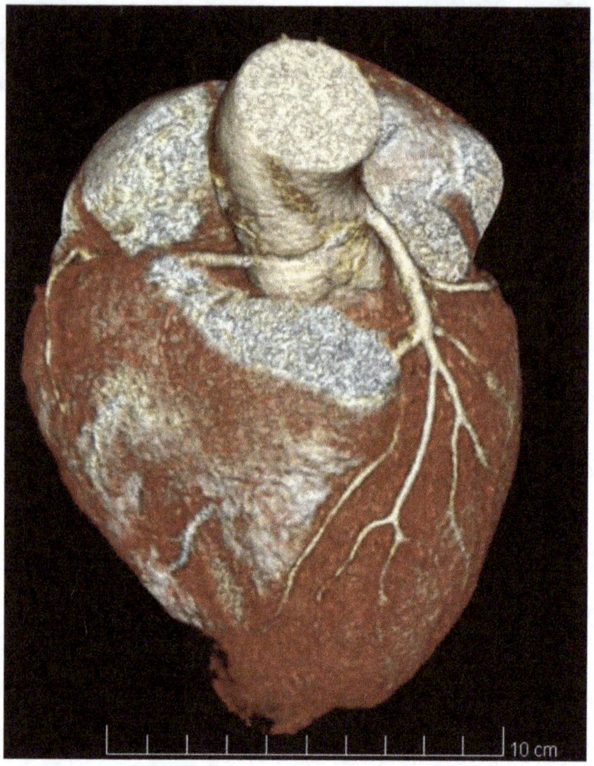

FIGURE 1: Coronary computed tomography showing the intramural path of the right coronary artery with origin close to the left coronary artery.

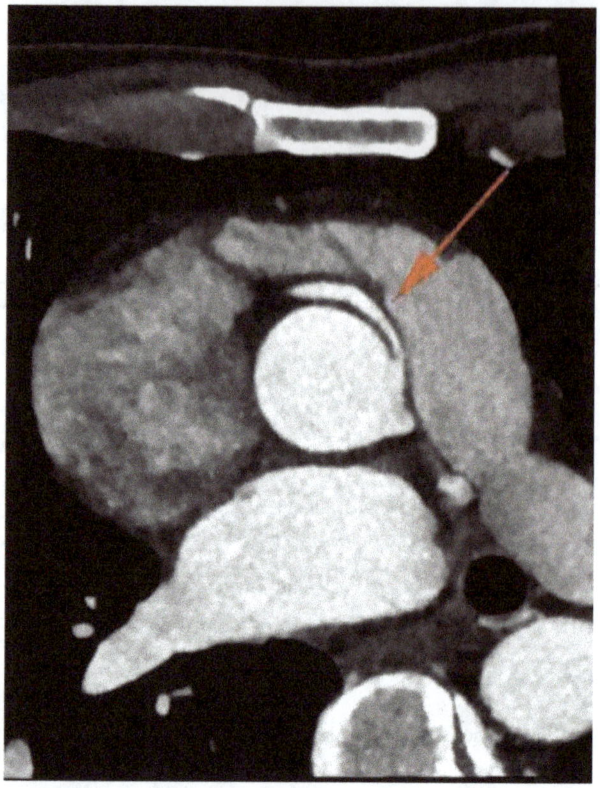

FIGURE 2: Coronary computed tomography showing the hypoplasic birth of right coronary artery (red arrow) originating close to the left sinus of Valsalva with further high-risk path between the aorta and the pulmonary artery.

intraluminal coronary atherosclerosis (Figure 3). The origin of the RCA was hypoplasic and followed a high-risk path between the aorta and the pulmonary artery with a short intramural path. Additionally, a positron electron tomography and contrast-enhanced computed tomography (PET-CT) showed discrete ischemia during physiological stress in the basal, inferobasal, and middle lateroapical segments, representing 10% of the left ventricle in the territory of the RCA, as well as in a part of the apex segment.

After multidisciplinary assessment, the patient underwent coronary artery bypass grafting. Postoperative course was uneventful, and the patient was discharged on postoperative day 6.

3. Discussion

Manifestations of a left-sided origin of the RCA are illustrated by our case report. This rare anomaly can be life-threatening, as such, we aim to discuss the prevalence of AAOCA, its variants, and its high-risk features.

As previously mentioned, anomalous coronary disease is the second most common cause of SCD in young athletes [2]. It is still a frequently neglected topic in cardiology. Autopsy series reveals that the majority of cases concern young patients (<35 years old) who die during or shortly after exercise [3] but can go unnoticed in the elderly patients until they present with myocardial infarction due to coronary atherosclerosis [4].

So far, there is no imaging test of choice for the diagnosis of AAOCA. When a coronary anomaly is assessed, nonpharmacological functional imaging such as echocardiography, nuclear study, or cardiovascular magnetic resonance with physical stress are recommended to be performed to measure myocardial ischemia (*class I* recommendation) [3].

There are multiple variants of AAOCA, and some of them are associated with a higher risk for SCD. AAOCA can be classified based on (i) the origin of the anomalous vessel: left coronary artery, right coronary artery, single coronary artery, or the circumflex coronary artery; (ii) the course of the anomalous vessel: intramural, intra-arterial, intramyocardial, prepulmonic, subpulmonic, and retroaortic; and (iii) the location, shape, and spatial relationship of the coronary ostia: two separate nonconfluent orifices arising from the same sinus, two confluent orifices located adjacent to each other, or one single orifice with bifurcation in the aortic wall and single orifice with bifurcation outside the aortic wall [5].

The exact prevalence of AAOCA in the general population, as well as the associated risk of SCD, remains unknown [6]. The prevalence of AAOCA in angiographic series has been reported between 0.6% and 1.3% and 0.3% in autopsies [7, 8]. In a prospective study by Yamanaka et al. based on 126,595 patients with coronary artery anomalies, 80% were benign and asymptomatic. However, 20% were life-threatening and presented with arrhythmia, syncope, myocardial infarction, or sudden cardiac death [9].

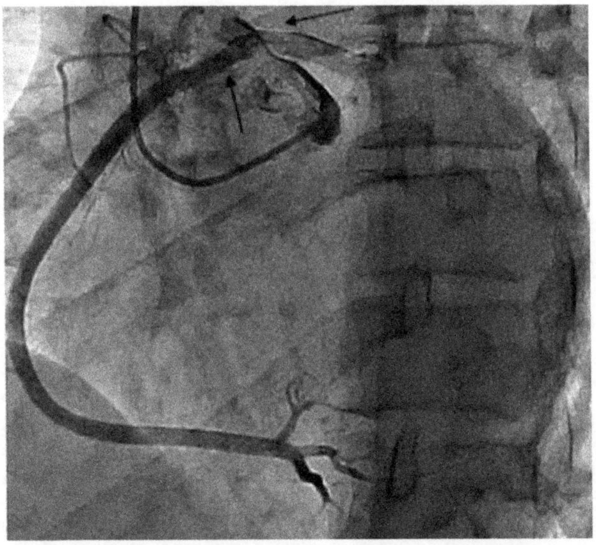

FIGURE 3: Coronary angiography revealing no atherosclerosis and the anomalous right coronary artery (left arrow) close to the origin of the left coronary artery (right arrow); with inter-aortico-pulmonary high-risk path.

In our case report, the patient presented an anomaly of the right coronary artery (ARCA) with an interarterial course as well as an intramural course arising just above the contralateral sinus of Valsalva. Of 8,522 patients referred for coronary computed tomography angiography, 72 (0.84%) had an anomalous coronary artery from opposite sinus of Valsalva, including right-sided origins of the left main coronary artery, left anterior descending coronary artery, left circumflex coronary artery, and left-sided origin of the right coronary artery [10]. In the latter study, 20 patients (0.22%) had left-sided origin of the RCA. Among patients with an anomalous coronary artery from the opposite sinus of Valsalva, 23 patients (0.28%) had an interarterial path. In this group, 6 patients (0.07%) had a high-risk course, defined in the review by a slit-like ostium, an acute angle take-off, an intramural route, and a significant compression between the aorta and the pulmonary trunk existing simultaneously. These high-risk features of an anomalous coronary artery from opposite sinus of Valsalva were only found in case of left-sided right coronary arteries, as was the case in our patient. Moreover, intra-arterial course is more frequent in ARCA, when compared to anomalous left coronary artery (0.23% versus 0.03%, respectively) [6].

The European Society of Cardiology's (ESC) identified risk factors for myocardial ischemia, such as high orifice, ostial stenosis, slit-like/fish-mouth-shaped orifice, acute angle take-off, intramural course and its length, interarterial path, and hypoplasia of the proximal coronary artery [3]. Our case presented several of these features, such as the hypoplastic ostium of the RCA, the interarterial course between the aorta and the pulmonary artery, and the short intramural path. Moreover, symptomatic patients such as the case we report is a *class I* recommendation for surgery [3]. Additionally, ischemia of 10% in the territory of the RCA found during PET-CT put him at higher risk for SCD.

Current guidelines do not support screening for AAOCA in asymptomatic athletes, given the low prevalence of this disease [6]. Further studies and clarification on the screening options of athletes remain an issue. Currently, the ESC and The American Heart Association and American Academy of Pediatrics both provide a recent consensus statement on cardiovascular screening of young college athletes [11, 12].

Surgery is indicated in case of symptomatic patients with left-sided origin of the right coronary artery with interarterial, intramural path and with hypoplasic ostia. Nevertheless, management of critical patients with intra-arterial course of an anomalous coronary artery is controversial.

Physicians should be aware of the symptoms of AAOCA, as these rare congenital abnormalities can lead to death. Appropriate imaging studies should be performed, and cases should be discussed with a multidisciplinary team.

References

[1] J. M. Laureti, K. Singh, and J. Blankenship, "Anomalous coronary arteries: a familial clustering," *Clinical Cardiology*, vol. 28, no. 10, pp. 488–490, 2005.

[2] A. P. Burke, A. Farb, R. Virmani, J. Goodin, and J. E. Smialek, "Sports-related and non-sports-related sudden cardiac death in young adults," *American Heart Journal*, vol. 121, no. 2, pp. 568–575, 1991.

[3] H. Baumgartner, J. De Backer, S. V. Babu-Narayan et al., "2020 ESC guidelines for the management of adult congenital heart disease," *European Heart Journal*, vol. 42, no. 6, pp. 563–645, 2020.

[4] H. R. Khan, H. Hashim, and M. Bhandari, "Anomalous origin of the epicardial left coronary artery from the right coronary sinus revealed in a patient presenting with acute myocardial infarction," *Journal of Ayub Medical College, Abbottabad*, vol. 28, no. 2, pp. 420–422, 2016.

[5] H. Agrawal, C. M. Mery, R. Krishnamurthy, and S. Molossi, "Anatomic types of anomalous aortic origin of a coronary artery: a pictorial summary," *Congenital Heart Disease*, vol. 12, no. 5, pp. 603–606, 2017.

[6] M. K. Cheezum, R. R. Liberthson, N. R. Shah et al., "Anomalous aortic origin of a coronary artery from the inappropriate sinus of Valsalva," *Journal of the American College of Cardiology*, vol. 69, no. 12, pp. 1592–1608, 2017.

[7] A. Yildiz, B. Okcun, T. Peker, C. Arslan, A. Olcay, and V. M. Bulent, "Prevalence of coronary artery anomalies in 12, 457 adult patients who underwent coronary angiography," *Clinical Cardiology*, vol. 33, no. 12, pp. E60–E64, 2010.

[8] G. Tuo, M. Marasini, C. Brunelli, L. Zannini, and M. Balbi, "Incidence and clinical relevance of primary congenital anomalies of the coronary arteries in children and adults," *Cardiology in the Young*, vol. 23, no. 3, pp. 381–386, 2013.

[9] O. Yamanaka and R. E. Hobbs, "Coronary artery anomalies in 126,595 patients undergoing coronary arteriography," *Catheterization and Cardiovascular Diagnosis*, vol. 21, no. 1, pp. 28–40, 1990.

[10] M. P. Opolski, J. Pregowski, M. Kruk et al., "Prevalence and characteristics of coronary anomalies originating from the opposite sinus of Valsalva in 8,522 patients referred for coronary computed tomography angiography," *The American Journal of Cardiology*, vol. 111, no. 9, pp. 1361–1367, 2013.

[11] A. Pelliccia, S. Sharma, S. Gati et al., "2020 ESC guidelines on sports cardiology and exercise in patients with cardiovascular disease," *European Heart Journal*, vol. 42, pp. 17–96, 2020.

[12] B. J. Maron, B. D. Levine, R. L. Washington, A. L. Baggish, R. J. Kovacs, and M. S. Maron, "Eligibility and disqualification recommendations for competitive athletes with cardiovascular abnormalities: task force 2: preparticipation screening for cardiovascular disease in competitive athletes: a scientific statement from the American Heart Association and American College of Cardiology," *Circulation*, vol. 132, no. 22, pp. e267–e272, 2015.

26

Cardiogenic Shock in a Hemodialyzed Patient on Flecainide: Treatment with Intravenous Fat Emulsion, Extracorporeal Cardiac Life Support and CytoSorb® Hemoadsorption

Nicolas De Schryver,[1] Philippe Hantson,[2,3] Vincent Haufroid,[3,4] and Mélanie Dechamps[5]

[1]*Department of Intensive Care, Clinique St-Pierre, 1340 Ottignies, Belgium*
[2]*Department of Intensive Care, Cliniques St-Luc, Université catholique de Louvain, 1200 Brussels, Belgium*
[3]*Louvain Centre of Toxicology and Applied Pharmacology, Université catholique de Louvain, 1200 Brussels, Belgium*
[4]*Department of Clinical Chemistry, Cliniques St-Luc, Université catholique de Louvain, 1200 Brussels, Belgium*
[5]*Cardiovascular Intensive Care, Cliniques St-Luc, Université catholique de Louvain, 1200 Brussels, Belgium*

Correspondence should be addressed to Philippe Hantson; philippe.hantson@uclouvain.be

Academic Editor: Assad Movahed

A 67-year-old woman with a history of end-stage renal disease on hemodialysis received a therapeutic dose (150 mg daily) of flecainide for three weeks. She was admitted to the Emergency Department for malaise and dizziness, and the electrocardiogram revealed ventricular tachycardia treated by amiodarone. Hemodynamic condition remained stable, and the toxicity of flecainide was initially not suspected until she developed within 8 hours a cardiogenic shock requiring vasopressors. The patient then received sodium bicarbonate (300 mmol) and dobutamine but experienced cardiac arrest two hours later. The administration of intravenous fat emulsion (IFE) was associated with return of spontaneous circulation, but there was a relapse of cardiovascular shock at the end of IFE infusion. The patient was placed on extracorporeal cardiac life support (ECLS), continuous hemofiltration, and hemoadsorption using the CytoSorb® cartridge. Serial determinations of serum flecainide concentration were obtained during the course of hemoadsorption, with a terminal half-life of 3.7 h during the first four hours and a global plasma clearance of 40.3 ml/min over the first 22 hours. The weaning of ECLS was possible on day 7. Intravenous fat emulsion infusion was followed by a significant increase in serum flecainide concentration. In addition, while conventional techniques of extrarenal epuration usually appear as poorly effective for flecainide removal, a mean plasma clearance of 40.3 ml/min was observed using the hemoadsorption technique based on CytoSorb® cartridge. However, the impact on the clinical course was probably extremely modest in comparison with ECLS.

1. Introduction

Flecainide is a Vaughan Williams class 1C antiarrhythmic drug influencing the fast inward sodium channel during the phase 0 of the action potential. Overdoses with flecainide have been associated with a high mortality rate (22.5%) in comparison with other class 1C molecules. Toxicity is less easily recognized in case of chronic therapy. Ventricular arrhythmias and decreased cardiac contractility in relationship with conduction disturbances are the main complications of flecainide overdose [1]. When the usual cardiopulmonary resuscitation with sodium bicarbonate and catecholamines is failing, rescue therapy with extracorporeal cardiac life support (ECLS) should be promptly considered. We report a case of flecainide toxicity following its therapeutic use in a patient with end-stage renal disease (ESRD). In addition to ECLS, the patient was also treated with intravenous fat emulsion (IFE) and an extrarenal epuration technique based on hemoadsorption (CytoSorb®).

2. Case Presentation

A 67-year-old woman (46 kg weight) underwent an aortic valve repair with aortic root replacement for severe dilation of the ascending aorta. In the postoperative period, she developed atrial fibrillation and was then prescribed flecainide two days before hospital discharge. Her other relevant medical history included ESRD requiring chronic hemodialysis, hypertension, and hypothyroidism. Her daily treatment included flecainide 150 mg od, losartan 100 mg od, acenocoumarol, levothyroxine 75 μg od, pantoprazole 40 mg od, calcitriol 0.25 mg od, and cinacalcet 30 mg od. Three weeks after hospital discharge, the patient suddenly felt dizzy and was referred at night to the Emergency Department. A 12 lead electrocardiogram showed an extremely broad QRS complex tachycardia at a rate of 115 bpm and without P waves. The negative concordance of the QRS complexes in the precordial leads, as well as the extreme right QRS axis deviation, was consistent with the diagnosis of ventricular tachycardia. The i.v. administration of 300 mg amiodarone resulted in a decrease of heart rate to 78 bpm with a blood pressure of 122/76 mmHg. A second ECG showed a regular rhythm without P waves and with broad QRS complexes (189 ms) and with diffuse repolarization abnormalities. Relevant laboratory investigations were arterial pH 7.44, bicarbonate 22 mmol/l, lactate 1.9 mmol/l, serum creatinine 9.57 mg/dl, urea 99 mg/dl, and hsTnI 40 ng/l. Liver function tests were normal. Blood was also drawn for toxicological investigations, but the results were not immediately available. The patient was admitted in the Intensive Care Unit (ICU) for further monitoring of blood pressure and heart rhythm. Systolic blood pressure remained initially above 100 mmHg, heart rate around 75/min, and arterial pH above 7.45. Eight hours after hospital admission, blood pressure progressively decreased and norepinephrine was started. The lactate level started to increase at the same time (7.7 mmol/l). The ICU physician on duty reconsidered the initial diagnosis of ventricular tachycardia as a sign of flecainide toxicity. Transthoracic echocardiography showed a marked interventricular dyssynchrony with severely decreased systolic function of both ventricles. Left ventricular ejection fraction was calculated using the biplane Simpson method at 36%. Cardiac output was calculated at 1920 ml/min. Administration of sodium bicarbonate (300 mmol), calcium gluconate (4 g), and dobutamine was initiated. Over the next 3 hours, the norepinephrine requirements rapidly increased up to 1.5 mcg/kg/min. Lactate levels increased up to 10 mmol/l, and neurological status worsened. The patient was intubated, and mechanical ventilation was started but cardiac arrest (pulseless electrical activity rapidly followed by asystole) occurred. Cardiopulmonary resuscitation (CPR) was immediately performed with 1 mg epinephrine administration every 3 minutes. CPR was briefly interrupted every 2 minutes for rhythm analysis but asystole persisted. Thirteen minutes after the initiation of CPR, intravenous fat emulsion (20% Intralipid®) (IFE) bolus (1.5 ml/kg) was given over 1 minute and was followed one minute later by return of spontaneous circulation. Continuous infusion of IFE was continued at a rate of 0.25 ml/kg/min immediately after bolus administration for a total of 450 ml administered. At the same time, hemodynamics dramatically improved with complete weaning of norepinephrine requirements but without perceptible shortening of the QRS complexes. Five minutes after the end of IFE administration, blood pressure again dropped and norepinephrine was restarted with increasing doses up to 1.5 mcg/kg/min. Initiation of an extracorporeal cardiac life support (ECLS) and transfer to a tertiary center were then decided. In the meantime, profound hypotension occurred (46/28 mmHg). A second bolus of IFE (1.5 ml/kg) was administered, followed by continuous infusion at a rate of 0.25 ml/kg/min. At the time of venoarterial cannulation for ECLS two hours later by the mobile team of the tertiary hospital, norepinephrine and epinephrine requirements peaked at 2.6 mcg/kg/min and 0.5 mcg/kg/min, respectively. The patient had received an additional dose of 200 mmol of sodium bicarbonate. The lactate level was 19.9 mmol/l. IFE administration was discontinued immediately after cannulation. A total volume of 20% IFE administration was 1500 ml (33 ml/body weight kg).

After transfer to the tertiary center, continuous venovenous hemodiafiltration (CVVHDF) and additional hemoadsorption using CytoSorb® cartridge were started with a blood flow of 200 milliliters per minute. The detailed toxicokinetics of flecainide in relationship with the epuration technique are presented in Figures 1 and 2. The serum flecainide concentration was 3477 ng/ml at the time of admission in the first hospital, well above the therapeutic range (200-1000).

Within 72 hours, norepinephrine requirement dropped to less than 0.2 μg/kg/min and QRS duration on ECG was reduced to 98 msec (atrial flutter). After 7 days, echocardiography showed a normal biventricular systolic function and ECLS could be weaned and removed. The patient maintained normal liver function tests over the ICU stay. Further clinical course was marked by pulmonary and abdominal infections, slow respiratory weaning, and gastrointestinal bleeding. The patient could be discharged to the ward on day 34, with an excellent neurological outcome and recovery of left ventricular function, and had a 6-month uneventful follow-up.

Genetic testing for CYP2D6 polymorphism was obtained. The investigated alleles were CYP2D6 *1, *2, *3, *4, *5, *6, *7, *8, *9, *10, *11, *15, *17, *29, *35, *41, duplication, and deletion. The patient genotype was confirmed to be CYP2D6*1/*4.

3. Discussion

Flecainide has similar characteristics to other medications for which IFE therapy has been successfully utilized. Flecainide has a large volume of distribution (V_D (4.9 L/kg)) and a high Log P (octanol/water) coefficient (3.8). This would predict a favorable response to IFE therapy in case of overdose with refractory shock [2]. The hypothesis of a "lipid sink" resulting in a sequestration of lipophilic medications from the receptors sites seems to be supported by some clinical observations contrasting with experimental data. Indeed, in a rabbit experimental model of flecainide poisoning, ILE administration did not result in an increase of plasma flecainide concentration [3]. Besides, IFE was not more effective

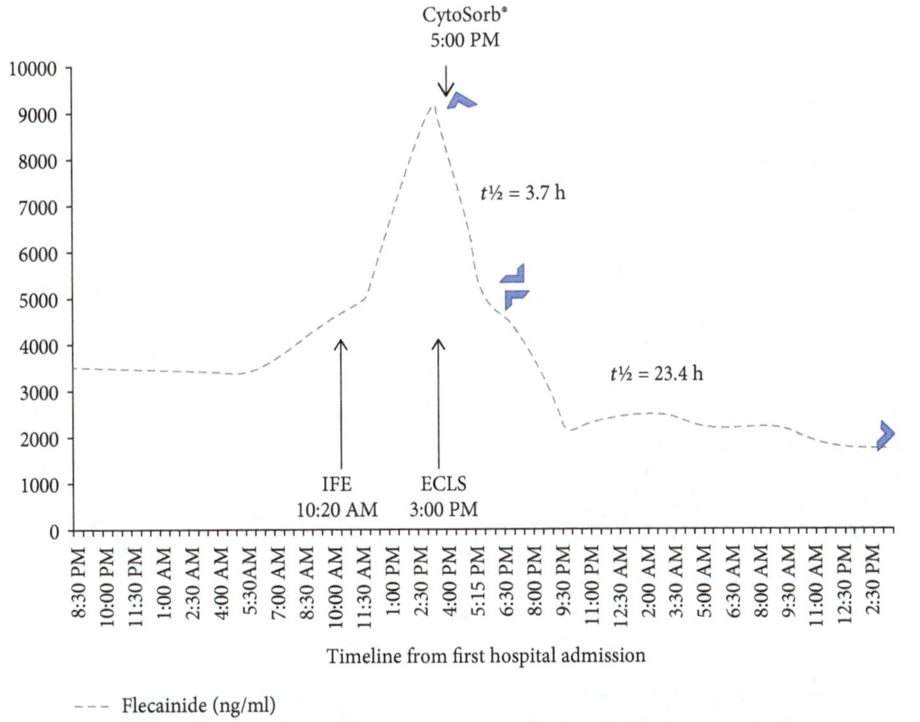

Figure 1: Evolution of serum flecainide concentration over time. IFE: intravenous fat emulsion. The terminal half-life (*t*½) elimination of flecainide was calculated over the first four hours (3.7 hours) following the introduction of CytoSorb® hemoadsorption and over the eighteen following hours (23.4 hours). Note that the terminal half-life was influenced by the combination of CytoSorb®, CVVHDF, and ECLS clearances and of metabolic (hepatic) clearance.

than hypertonic sodium bicarbonate on the correction of QRS widening [3]. In a case of 2.5 g flecainide overdose, the intravenous infusion of a total of 1 L of 20% IFE was followed by an increase of serum flecainide concentration from 1800 ng/ml 100 minutes pre-IFE administration to 2760 ng/ml 7 hours post-IFE administration. In another patient admitted 90 minutes after a mixed overdose with 25 mg bisoprolol, 900 mg flecainide, and 225 mg aspirin, IFE therapy was administered soon after admission after that the patient had developed ventricular fibrillation. The total flecainide concentration rose from 1512 ng/ml on admission to 2699 ng/ml 9 hours postingestion. However, in both cases, the interpretation of the increase of flecainide concentrations should be cautious as the second sample could have been drawn during the absorption phase of flecainide. In our patient, the increase of serum flecainide concentration could not be ascribed to a prolonged intestinal absorption and the close temporal relationship with IFE administration suggests a sequestration into the intravascular lipid compartment. However, as in other publications, we were not able to determine free flecainide levels as the only pharmacologically active concentrations. We recognize also that the dosage regimen for IFE therapy was excessive in our patient.

Approximately 30% of an oral dose of flecainide is excreted in urine as unchanged drug, and in patients with renal impairment, the total clearance of this drug might fall by approximately 40% [1]. Our patient had ESRD requiring intermittent hemodialysis, and a daily dose of 150 mg flecainide was likely excessive. In addition, genetic factors could also reduce flecainide metabolic clearance. Flecainide is primarily metabolized by hepatic cytochrome P450 CYP2D6 and CYP1A enzymes. The patients with the CYP2D6*1/*1 (two functioning alleles) genotype are considered as extensive metabolizers. Our patient was genotyped CYP2D6* 1/*4 (*4 as an inactive allele) and should be classified as an intermediate metabolizer. Impaired CYP2D6 activity reduces flecainide clearance by 21% in intermediate metabolizers [4]. The restoration of hemodynamic conditions by ECLS, and particularly of liver blood flow, was likely associated with a relative preservation of hepatic clearance.

Due to its pharmacological properties, flecainide is not effectively removable by different extrarenal epuration techniques (hemodialysis, hemofiltration, and hemoperfusion), and this has been verified by isolated case reports [5, 6]. Flecainide overdose had not been previously treated with the hemoperfusion cartridge CytoSorb®. The cartridge is characterized by a biocompatible porous polymer absorber with a total surface of exchange of 45,000 m^2. It mainly absorbs hydrophobic low and middle molecular substances in a concentration-dependent manner. In vitro data suggest that among cardiovascular drugs, digoxin, amlodipine, and verapamil could be effectively removed, while no data were available for flecainide [7]. The total serum flecainide was well above the therapeutic range at the beginning of hemoadsorption. As expected, the maximal extraction ratio was observed over the first hours. With a mean blood flow of 200 ml/min and a mean extraction ratio of 31%, we can estimate that the clearance of the circuit expressed as plasma clearance was 40.3 ml/min over the first 22 hours. However, we agree that the total plasma clearance of flecainide is

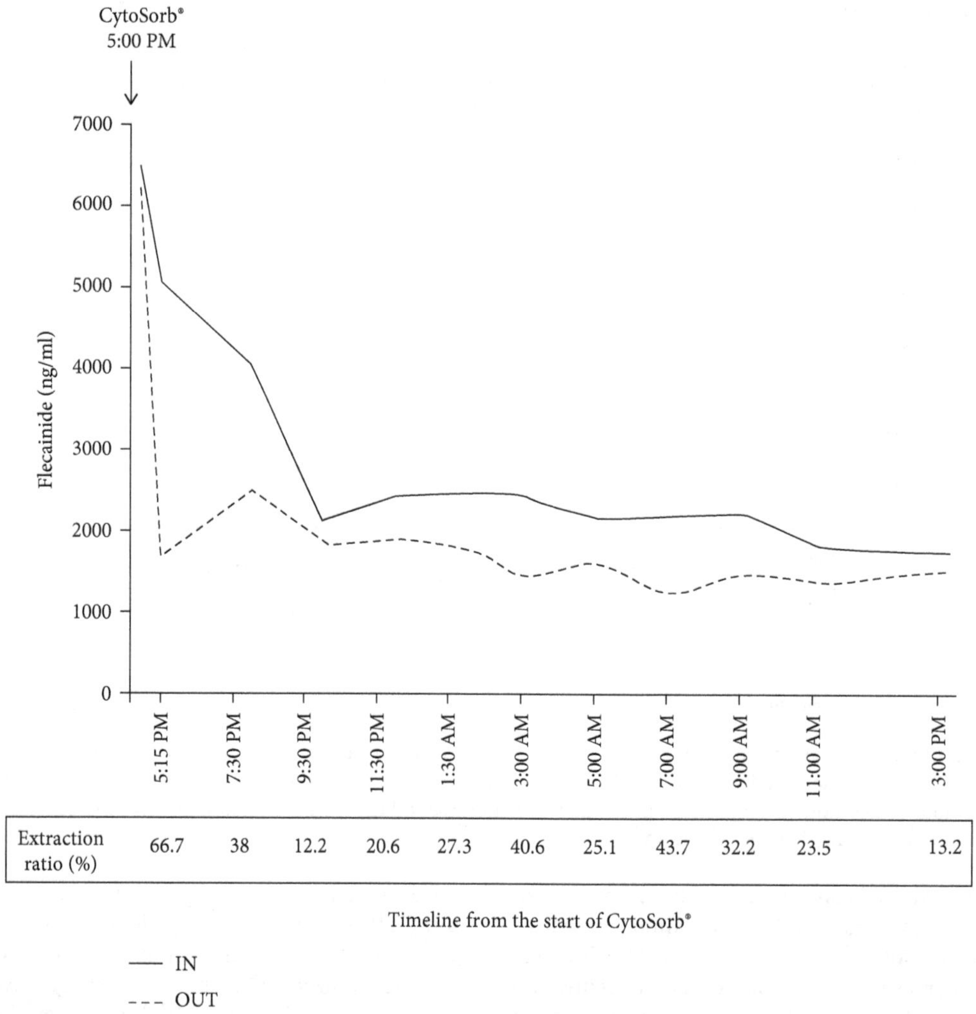

Figure 2: Determination of the serum flecainide concentration at the inlet (IN) and outlet (OUT) of the CytoSorb® hemoadsorption circuit. The extraction ratio (%) could be expressed as (concentration IN-concentration OUT/concentration IN). Blood flow in the circuit was 200 ml/min. Plasma flow rate was expressed as blood flow rate × (1-haematocrit).

represented by the sum of the metabolic (hepatic) clearance and of the clearance related to CVVHDF and CytoSorb®. The exact contribution of hemoadsorption to the clinical improvement could not be easily assessed as other therapies were simultaneously applied. This is particularly true for ECLS that has been applied with success in several cases of refractory (but transient) cardiogenic shock [8–10]. The concurrent or sequential use of both IFE and ECLS in case of drug-related cardiovascular toxicity is still uncommon with a possible negative influence of IFE on the tubing, valves, and circuits [11]. The influence of IFE on the CytoSorb® cartridge is also not known. It is also likely that the efficacy of CytoSorb® on flecainide epuration could decrease with time following cartridge saturation.

The limitations of this single observation have to be acknowledged. First, sodium bicarbonate should have been administered earlier, as soon as flecainide toxicity is suspected, and the total amount of IFE here exceeded the recommended dose. As IFE was not the sole medication used during resuscitation, the apparent clinical improvement could not be ascribed to IFE therapy only. Second, the respective role of each intervention (ECLS, CVVHDF, and hemoadsorption) for the hemodynamic improvement remains difficult to establish, but ECLS was undoubtedly the most saving technique. Third, the effectiveness of the CytoSorb® cartridge for flecainide removal cannot be fully appreciated by the calculations of blood extraction as the amount of drug coated on the cartridge cannot be determined.

Additional Points

Learning Objective. Therapeutic use of flecainide in patients with end-stage renal disease may be associated with serious toxicity. When standard therapy is failing following refractory cardiogenic shock, extracorporeal cardiac life support combined with sequestration of flecainide in a lipid phase followed by hemoadsorption could be helpful in selected cases.

Consent

A written consent was obtained from the patient.

References

[1] R. Subedi, R. K. Dean, A. Chaudhary, and T. Szombathy, "Flecainide toxicity in renal failure," *Baylor University Medical Center Proceedings*, vol. 31, no. 3, pp. 328–330, 2018.

[2] P. E. Moussot, F. Marhar, V. Minville et al., "Use of intravenous lipid 20% emulsion for the treatment of a voluntary intoxication of flecainide with refractory shock," *Clinical Toxicology*, vol. 49, no. 6, p. 514, 2011.

[3] G. Cave, M. Harvey, P. Quinn, and D. Heys, "Hypertonic sodium bicarbonate versus intravenous lipid emulsion in a rabbit model of intravenous flecainide toxicity: no difference, no sink," *Clinical Toxicology*, vol. 51, no. 5, pp. 394-397, 2013.

[4] K. Doki, M. Homma, K. Kuga et al., "Effect of CYP2D6 genotype on flecainide pharmacokinetics in Japanese patients with supraventricular tachyarrhythmia," *European Journal of Clinical Pharmacology*, vol. 62, no. 11, pp. 919–926, 2006.

[5] R. Wurzberger, E. Witter, H. Avenhaus, H. Henneman, and J. U. Becker, "Hämoperfusion bei Flecainidintoxikation," *Klinische Wochenschrift*, vol. 64, no. 9, pp. 442–444, 1986.

[6] M. Steinmetz, G. Nickenig, T. Sauerbruch, F. Eyer, and C. Rabe, "Effect of hemoperfusion on flecainide serum concentration - a case report," *Clinical Toxicology*, vol. 55, no. 2, pp. 153-154, 2017.

[7] E. C. Poli, T. Rimmelé, and A. G. Schneider, "Hemoadsorption with CytoSorb®," *Intensive Care Medicine*, vol. 45, no. 2, pp. 236–239, 2019.

[8] E. Brumfield, K. R. Bernard, and C. Kabrhel, "Life-threatening flecainide overdose treated with intralipid and extracorporeal membrane oxygenation," *The American Journal of Emergency Medicine*, vol. 33, no. 12, pp. 1840.e3–1840.e5, 2015.

[9] A. Mandawat, S. A. McCullough, L. G. Gilstrap, and R. W. Yeh, "Successful treatment of flecainide overdose with sustained mechanical circulatory support," *HeartRhythm Case Reports*, vol. 1, no. 3, pp. 137–140, 2015.

[10] S. K. Sivalingam, V. T. Gadiraju, M. V. Hariharan, A. R. Atreya, J. E. Flack, and H. Aziz, "Flecainide toxicity—treatment with intravenous fat emulsion and extra corporeal life support," *Acute Cardiac Care*, vol. 15, no. 4, pp. 91-92, 2013.

[11] K. Shekar, J. A. Roberts, C. I. Mcdonald et al., "Sequestration of drugs in the circuit may lead to therapeutic failure during extracorporeal membrane oxygenation," *Critical Care*, vol. 16, no. 5, article R194, 2012.

27

Incidental Anomalous Left Coronary Artery in a Transplanted Heart

Sri Harsha Patlolla, Saraschandra Vallabhajosyula, and Malcolm R. Bell

Department of Cardiovascular Medicine, Mayo Clinic, Rochester, Minnesota, USA

Correspondence should be addressed to Malcolm R. Bell; bell.malcolm@mayo.edu

Academic Editor: Assad Movahed

Anomalous coronary artery is an uncommon congenital cardiac anomaly that is often detected incidentally on coronary angiography. It has rarely been reported in the donor heart of patients who have undergone cardiac transplantation. Here, we report a case of a 72-year-old patient who received a second heart transplant and has been identified to have an anomalous left main coronary artery originating from the right coronary sinus on postoperative coronary angiography.

1. Introduction

Anomalous coronary artery arising from the opposite sinus has been reported in less than 2% of the population [1], and the reported frequency of a left main coronary artery arising from the right coronary sinus is less than 0.2% [2, 3]. The anomalous origin of coronary arteries has been infrequently noted in patients with prior cardiac transplantation. Herein, we report a case of an anomalous left coronary artery in a patient with a prior cardiac transplantation.

2. Case Report

A 72-year-old male presented to the Mayo Clinic Cardiac Catheterization Laboratory for routine posttransplant surveillance coronary angiography after undergoing a second orthotopic heart transplantation at another institution four months ago. He received his first heart transplant 30 years ago for dilated cardiomyopathy which was complicated by progressive cardiac allograft vasculopathy. In 2019, he was listed and received a second cardiac transplantation at an outside medical center. The early postoperative course was uneventful, and he was on a stable immunosuppressive regimen with prednisone, tacrolimus, and mycophenolate mofetil. A postoperative coronary angiography was attempted four weeks following the transplantation, but the left coronary artery could not be selectively engaged due to the reported inferior origin of the left main artery with likely posterior rotation. He reported being told by his physicians that they "were unable to find his heart arteries." He subsequently transferred his posttransplant care to the Mayo Clinic. As a part of the routine postoperative surveillance, he was scheduled for a coronary angiogram, right heart catheterization, and endomyocardial biopsy.

The review of the earlier angiogram had raised the suspicion of an anomalous left coronary artery. During coronary angiography, the right coronary artery was engaged without difficulty using a 6Fr Williams right catheter and looked normal in appearance (Figure 1 and Online Video 1); the left coronary artery was also seen arising posterior-inferiorly adjacent to the right coronary ostium. Selective injection from this position using a 6Fr multipurpose catheter revealed an anomalous left coronary artery arising from the right coronary sinus (Figures 2(a), 2(b), and 3 and Online Videos 2A, 2B, and 3). The long left main artery followed a retroaortic course before bifurcating into the left anterior descending and left circumflex arteries which otherwise appeared normal in appearance. We had discussed obtaining a dedicated coronary computerized tomographic scan to delineate his coronary anatomy; however, given his advanced renal disease,

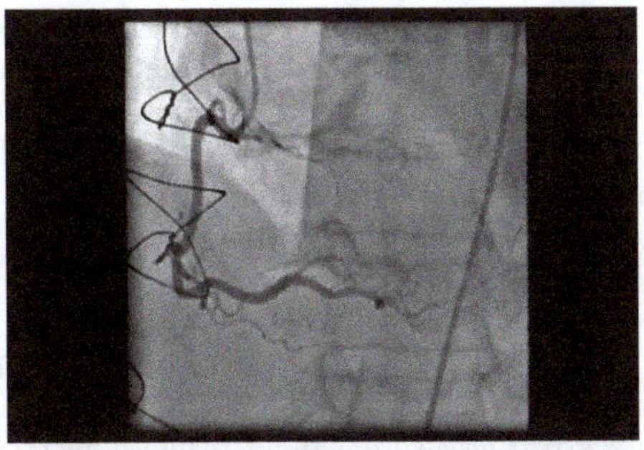

FIGURE 1: Right coronary artery arising from the right coronary sinus. Left anterior oblique cranial view showing a dominant right coronary artery arising from the right coronary sinus.

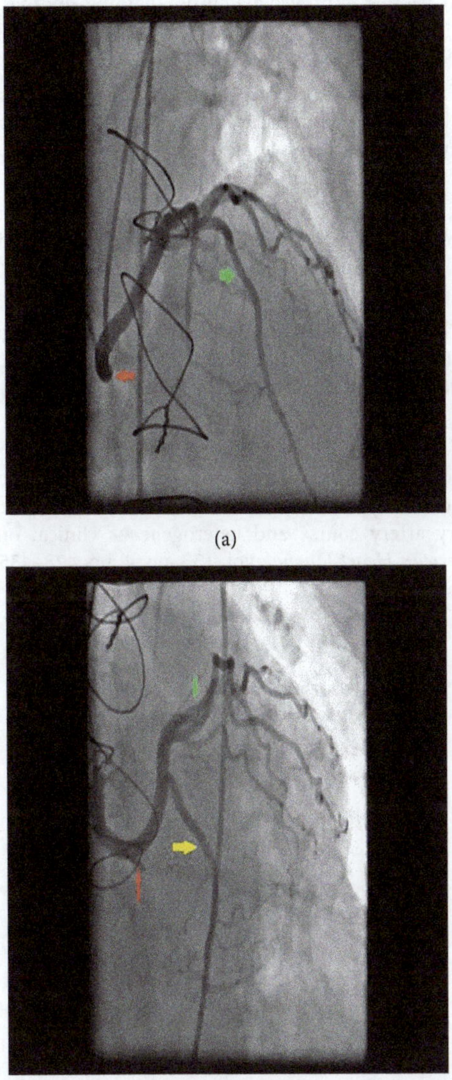

(a)

(b)

FIGURE 2: Anomalous left coronary artery arising from the right coronary sinus. Right anterior oblique cranial view (a) and left anterior oblique caudal view (b) showing an anomalous left coronary artery arising from the right coronary sinus with a long left main artery (red arrows) that bifurcates into a left anterior descending (green arrows) and left circumflex coronary artery (yellow arrow).

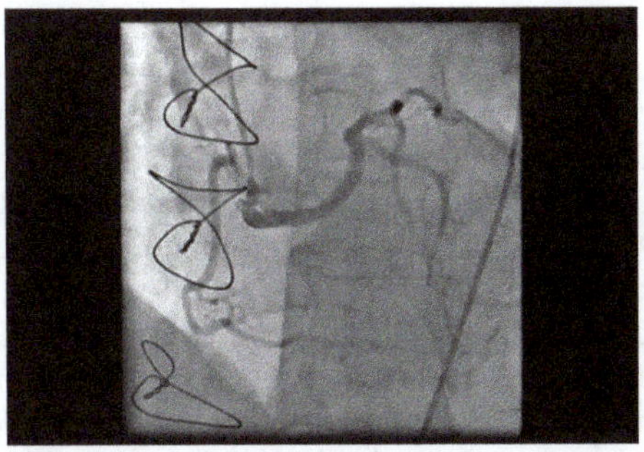

FIGURE 3: Right coronary artery and anomalous left coronary artery arising from the right coronary sinus. Left anterior oblique view showing a semiselective injection of the right coronary sinus with two discrete origins for the right coronary artery and anomalous left coronary artery.

this was deferred after discussion with colleagues in heart failure and cardiac transplantation. Given his asymptomatic status, he was managed conservatively with routine post-transplant surveillance.

3. Discussion

Though coronary anomalies are mostly benign, in some cases, they are known to cause ischemic changes that can precipitate myocardial infarction or sudden cardiac death [4]. A nationwide study reported coronary anomalies originating from the opposite sinus as the second most common cause of sudden cardiac death in young athletes [5]. Such clinically significant events are mostly dependent on the course taken by the anomalous left coronary artery when arising from the opposite sinus [6]. An interarterial course between the aorta and pulmonary artery is often associated with sudden cardiac death. Retroaortic, anterior, and trans-septal courses of the anomalous left coronary artery have less frequently been associated with adverse events [4, 7]. Although a retroaortic course is generally considered to have a minimal risk of sudden cardiac death, there have been reports of its association with sudden death and ischemic events [2, 8, 9]. Our patient did not have any clinical symptoms necessitating intervention.

Coronary artery anomalies are a rare finding especially in heart transplant recipients and are mostly benign. They are usually identified on postoperative coronary angiograms [1, 4]. As most heart donors are young patients who are unlikely to have any preexisting indications for angiography, it is difficult to detect such anomalies prior to transplant. However, if coronary anomalies are suspected, it is important to consider the future risk of complications before rejecting the donor heart. A careful evaluation of the coronary ostia on transthoracic echocardiography should be able to identify most coronary anomalies. Computerized tomographic coronary angiography and magnetic resonance coronary angiography have been suggested as a class IIA/B recommendation for the evaluation of anomalous coronary arteries by the American Heart Association Committee on Cardiovascular Imaging [10]. Our patient had stage III chronic kidney disease, and thus, follow-up confirmatory computerized tomographic coronary angiography was deferred. Currently, there is limited evidence on the role of cross-sectional imaging for coronary anomalies in donor hearts. Coronary anomalies in native hearts are prone to spontaneous coronary spasm in 1/3 of the cases [11]. However, this may not be perceived in a donor heart but spasm may be considered, along with appropriate testing, if there is suspicion of angina and/or ischemia [12]. Coronary anomalies can be managed either medically or surgically depending on the presentation. In general, an individualized approach based on the patient's age group, clinical presentation, and consideration of the risk of sudden cardiac death is advocated [1, 13–17].

Authors' Contributions

SV and MRB are responsible for the case evaluation, management, and clinical follow-up. SHP and SV are assigned to the conception and design, literature review, and draft write-up. SV and MRB are assigned to the critical revisions and mentoring. SHP, SV, and MRB approved the final manuscript.

References

[1] J. C. E. Lim, A. Beale, and S. Ramcharitar, "Anomalous origination of a coronary artery from the opposite sinus," *Nature Reviews Cardiology*, vol. 8, no. 12, pp. 706–719, 2011.

[2] N. K. Kejriwal, J. Tan, S. P. Gordon, and M. A. J. Newman, "Retroaortic course of the anomalous left main coronary artery: is it a benign anomaly?: a case report and review of literature," *Heart, Lung & Circulation*, vol. 13, no. 1, pp. 97–100, 2004.

[3] D. Kimbiris, "Anomalous origin of the left main coronary artery from the right sinus of Valsalva," *The American Journal of Cardiology*, vol. 55, no. 6, pp. 765–769, 1985.

[4] P. P. Agarwal, C. Dennie, E. Pena et al., "Anomalous coronary arteries that need intervention: review of pre- and postoperative imaging appearances," *Radiographics*, vol. 37, no. 3, pp. 740–757, 2017.

[5] B. J. Maron, J. J. Doerer, T. S. Haas, D. M. Tierney, and F. O. Mueller, "Sudden deaths in young competitive athletes: analysis of 1866 deaths in the United States, 1980-2006," *Circulation*, vol. 119, no. 8, pp. 1085–1092, 2009.

[6] O. Yamanaka and R. E. Hobbs, "Coronary artery anomalies in 126, 595 patients undergoing coronary arteriography," *Catheterization and Cardiovascular Diagnosis*, vol. 21, no. 1, pp. 28–40, 1990.

[7] P. Angelini, "Coronary artery anomalies–current clinical issues: definitions, classification, incidence, clinical relevance, and treatment guidelines," *Texas Heart Institute Journal*, vol. 29, no. 4, pp. 271–278, 2002.

[8] F. K. Patterson, "Sudden death in a young adult with anomalous origin of the posterior circumflex artery," *Southern Medical Journal*, vol. 75, no. 6, pp. 748-749, 1982.

[9] B. Madea and R. Dettmeyer, "Sudden death in cases with anomalous origin of the left coronary artery," *Forensic Science International*, vol. 96, no. 2-3, pp. 91–100, 1998.

[10] D. A. Bluemke, S. Achenbach, M. Budoff et al., "Noninvasive coronary artery imaging: magnetic resonance angiography and multidetector computed tomography angiography: a scientific statement from the american heart association committee on cardiovascular imaging and intervention of the council on cardiovascular radiology and intervention, and the councils on clinical cardiology and cardiovascular disease in the young," *Circulation*, vol. 118, no. 5, pp. 586–606, 2008.

[11] P. Angelini and C. Uribe, "Anatomic spectrum of left coronary artery anomalies and associated mechanisms of coronary insufficiency," *Catheterization and Cardiovascular Interventions*, vol. 92, no. 2, pp. 313–321, 2018.

[12] R. J. Widmer, B. Samuels, H. Samady et al., "The functional assessment of patients with non-obstructive coronary artery disease: expert review from an international microcirculation working group," *EuroIntervention*, vol. 14, no. 16, pp. 1694–1702, 2019.

[13] E. Erez, V. K. Tam, N. A. Doublin, and J. Stakes, "Anomalous coronary artery with aortic origin and course between the great arteries: improved diagnosis, anatomic findings, and surgical treatment," *The Annals of Thoracic Surgery*, vol. 82, no. 3, pp. 973–977, 2006.

[14] S. E. Moustafa, K. Zehr, M. Mookadam, E. C. Lorenz, and F. Mookadam, "Anomalous interarterial left coronary artery: an evidence based systematic overview," *International Journal of Cardiology*, vol. 126, no. 1, pp. 13–20, 2008.

[15] J. A. Davis, F. Cecchin, T. K. Jones, and M. A. Portman, "Major coronary artery anomalies in a pediatric population: incidence and clinical importance," *Journal of the American College of Cardiology*, vol. 37, no. 2, pp. 593–597, 2001.

[16] J. E. Davies, H. M. Burkhart, J. A. Dearani et al., "Surgical management of anomalous aortic origin of a coronary artery," *The Annals of Thoracic Surgery*, vol. 88, no. 3, pp. 844–848, 2009, discussion 847-848.

[17] A. J. Taylor, J. P. Byers, M. D. Cheitlin, and R. Virmani, "Anomalous right or left coronary artery from the contralateral coronary sinus: "high-risk" abnormalities in the initial coronary artery course and heterogeneous clinical outcomes," *American Heart Journal*, vol. 133, no. 4, pp. 428–435, 1997.

28

Camrelizumab-Related Lethal Arrhythmias and Myasthenic Crisis in a Patient with Metastatic Thymoma

Bo Zhang, Laxman Gyawali, Zengzhang Liu, Huaan Du, and Yuehui Yin

Department of Cardiology, The Second Affiliated Hospital of Chongqing Medical University, No. 288 Tian Wen Avenue, Nan'an District, Chongqing 401336, China

Correspondence should be addressed to Huaan Du; duhuaan20@126.com

Academic Editor: Tong Liu

Immune checkpoint inhibitors (ICIs) have emerged in recent years as promising treatment options for several malignant tumors. However, ICI therapy has also been associated with various immune-related adverse events (irAEs), especially for patients with preexisting autoimmune status, which sometimes can be life-threatening. A 68-year-old woman diagnosed with metastatic thymoma was treated with camrelizumab, a new ICI, as her antitumor protocol. Eleven days after the first dose of camrelizumab, the patient was admitted to our hospital with symptoms of dyspnea, fatigue, and poor appetite. Workups on admission indicated dramatically elevated transaminase, troponin I, creatine kinase, and a new-onset conduction abnormality on electrocardiography. After detailed evaluation, ICI-related myocarditis, myositis, and hepatitis were diagnosed, and therapies including intravenous methylprednisolone were administered. Coronary angiography was performed to exclude acute coronary syndrome due to dynamic electrocardiography changes on day 3. She lapsed into a coma with respiratory muscle failure on the next day, which was highly suspected of myasthenic crisis. Mechanical ventilation and higher dose of methylprednisolone plus intravenous immunoglobulin were applied immediately. However, the third atrioventricular block occurred within the same day, and an urgent temporary pacemaker was placed. More seriously, refractory ventricular tachycardia (VT) occurred subsequently, and even multiple antiarrhythmic drugs used in combination failed to alleviate the VT storm. On day 5 of hospitalization, she suffered from ventricular fibrillation and died of cardiac arrest. In clinical practice, close follow-up should be conducted after ICI treatment, especially for patients already with or at high risk for autoimmune disorders. A multidisciplinary team approach is of importance for better management of patients with multiple organ involvement.

1. Introduction

Immune checkpoint inhibitors (ICIs) are widely used for treatment of diverse types of malignances. ICIs block the interaction between cytotoxic T lymphocyte-associated antigen-4 (CTLA-4), programmed cell death protein 1 (PD-1), and their cognate ligands and thus generate immune responses to tumor cells. However, immune-related adverse events (irAEs) become an inevitable issue, among which colitis, dermatitis, myositis, hepatitis, and endocrinopathies are most frequent [1]. Cardiac and neuromuscular irAEs are rare but potentially life-threatening [2].

The thymus is an immune organ, which means that thymoma may be accompanied by autoimmune disorders or paraneoplastic syndrome. However, cardiovascular involvement occurs with a low incidence of less than 1% [3]. Theoretically, ICIs working as immunotherapy can trigger irAEs in thymoma patients. Here, we report a thymoma patient with multiple organ damage after the first dose of camrelizumab, a newly approved ICI [4].

2. Case Presentation

A 68-year-old woman presented to her local hospital in April 2020 with a 1-week history of increasing exertional dyspnea. Chest computed tomography (CT) revealed an anterior mediastinal mass (44 × 51 mm) with pleural invasion and a large volume of left pleural effusion fluid. The

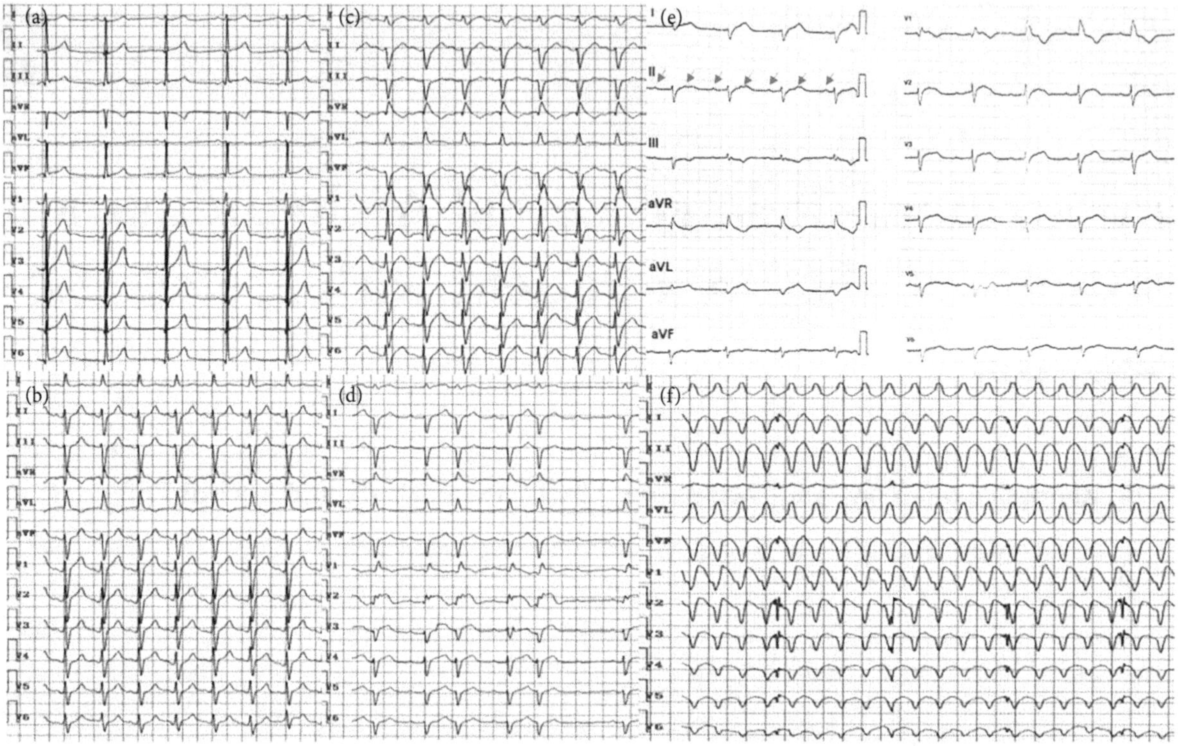

FIGURE 1: Progressive alterations on ECG. (a) Sinus rhythm and normal cardiac conduction before immune checkpoint inhibitor use. (b) New-onset left anterior fascicular branch block on admission. (c) New-onset complete right branch block plus left anterior fascicular branch block, namely bifascicular branch block. (d) Intermittent second degree atrioventricular block, with frequent premature atrial contractions, ST segment elevation, and poor R-wave progression in precordial leads. (e) Third degree atrioventricular block. Blue arrows indicating regular P waves. (f) Ventricular tachycardia (VT) with heart rate of 230 beats/min.

patient was diagnosed with type B2 thymoma (T4N0M1 stage IV) with pleural and left paranephros metastases detected by chest and abdominal enhanced CT, as well as pleural fluid cytology and pleural biopsy. Symptoms were significantly improved by left thoracic pleural drainage. However, due to the late diagnosis and metastasis, she lost her best opportunity for surgery. The patient declined chemotherapy and radiotherapy because of concerns about the side effects. One week after diagnosis, the patient was prescribed with camrelizumab at a dose of 200 mg, with intravenous delivery every 3 weeks. She had no history or positive familial history of cardiovascular disease, neurological disorder, or any other chronic diseases. Indicators including blood cell count, transaminase, creatinine, troponin I (TnI), creatine kinase (CK), creatine kinase MB (CK-MB), thyroid function, electrocardiography (ECG, Figure 1(a)), and echocardiography were unremarkable before initiation of camrelizumab treatment.

However, the patient was admitted to our hospital with complaints of dyspnea, fatigue, muscle weakness, palpitation, and poor appetite 11 days following camrelizumab therapy. Vital signs on admission were stable except for increased respiratory rate of 26 breaths/min and heart rate of 120 beats/min. Manual muscle test indicated slight weakness of the arm and leg skeletal muscles. No other positive signs were detected. Laboratory studies indicated TnI 13.94 ng/mL (normal < 0.030), CK-MB 213.70 ng/mL (normal < 6.30), and CK 8811.40 U/L (normal < 174.0). Alanine aminotransferase (ALT) and aspartate aminotransferase (AST) reached 290 U/L (normal < 40) and 805 U/L (normal < 35), respectively. Serum inflammatory markers, including white blood cell (WBC) count, C-reactive protein (CRP), erythrocyte sedimentation rate (ESR), and procalcitonin (PCT), were all elevated by varying degrees. The thyroid function was normal. Arterial blood gas analysis indicated normal partial pressure of carbon dioxide and decreased oxygen partial pressure of 76 mmHg. Plasma D-dimer and N-terminal pro-brain natriuretic peptide (NT-proBNP) increased, with limited clinical significance, to 690.2 ng/mL (normal < 550.0) and 1169.5 pg/mL (normal < 900.0), respectively (Table 1). Detections for pathogen infections and autoimmune disorders were both negative (Table 2). Transthoracic echocardiography (TTE) revealed preserved left ventricular ejection fraction (LVEF) of 65% with no abnormality of chamber size and ventricular wall motion. ECG on admission showed a new-onset left anterior fascicular branch block (Figure 1(b)), followed by bifascicular branch block on the next day (Figure 1(c)). Cardiac magnetic resonance imaging (MRI) failed to be successfully achieved due to substandard heart rate and breathing rate controlling. In view of the absence of underlying cardiovascular diseases, chemotherapy, radiotherapy, statin use, evidence of virus or other pathogen infections, and a history of ICI administration a few days prior to hospitalization, as well

TABLE 1: Results of routine laboratory test.

Parameter	Normal range	Before ICI use	On admission	Day 2	Day 3	Day 4	Day 5
TnI (ng/mL)	<0.030	0.01	13.94	36.05	63.0	46.0	20.8
CK-MB (ng/mL)	0.60-6.30	1.10	213.70	233.6	135.1	71.2	33.8
CK (U/L)	38.0-174.0	20.4	8811.4	4051.3	2245.9	1259.5	867.9
ALT (U/L)	7-40	12	290		273		183
AST (U/L)	13-35	18	805		566		155
Serum K (mmol/L)	3.5-5.3	3.65	4.19	3.74	4.58	4.87	4.92
Serum Mg (mmol/L)	0.75-1.02	0.82	0.85	0.85	0.99	1.01	1.04
Scr (μmol/L)	41.0-81.0	58.4	73.4	43.2	96.2	96.2	105.6
GFR (mL/min)	75.0-300.0	94.1	72.2	141.2	52.9	60.5	47.5
Arterial pH	7.37-7.45		7.46	7.40	7.39	7.01	7.37
PaO_2 (mmHg)	83-108		76	78	81	48	64
$PaCO_2$ (mmHg)	35-48		37	40	38	104	36
BE (mmol/L)	-3.0-3.0		2.3	1.8	1.3	-7.3	-4.1
D-dimer (ng/mL)	<550.0	586.2	690.2	780.1		890.5	900.4
NT-proBNP (pg/mL)	<900.0	308.8	1169.5	1208.2		2230.4	2508.5
WBC ($\times 10^9$/L)	3.50-9.50	7.52	18.8	19.3	21.4	22.6	20.5
Neu (%)	45.0-75.0	71.8	88.2	89.8	89.6	90.1	89.8
RBC ($\times 10^{12}$/L)	3.80-5.10	4.0	3.98	3.91	3.82	3.56	3.81
Platelet ($\times 10^9$/L)	100-300	149	100	105	98	91	89
CRP (mg/L)	<10	<5.0	15.03	20.0	23.26	24.00	26.80
ESR (mm/h)	<20	12	30	38			57
PCT (ng/mL)	<0.0500	0.0100	0.18		0.20		0.04
Free T3 (pmol/L)	3.1-6.8	3.8	3.3				
Free T4 (pmol/L)	9.5-24.5	13.3	16.1				
TSH (μIU/mL)	0.35-5.00	2.56	2.75				

ICI: immune checkpoint inhibitor; TnI: troponin I; CK-MB: creatine kinase MB; CK: creatine kinase; ALT: alanine aminotransferase; AST: aspartate aminotransferase; K: potassium; Mg: magnesium; Scr: serum creatinine; GFR: glomerular filtration rate; PaO_2: partial pressure of arterial oxygen; $PaCO_2$: partial pressure of arterial carbon dioxide; BE: base excess; NT-proBNP: N-terminal pro-brain natriuretic peptide; WBC: white blood cell; Neu: neutrophil; RBC: red blood cell; CRP: C-reactive protein; ESR: erythrocyte sedimentation rate; PCT: procalcitonin; T3: triiodothyronine; T4: hyroxine, TSH: thyroid-stimulating hormone.

TABLE 2: Results of pathogen test and autoantibody detection.

Category	Result	Category	Result
CVB3-IgM	Neg	Anti-dsDNA	Neg
PVB19-IgM	Neg	Anti-Sm	Neg
ADV-IgM	Neg	Anti-SSA	Neg
HSV-IgM	Neg	Anti-SSB	Neg
Influenza A-IgM	Neg	Anti-Scl-70	Neg
COVID-19 test	Neg	Anti-PM-Scl	Neg
RV-IgM	Neg	Anti-Ro-52	Neg
RSV-IgM	Neg	Anti-mi-2a	Neg
Chlamydia pneumoniae-IgM	Neg	Anti-PL-7	Neg
Mycoplasma pneumoniae-IgM	Neg	Anti-PL-12	Neg
Toxoplasma gondii-IgM	Neg	Anti-SRP	Neg
Blood culture	Neg		
Sputum culture	Neg		
Stool culture	Neg		

CVB3: coxsackievirus B3; PVB19: parvovirus B19; ADV: adenovirus; HSV: herpes simplex virus; COVID: coronavirus disease; RV: rubella virus; RSV: respiratory syncytial virus; Neg: negative.

as multiple organ involvement simultaneously, ICI-related myocarditis, myositis, and hepatitis were diagnosed. Intravenous methylprednisolone (80 mg/day), polyene phosphatidylcholine (465 mg/day), reduced glutathione (1.8 g/day), and supportive therapies (including glucose, potassium, and magnesium supplements) were prescribed. In addition, empirical treatment with intravenous antibiotic (piperacillin/tazobactam 4.5 g three times daily) was given to the patient, as concomitant bacterial infection could not be ruled out completely in that stage because of increased inflammatory markers. The patient declined to undergo biopsy of the associated organs due to the potential complications.

On day 3 of hospitalization, ECG revealed an intermittent second-degree atrioventricular block, with frequent premature atrial contractions, ST segment elevation, and poor R-wave progression in precordial leads (Figure 1(d)). Considering the elevated biomarkers of myocardial damage and dynamic ECG alterations, coronary angiography was performed to exclude myocardial infarction even without typical clinical presentations, which revealed normal coronary artery anatomy (Figure 2). Unfortunately, the patient lapsed into a coma with extremely weak respiratory

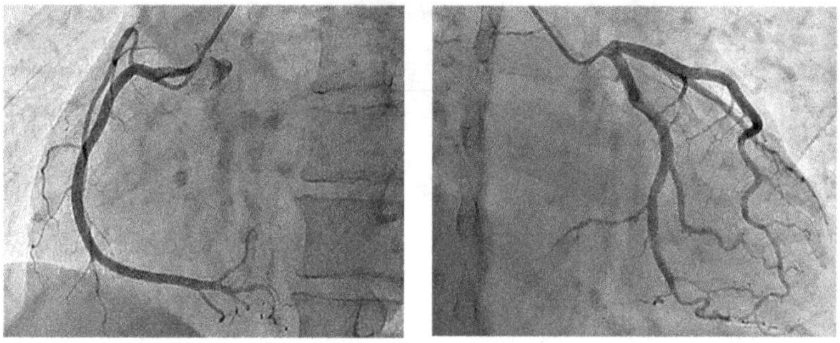

(a) (b)

FIGURE 2: Coronary angiography showing a normal coronary artery anatomy.

TABLE 3: Timeline.

18 days prior to admission	Patient diagnosed with type B2 thymoma with pleural and left paranephros metastases at her local hospital, treated with thoracic pleural drainage
11 days prior to admission	First dose of intravenous camrelizumab administered
On admission	Symptoms of dyspnea, fatigue, and poor appetite New-onset left anterior fascicular branch block Elevated CK, CK-MB, TnI, ALT, and AST
Day 2 of hospitalization	Bifascicular branch block Diagnosed with ICI-related myocarditis, myositis, and hepatitis Intravenous methylprednisolone (80 mg/day) Intravenous piperacillin/tazobactam (4.5 g three times daily) Intravenous polyene phosphatidylcholine (465 mg/day) Intravenous reduced glutathione (1.8 g/day) Intravenous glucose, potassium, and magnesium supplements
Day 3 of hospitalization	Intermittent second-degree atrioventricular block and ST segment elevation and poor R-wave progression in precordial leads Coronary angiography confirming normal anatomy of coronary artery
Day 4 of hospitalization	Coma due to respiratory muscle paralysis Mechanical ventilation and higher dose of methylprednisolone (1 g/day) plus IVIG (20 g/day) applied Third degree atrioventricular block Urgent temporary pacemaker placed Ventricular tachycardia Direct current defibrillation and multiple antiarrhythmic drugs used
Day 5 of hospitalization	Ventricular fibrillation followed by cardiac arrest, and finally died

CK: creatine kinase; CK-MB: creatine kinase MB; TnI: troponin I; ALT: alanine aminotransferase; AST: aspartate aminotransferase; ICI: immune checkpoint inhibitor; IVIG: intravenous immunoglobulin.

movement on the next day. Arterial blood gas analysis showed fatal carbon dioxide retention with partial pressure of 104 mmHg, with a decreased oxygen partial pressure of 48 mmHg in parallel. Myasthenic crisis was clinically diagnosed for the underlying disease of thymoma and a rapid progression to life-threatening respiratory failure due to respiratory muscle involvement. Tracheal intubation and mechanical ventilation were applied immediately, by which hypercapnia and hypoxia were corrected promptly and consciousness was regained. A higher dose of methylprednisolone (1 g/day) was administered, and intravenous immunoglobulin (IVIG, 20 g/day) was initiated after neurological consultation. Third-degree atrioventricular block occurred abruptly within the same day (Figure 1(e)) even with stable gas exchange and serum electrolyte levels, and then, an urgent temporary pacemaker was inserted. Although multiple therapeutic measures were administered, clinical status deteriorated after the occurrence of ventricular tachycardia (VT) with heart rate of 230 beats/min (Figure 1(f)). The patient presented with loss of consciousness and emergency electrical cardioversion was performed to terminate the lethal arrhythmia. However, even though intravenous administration of high doses of amiodarone, lidocaine, β-blocker, and diazepam were used successively, they failed to relieve the VT storm completely. One day after VT, the patient suffered from ventricular fibrillation followed by cardiac arrest, from which she could not be resuscitated (Table 3). Postmortem examination was suggested but was refused by her family members.

3. Discussion

ICIs are increasingly used in clinical practice, which in turn can potentially activate autoactive T cells causing immune attack to multiple organs sequentially or simultaneously.

The prevalence of myocarditis caused by ICIs has been reported previously. Data from Bristol-Myers Squibb corporate safety databases showed a rate of 0.09% after administration of nivolumab or ipilimumab and a higher rate of 0.27% when in combination [5]. A multicenter registry reported a prevalence of 1.14% with a median time of onset of 34 days after starting ICIs [6]. Although ICI-related myocarditis seems to be rare, prognosis can be poor and a mortality rate of 50% was reported by Salem and colleagues [7]. In the present case, the patient suffered from ICI-related myocarditis with normal LVEF, but progressive conduction abnormalities and fatal ventricular arrhythmias, and this situation may be even more rare [7]. Endomyocardial biopsy (EMB) is the gold standard to diagnose myocarditis, but this method is rarely conducted due to its invasive nature and possible complications. Lymphocytic infiltration within the myocardium, mainly positive for CD3 or the macrophage marker CD68, is the common pathological presentation of ICI-related myocarditis. Apart from the myocardium, the sinus and atrioventricular nodes can also be infiltrated with lymphocytes, which are potential targets of the activated T cells, so different arrhythmias and conduction abnormalities may occur as a result [5]. Cardiac MRI, which is of high sensitivity and specificity and is usually considered a surrogate to EMB, plays an important role in the diagnosis of myocarditis with traditional causes. However, the diagnostic value of this non-invasive technique in ICI-related myocarditis seems to be not so high as in other common types of myocarditis [8]. In the present case, neither EMB nor cardiac MRI was performed due to subjective and objective reasons. Even without support of the aforementioned examinations, it was reasonable to be diagnosed as ICI-related myocarditis because of the recent medication history of ICI, typical progression of clinical features, elevated myocardial injury biomarkers, dynamic ECG changes, and the exclusion of other confusing causes, which also met the criteria proposed by International Cardio-Oncology Society for clinical diagnosis of ICI-related myocarditis [9]. Intravenous glucocorticoid was prescribed immediately after diagnosis of ICI-related myocarditis, but it could not stop the progression of cardiac conduction disturbance.

The thymus is a central immune organ that is responsible for T-cell development by positive and negative selection. Thymic epithelial tumors (TETs) include thymic carcinoma and thymoma. Thymoma is more likely accompanied by autoimmune disorders, among which myasthenia gravis (MG) is the most common, with a high rate of 30-44% [3]. Other immunological disorders, such as myositis, myocarditis, colitis, hepatitis, and Graves' disease, can also be involved at relatively lower frequencies. Generally, chemotherapy or chemoradiotherapy is recommended for metastatic thymoma, while unsatisfactory responses are often observed in clinical settings. Studies have shown abundant programmed death ligand 1 (PD-L1) expression using immunohistochemistry in TETs [10, 11], which support the potential clinical efficacy of ICIs in TETs. Case series and phase II trials have further demonstrated that ICIs are effective in advanced TETs and thymoma [12–14]. More importantly, the prevalence of ICI-related myocarditis and other irAEs is markedly higher in patients with TETs than with other types of cancers. In one phase II trial, investigating the use of pembrolizumab in patients with recurrent or relapsed TETs, 9.1%, 6.1%, 12.1%, and 3.0% of the patients developed myocarditis, MG, hepatitis, and thyroiditis, respectively [14]. There is a case report of a fatal immune-related storm in a thymoma patient treated with pembrolizumab, leading to hepatotoxicity accompanied by lymphocytosis, thrombocytopenia, and thyroid dysfunction [15]. Multiple organ damage was also involved in our case. Apart from the rapid progression of cardiac adverse events, myasthenic crisis is another fatal complication. The literature suggests that ICI-related MG can be exemplified by *de novo* presentations and exacerbation of preexisting or subclinical MG, with a high proportion of 72.7% for the former [16]. With no MG manifestation prior to the administration of camrelizumab, ICI-related *de novo* MG may be the most likely diagnosis of our patient, although exacerbation of subclinical MG could not be excluded. Immature and TET-derived thymocytes that have escaped self-tolerance and become autoactive may be the mechanism for the development of MG in patients with TETs [17]. ICI therapy can further activate T lymphocytes and strength the autoimmune activity of the cells, given the fact that TET patients are more susceptible to developing autoimmune disorders, which makes thymoma patients more likely than patients with other cancers to experience multiple irAEs [3, 14]. Even a higher dose of glucocorticoid and IVIG were administered immediately after diagnosis of myasthenic crisis, and they could not reverse the outcome due to the extremely worsening situation.

To the best of our knowledge, this is the first report of a thymoma patient developing ICI-related myocarditis, concomitant with MG, myositis, and hepatitis, after the first dose of camrelizumab. Some attention should be paid by clinicians to the following: (1) Complete evaluation must be performed before initiation of ICI, and patients already with or at high risk for autoimmune disorders may not be suitable candidates. (2) Sometimes irAEs can be nonspecific or even asymptomatic, so close regular follow-up with ECG, echocardiography, and routine laboratory tests should be conducted within the first week after ICI treatment, especially for new drugs we are not familiar with. (3) Since irAEs are often characterized by multiple organ involvement, a multidisciplinary approach is important for better management of that group of patients. The manuscript has been previously posted on a preprint server as a preprint [18].

Consent

No written consent has been obtained from the patients as there is no patient identifiable data included in this case report.

References

[1] J. A. Thompson, B. J. Schneider, J. Brahmer et al., "Management of immunotherapy-related toxicities, version 1.2019," *Journal of the National Comprehensive Cancer Network: JNCCN*, vol. 17, no. 3, pp. 255–289, 2019.

[2] D. Y. Wang, J. Salem, J. V. Cohen et al., "Fatal toxic effects associated with immune checkpoint inhibitors: a systematic review and meta-analysis," *JAMA Oncology*, vol. 4, no. 12, pp. 1721–1728, 2018.

[3] E. A. Lippner, D. B. Lewis, W. H. Robinson, and T. R. Katsumoto, "Paraneoplastic and therapy-related immune complications in thymic malignancies," *Current Treatment Options in Oncology*, vol. 20, no. 7, p. 62, 2019.

[4] A. Markham and S. J. Keam, "Camrelizumab: first global approval," *Drugs*, vol. 79, no. 12, pp. 1355–1361, 2019.

[5] D. B. Johnson, J. M. Balko, M. L. Compton et al., "Fulminant myocarditis with combination immune checkpoint blockade," *New England Journal of Medicine*, vol. 375, no. 18, pp. 1749–1755, 2016.

[6] S. S. Mahmood, M. G. Fradley, J. V. Cohen et al., "Myocarditis in patients treated with immune checkpoint inhibitors," *Journal of the American College of Cardiology*, vol. 71, no. 16, pp. 1755–1764, 2018.

[7] J. E. Salem, A. Manouchehri, M. Moey et al., "Cardiovascular toxicities associated with immune checkpoint inhibitors: an observational, retrospective, pharmacovigilance study," *The Lancet. Oncology*, vol. 19, no. 12, pp. 1579–1589, 2018.

[8] L. Zhang, M. Awadalla, S. S. Mahmood et al., "Cardiovascular magnetic resonance in immune checkpoint inhibitor-associated myocarditis," *European Heart Journal*, vol. 41, no. 18, pp. 1733–1743, 2020.

[9] J. Herrmann, D. Lenihan, S. Armenian et al., "Defining cardiovascular toxicities of cancer therapies: an international cardio-oncology society (IC-OS) consensus statement," *European Heart Journal*, vol. 43, pp. 280–299, 2022.

[10] S. Yokoyama and H. Miyoshi, "Thymic tumors and immune checkpoint inhibitors," *Journal of Thoracic Disease*, vol. 10, no. S13, pp. S1509–S1515, 2018.

[11] K. C. Arbour, J. Naidoo, K. E. Steele et al., "Expression of PD-L1 and other immunotherapeutic targets in thymic epithelial tumors," *PLoS One*, vol. 12, no. 8, article e0182665, 2017.

[12] A. Rajan, C. R. Heery, A. Thomas et al., "Efficacy and tolerability of anti-programmed death-ligand 1 (PD-L1) antibody (avelumab) treatment in advanced thymoma," *Journal for Immunotherapy of Cancer*, vol. 7, no. 1, p. 269, 2019.

[13] G. Giaccone, C. Kim, J. Thompson et al., "Pembrolizumab in patients with thymic carcinoma: a single-arm, single-centre, phase 2 study," *The Lancet Oncology*, vol. 19, no. 3, pp. 347–355, 2018.

[14] J. Cho, H. S. Kim, B. M. Ku et al., "Pembrolizumab for patients with refractory or relapsed thymic epithelial tumor: an open-label phase II trial," *Journal of Clinical Oncology*, vol. 37, no. 24, pp. 2162–2170, 2019.

[15] A. Argentiero, A. G. Solimando, V. Ungaro et al., "Case report: lymphocytosis associated with fatal hepatitis in a thymoma patient treated with anti-PD1: new insight into the immune-related storm," *Frontiers in Oncology*, vol. 10, article 583781, 2020.

[16] D. Makarious, K. Horwood, and J. Coward, "Myasthenia gravis: an emerging toxicity of immune checkpoint inhibitors," *European Journal of Cancer*, vol. 82, pp. 128–136, 2017.

[17] S. Shahar, A. Nancy, A. Arie, and S. Yehuda, "Thymoma and autoimmunity," *Cellular & Molecular Immunology*, vol. 8, no. 3, pp. 199–202, 2011.

[18] B. Zhang, L. Gyawali, Z. Z. Liu, H. A. Du, and Y. H. Yin, *Caremlizumab-related lethal arrhythmias and myasthenic crisis in a patient with metastatic thymoma: a case report*, Research Squre, Preprint, 2021, https://www.researchsquare.com/article/rs-305090/v1.

29

A Case of Contralateral Pneumothorax, Pneumomediastinum and Pneumopericardium after Dual-Chamber Pacemaker Implantation

Wajeeh ur Rehman[1], **Altif Muneeb**,[1] **Usama Sakhawat**,[1] **Pranava Ganesh**,[2] **Nabil Braiteh**[2], **Vince Skovira**,[2] **Waseem Sajjad**,[2] **and Afzal ur Rehman**[2]

[1]*Department of Internal Medicine, United Health Services Hospitals, Wilson Regional Medical Center, Johnson City, NY, USA*
[2]*Department of Cardiology, United Health Services Hospitals, Heart and Vascular Institute, Wilson Regional Medical Center, Johnson City, NY, USA*

Correspondence should be addressed to Wajeeh ur Rehman; wajeeh.rehman9@gmail.com

Academic Editor: Christopher Snyder

As permanent pacemaker implantation is increasingly becoming a common practice, it is important to understand potential complications associated with the procedure. We present a 78-year-old Caucasian female who developed contralateral pneumomediastinum, pneumothorax, and pneumopericardium after undergoing implantation of a dual-chamber pacemaker.

1. Case Summary

A 79-year-old Caucasian female with significant past medical history of atrial fibrillation not on oral anticoagulation, chronic obstructive pulmonary disease, gastroesophageal reflux disease, hypothyroidism, hyperlipidemia, and congestive heart failure with low ejection fraction presented with severe fatigue and dizziness. According to the patient, she was in a normal state of health one month ago when she started developing shortness of breath on exertion and orthopnea. Over the past week, her symptoms had gotten progressively worse. In addition to these complaints, she also had developed new substernal chest discomfort over the past week. The patient was planning to undergo elective colonoscopy when pre-procedural electrocardiogram (EKG) revealed a complete third-degree heart block. The patient was brought to the emergency department (ED) by emergency medical services (EMS). At the time of presentation in the ED, the patient was feeling dizzy and weak. The patient has also had associated symptoms of palpitations and lightheadedness. The patient denied having any loss of consciousness or syncope.

EKG was repeated, which again confirmed normal sinus rhythm with a third-degree atrioventricular (AV) block with stable ventricular escape rhythm at a ventricular rate of approximately 23 bpm.

On subsequent EKGs, there was found to be changing ectopic ventricular foci; on one EKG, it appeared to be localizing to Left ventricular (LV) basal anteroseptal region; on another, to the basal inferoseptal region.

The patient was admitted to telemetry. Overnight, the patient had a long 10-second AV block without any ventricular escape rhythm associated with syncope. Therefore, the patient underwent transvenous temporary pacemaker insertion via right femoral vein with a rate of 80, output of 10 mg, and sensitivity of 5 mV.

The next morning, the patient underwent implantation of dual-chamber permanent pacemaker with removal of temporary venous pacemaker for complete third-degree heart block [1].

The pacemaker pocket was created by an infraclavicular incision in pectoralis major for Boston Scientific ESSENTIO ELDR, Delaware, USA pacemaker generator.

Access was obtained in the left axillary vein after which the right ventricular pacing lead was placed followed by a

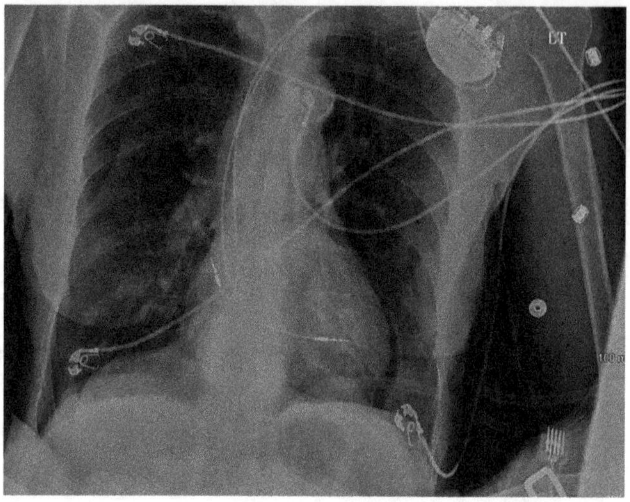

Figure 1: Anteroposterior chest radiograph revealing pneumopericardium.

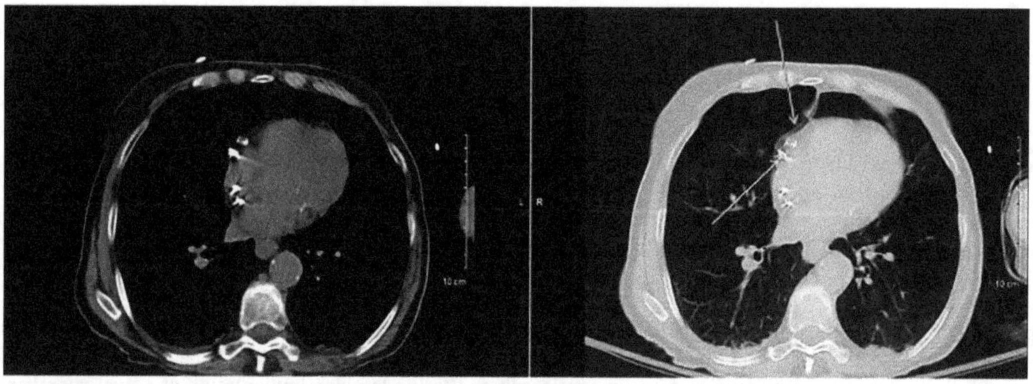

Figure 2: Yellow arrow showing the RA lead penetrating the atrial wall and green arrow showing the pneumopericardium.

right atrial pacing lead using single-plane fluoroscopy. At the time of implantation, the right atrial lead pacing threshold was 0.7 V at 0.5 ms, sensing at 3.5 mV, and impedance of 519 Ω, (Medtronic 4076, Minneapolis, Minnesota, USA). The right ventricular lead pacing threshold was 0.5 V at 0.5 ms, sensing at 11.2 mV, and impedance of 790 Ω (Medtronic 4076).

The initial chest X-ray after implantation showed right lower lobe anterior pneumothorax and pneumopericardium (Figure 1). A computerized tomography (CT) scan of the chest was done to investigate the etiology of the contralateral pneumothorax that revealed right atrial lead projecting through the right atrial wall and right ventricular lead at the wall (Figure 2). There was moderate right pneumothorax and small right effusion and moderate pneumopericardium anteriorly, about 2.3 cm thick. Small amount of air was also visualized anterior and posterior to aorta likely mild pneumomediastinum (Figures 2–4). Transthoracic echocardiogram was also repeated after the procedure that revealed pneumopericardium and normal right ventricular function (Figure 5).

Cardiothoracic surgery was consulted, and a 14 Fr pigtail chest tube was inserted in the sixth intercostal space. Device interrogation demonstrated no change in pacing threshold, sensing, normal impedance of both leads, and no issues with the functionality of pacemaker; therefore, right atrial (RA) lead repositioning was not required. Chest X-ray was repeated the next morning, following chest tube placement that revealed significant improvement in pneumothorax and pneumopericardium. A CT of the chest was repeated 4 days later and revealed complete resolution of the pneumothorax, pneumopericardium, and pneumopericardium. The patient was discharged home safely and had been symptom free for a 1-month follow-up.

2. Discussion

Despite a relatively low rate of complications ranging from less than 1 to 6% with cardiac pacemaker implantation, it is pertinent to early recognition and timely management of these complications [2]. The most common complications include risk of bleeding, phlebitis, lead dislodgement, infection, hemothorax, pneumothorax, pneumopericardium, and even cardiac perforation [3].

The rate of some specific early complications like subclavian vein rupture and pneumothorax has been found to be

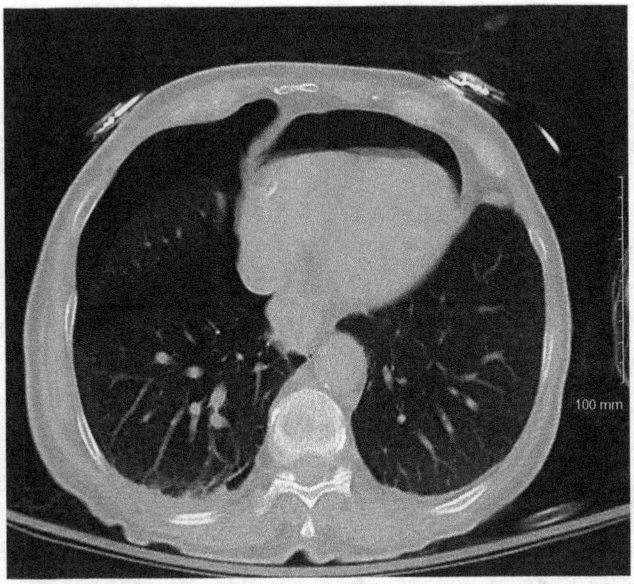

FIGURE 3: Noncontrast chest CT scan showing pneumopericardium, pneumothorax, and pericardial effusion.

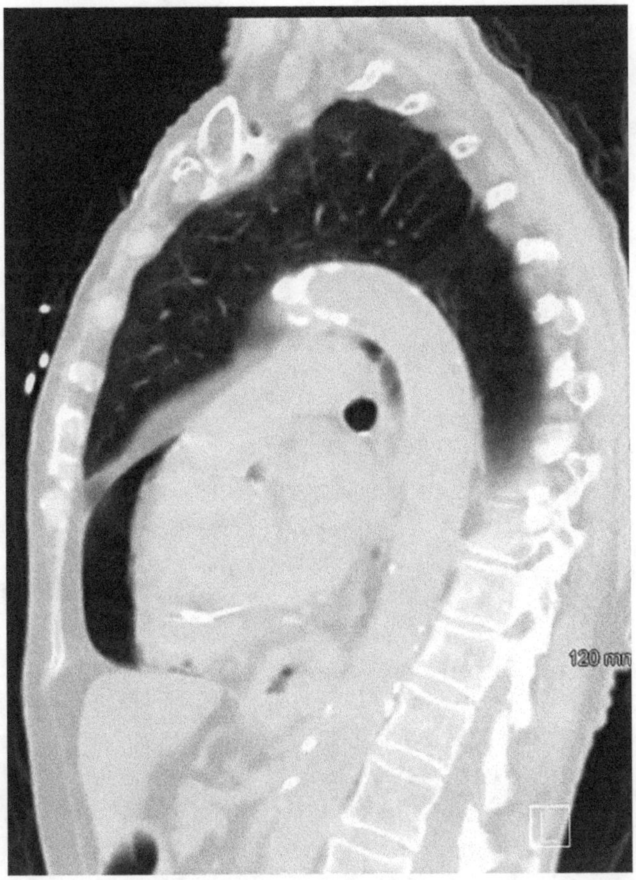

FIGURE 4: CT chest sagittal view demonstrating pneumopericardium.

higher with dual chambers when compared to single chamber devices [4].

Chest X-ray, echocardiogram, and device interrogation are all helpful modalities in determining immediate post-implantation complications. A CT of the chest [3] has the highest sensitivity in revealing all complications associated with pacemaker implantation including pneumomediastinum.

Commonly, pneumothorax is a complication visualized on the ipsilateral side of Permanent pacemaker (PPM) insertion; however, in rare instances, contralateral pneumothorax can also develop as seen in this case. Possible mechanisms for contralateral pneumothorax include the injury to pleura by the RA lead extrusion through the atrial appendage or pleural injury by guide-wire during Seldinger set introduction.

Development of pneumopericardium and pneumomediastinum on the contralateral side of PPM placement is likely due to perforation of the atrial lead through the wall of the atrial appendage. Penetration of the RA lead does not change lead parameters due to penetration of the helix of the lead, which is not part of the electrode, and the electrode remains in contact with the myocardium. The lead may plug the micro-defect and, therefore, no pericardial effusion [5].

Management of such rare complications after pacemaker implantation depends on the patient's hemodynamic status, device interrogation, and amount of air and blood leak.

Srivathsan et al. performed both chest tube insertion and atrial lead extraction and had a successful outcome [6]. At the same time, in other cases of similar complications, chest

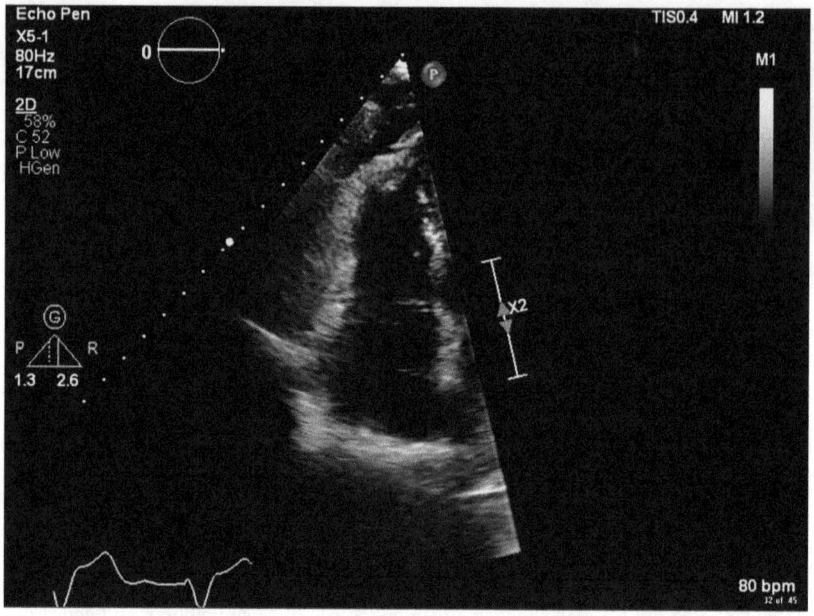

Figure 5: Transthoracic echocardiogram revealing pneumopericardium.

tube insertion without right atrial lead extraction management resulted in resolution of both pneumothorax and pneumopericardium [5, 7].

References

[1] M. Glikson, J. C. Nielsen, M. B. Kronborg et al., "2021 ESC guidelines on cardiac pacing and cardiac resynchronization therapy," *European Heart Journal*, vol. 42, no. 35, pp. 3427–3520, 2021.

[2] S. K. Mulpuru, M. Madhavan, C. J. McLeod, Y. M. Cha, and P. A. Friedman, "Cardiac pacemakers: function, troubleshooting, and management: part 1 of a 2-part series," *Journal of the American College of Cardiology*, vol. 69, no. 2, pp. 189–210, 2017.

[3] S. Aktaa, K. Fatania, C. Gains, and H. White, "Chest pain following permanent pacemaker insertion… a case of pneumopericardium due to atrial lead perforation," *BMJ Case Reports*, 2018, https://casereports.bmj.com/content/casereports/2018/bcr-2018-226318.full.pdf.

[4] F. Eberhardt, F. Bode, H. Bonnemeier et al., "Long term complications in single and dual chamber pacing are influenced by surgical experience and patient morbidity," *Heart*, vol. 91, no. 4, pp. 500–506, 2005.

[5] N. K. Parashar, "An unexpected complication of intracardiac device implantation: contralateral pneumothorax and pneumopericardium," *ScienceDirect*, vol. 11, p. 2, 2019, https://www.sciencedirect.com/science/article/pii/S0972629219300373.

[6] K. Srivathsan, R. A. Byrne, C. P. Appleton, and L. R. Scott, "Pneumopericardium and pneumothorax contralateral to venous access site after permanent pacemaker implantation," *Europace*, vol. 5, no. 4, pp. 361–363, 2003.

[7] T. Nantsupawat, J. M. Li, D. G. Benditt, and S. Adabag, "Contralateral pneumothorax and pneumopericardium after dual-chamber pacemaker implantation: mechanism, diagnosis, and treatment," *HeartRhythm Case Reports*, vol. 4, no. 6, pp. 256–259, 2018.

30

Peri-Contrast Staining as a Marker of Stent Failure: Restenosis, Thrombosis and Fracture

Fakilahyel S. Mshelbwala[1] **Brittany Fuller**[2] **Khaldoon Alaswad**[2] **and Mir B. Basir**[2]

[1]*Cardiology Fellow PGY4, Henry Ford Hospital, K-14 Cardiology, 2799 W. Grand Blvd, Detroit, MI 48202, USA*
[2]*Department of Cardiology, Henry Ford Hospital, Detroit, Michigan, USA*

Correspondence should be addressed to Fakilahyel S. Mshelbwala; fmshelb1@hfhs.org

Academic Editor: Ertugurul Ercan

Peri-stent contrast staining (PSS), defined as contrast staining around the stent struts, has been identified as an indicator of future stent failure in first generation, sirolimus-eluting coronary stents. 1 PSS has been associated with in-stent restenosis, stent thrombosis, stent fracture, and the development of coronary aneurysm. As the frequency of patients with first generation sirolimus-eluting coronary stents becomes infrequent; PSS may go unrecognized. Herein, we present a patient with a decade of longitudinal follow-up, who developed PSS identified on coronary angiogram with recurrent stent failure.

1. Introduction

First generation, sirolimus-eluting coronary stents, such as the Cypher stent (Cordis Corp., Miami Lakes, Florida), were approved for use by the FDA in 2003. Peri-stent contrast staining (PSS), defined as contrast staining around the stent struts, has been identified as an indicator of future stent failure in such stents. 1 PSS has been associated with in-stent restenosis, stent thrombosis, stent fracture, and the development of coronary aneurysm. As the frequency of patients with first generation sirolimus-eluting coronary stents becomes infrequent, PSS may go unrecognized. Herein, we present a patient with a decade of longitudinal follow up, who developed PSS which was identified on coronary angiogram with recurrent stent failure.

2. Case Report

A 64-year-old male presented with substernal chest pain an hour prior to arrival in the emergency department. Vital signs included a blood pressure of 140/81, heart rate of 69, respiration at 17 beats/min, and oxygenation at 89% on room air. Physical examination was unremarkable; however, the patient was in mild distress and diaphoretic. Electrocardiography (ECG) revealed ST elevation in leads V3-V6 (Figure 1(a)).

Our patient has a history of coronary artery disease with multivessel percutaneous coronary intervention (PCI), heart failure with reduced ejection fraction, hypertension, and hyperlipidemia. The patient had his first myocardial infarction in 2008 in the setting of an inferior wall myocardial infarction and underwent primary PCI of the RCA. He thereafter underwent staged PCI of the circumflex and subsequent staged PCI of the left anterior descending artery (LAD) using a 3.5 mm × 28 mm Cypher stent in the proximal segment and overlapping 3 mm × 28 mm and 2.75 mm × 18 mm Cypher stents in the mid to distal LAD (Figures 1(b) and 1(c)). The patient subsequently presented in 2011 with a non-ST segment elevation myocardial infarction secondary to a thrombotic diagonal lesion which was treated using a 2.5 mm × 12 mm Xience stent. The final angiogram revealed PSS in the proximal and distal LAD (Figure 1(d)). A few months later, the patient presented with chest pain after stopping his clopidogrel prior to a procedure. He was found to have stent thrombosis within the mid LAD and second diagonal and was treated with angioplasty and a

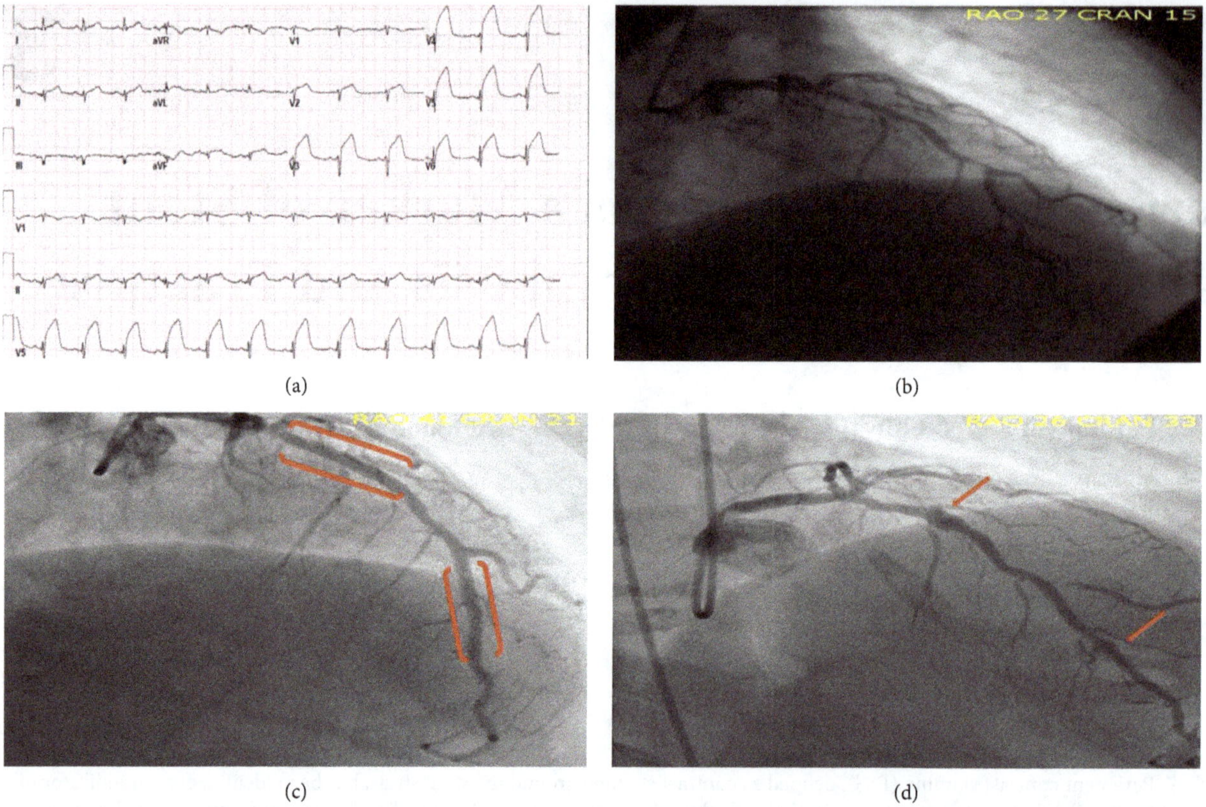

Figure 1: (a) ECG on presentation for the current admission showing ST segment elevation in V3-V6. (b) Initial angiogram on presentation in 2008. The patient had presented with an inferior wall myocardial infarction and underwent primary PCI of the RCA and subsequent staged PCI of the LAD one month later. (c) Angiogram after staged PCI of the LAD using 3.5 mm × 28 mm Cypher stent in the proximal segment of the LAD and overlapping 3 mm × 28 mm and 2.75 mm × 18 mm Cypher stents in the mid to distal LAD (stent locations marked with red brackets). (d) NSTEMI in 2011 secondary to thrombotic diagonal lesion which was ultimately treated with 2.5 mm × 12 mm Xience stent. Coronary angiogram revealed PSS in the proximal and distal LAD (red arrows).

3.5 mm × 15 mm BMS in the mid LAD. Again, PSS was noted in the proximal and distal LAD (Figure 2(a)). In 2013, the patient presented with anterior STEMI and was found to have late stent thrombosis of his proximal LAD, at the site of previous PSS (Figure 2(b)). The proximal LAD lesion was treated with balloon angioplasty, and 2.5 mm × 23 mm BMS was placed in the distal LAD. PSS was noted in the proximal LAD on final angiogram (Figure 2(c)).

Due to the nature of the chest pain on presentation and ECG changes, the cardiac catheterization laboratory was activated. Emergent coronary angiography demonstrated acute stent thrombosis of the proximal LAD at the site of previous PSS, with evidence of stent fracture and aneurysm (Figure 3(a)). Additionally, stent fracture in the distal LAD was also demonstrated at the site of previous PSS.

The patient initially presented to an outside hospital, and despite multiple attempts, the lesion could not be wired due to the fracture and aneurysm (Figure 3(b)). An intra-aortic balloon pump (IABP) was placed, and the patient was transferred to our institution. Intravascular ultrasound (IVUS) of the proximal LAD demonstrated an undersized stent, aneurysmal dilation with intramural hematoma in the area of stent fracture (see Supplementary Material for media file—Media 1). The lesion was successfully crossed using a Sasuke microcatheter and Gaia Next wire (Ashahi, Japan); however, there was significant difficulty in passing equipment leading to wire loss and aborting the procedure. The patient was brought back a few hours later due to recurrent symptoms with successful placement of DES; however, his procedure was complicated by no reflow and overall unsuccessful revascularization (Figures 3(c) and 3(d)). After initial recovery in the hospital, the patient was safely discharged home on goal directed medical therapy. After >6 months of outpatient follow-up and uptitration of his medication, the patient had improvement of his left ventricular ejection fraction to >45% without recurrent admission to the hospital. We recommended prolonged dual antiplatelet given the patients low bleeding risk.

3. Discussion

PSS is defined as contrast staining outside of the stent contour extending >20% of the stent diameter measured by quantitative coronary angiography [1]. PSS has been associated with stent fracture, target lesion revascularization, and late stent thrombosis [1]. Imai et al. evaluated 3081 lesions in 1998 subjects, for angiographic evidence of PSS 12 months after sirolimus-eluting stent implantation. They found that stent fracture was more frequent in lesions with

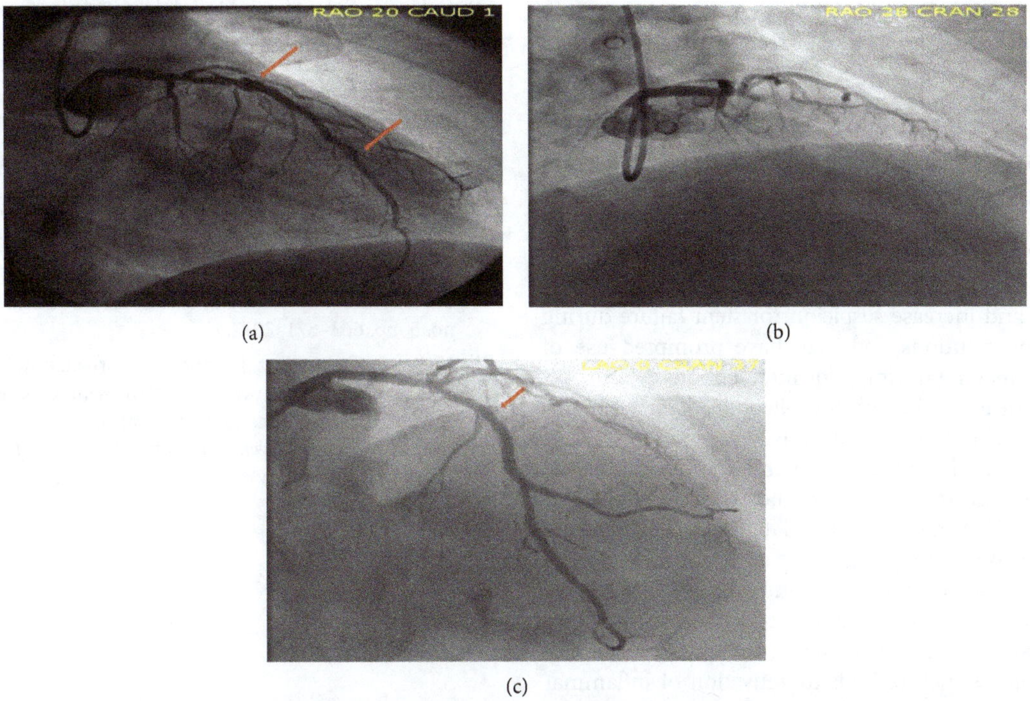

Figure 2: (a) 3 months later, also in 2011, the patient presented with chest pain after clopidogrel interruption prior to surgery. He was found to have acute stent thrombosis in the mid LAD and second diagonal artery. Patient was treated with angioplasty and 3.5 mm × 15 mm BMS in mid LAD. A BMS was used due to the need for an upcoming surgery. Again, PSS was seen in the proximal and distal LAD (red arrows). (b) In 2013, the patient presented with an anterior STEMI and was found to have late stent thrombosis of the proximal LAD at site of previously identified PSS. The proximal LAD lesion was treated with angioplasty, and a 2.5 mm × 23 mm BMS was placed in the distal LAD. (c) PSS was noted in the proximal LAD on final angiogram (red arrow).

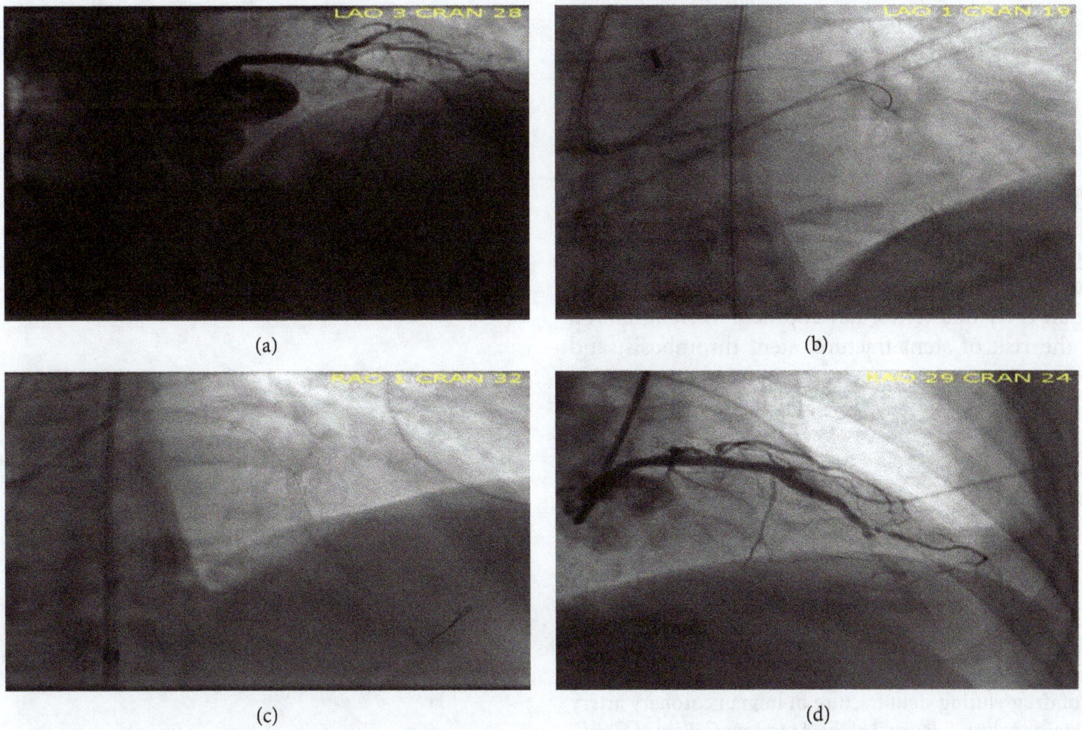

Figure 3: (a) During the index procedure, coronary angiogram revealed acute stent thrombosis of proximal LAD and stent fracture with aneurysm formation at site of previously identified PSS. (b) Failed attempt at advancing wire beyond fractured stent in the proximal LAD, outline the coronary aneurysm. (c) Successful crossing of Cypher stent in proximal LAD on a third attempt given recurrent symptoms. (d) Final coronary angiogram with the inability to establish TIMI 3 flow in distal LAD.

PSS (43.1% vs. 5.4%, $P < 0.0001$). Several mechanisms have been postulated to be predictors of stent fracture including stents placed in the RCA, the use of overlapping stents, longer stent length, and vessel tortuosity [2, 4]. The presence of chronic total occlusion has been identified as an independent risk factor for PSS as well [1]. On review of previous coronary angiograms of our patient, we noted PSS at the site of stent fracture and at the site of previously implanted Cypher stents. The PSS preceded the development of stent fracture. Recognizing the appearance of PSS may have led to further investigation and increase suspicion for stent failure during preceeding interventions and may have prompted use of intravascular imaging during prior interventions.

Stent fracture is a known complication of first-generation, sirolimus-eluting stents and was first reported in 2004 [4]. Several studies have reported increase in occurrence of in-stent restenosis and stent thrombosis in the setting of stent fracture [5]. It has been speculated that stent fracture results in decrease in drug availability at the location of fracture, leading to abnormal proliferation of smooth muscle lining the coronary vessel and subsequent impairment of endothelialization [6]. Furthermore, the presence of the exposed metallic structure leads to activation of inflammatory cytokines and triggers platelet activation that subsequent stent thrombosis [1, 7]. It has been hypothesized that aneurysmal dilation of coronary vessels after placement of drug eluting stents may be due to immunologic reaction from the drug which can cause intimal remodeling and dilation of the vessel [3]. Imaging techniques such as fluoroscopy with or without contrast, intravascular ultrasound, multislice CT, and optical coherence imaging are important modalities to identify stent fracture [5]. PSS can also be easily identified on by fluoroscopy and is an important marker of possible future stent failure.

4. Conclusion

PSS is most commonly associated with first generation sirolimus-eluting coronary stents such as the Cypher stent and can be an early marker for development of stent failure; increasing the risk of stent fracture, stent thrombosis, and in-stent restenosis.

References

[1] M. Imai, K. Kadota, T. Goto et al., "Incidence, risk factors, and clinical sequelae of angiographic peri-stent contrast staining after sirolimus-eluting stent implantation," *Circulation*, vol. 123, no. 21, pp. 2382–2391, 2011.

[2] G. Nakazawa, A. V. Finn, M. Vorpahl et al., "Incidence and predictors of drug-eluting stent fracture in human coronary artery a pathologic analysis," *Journal of the American College of Cardiology*, vol. 54, no. 21, pp. 1924–1931, 2009.

[3] H. Doi, A. Maehara, G. S. Mintz et al., "Classification and potential mechanisms of intravascular ultrasound patterns of stent fracture," *The American journal of cardiology*, vol. 103, no. 6, pp. 818–823, 2009.

[4] G. Sianos, S. Hofma, J. M. R. Ligthart et al., "Stent fracture and restenosis in the drug-eluting stent era," *Catheterization and cardiovascular interventions: official journal of the Society for Cardiac Angiography & Interventions*, vol. 61, no. 1, pp. 111–116, 2004.

[5] M. Chinikar and P. Sadeghipour, "Coronary stent fracture: a recently appreciated phenomenon with clinical relevance," *Current cardiology reviews*, vol. 10, no. 4, pp. 349–354, 2014.

[6] S. Kuramitsu, M. Iwabuchi, T. Haraguchi et al., "Incidence and clinical impact of stent fracture after everolimus-eluting stent implantation," *Circulation: Cardiovascular Interventions*, vol. 5, no. 5, pp. 663–671, 2012.

[7] M. S. Lee, D. Jurewitz, J. Aragon, J. Forrester, R. R. Makkar, and S. Kar, "Stent fracture associated with drug-eluting stents: clinical characteristics and implications," *Catheterization and cardiovascular interventions: official journal of the Society for Cardiac Angiography & Interventions*, vol. 69, no. 3, pp. 387–394, 2007.

31

Right Coronary Artery STEMI following Blunt Thoracic Trauma

Saad Sikanderkhel,[1] Jon-Austin Ash,[2] Kimberly O'Dell,[2] Jacob Mok,[2] Harish Manyam,[1] and John Golding[3]

[1]*Department of Cardiovascular Medicine, University of Tennessee College of Medicine Chattanooga, USA*
[2]*Department of Internal Medicine, University of Tennessee College of Medicine Chattanooga, USA*
[3]*Heart and Lung Institute, Erlanger Baroness Hospital, Chattanooga, Tennessee, USA*

Correspondence should be addressed to Jon-Austin Ash; jonaustinash@gmail.com

Academic Editor: Ertugurul Ercan

We present a case report of an otherwise healthy 37-year-old male without pertinent cardiac history or risk factors, who presented with cardiac trauma after a motor vehicle collision (MVC). Initial workup including electrocardiogram (ECG), transthoracic echocardiogram (TTE), and uptrending serial troponins warranted coronary angiography, during which occlusive thrombi were discovered in the proximal right coronary artery (pRCA), the right posterolateral vessel (rPL), and the right posterior descending artery (PDA). Subsequently, the patient underwent percutaneous coronary intervention of the RCA and PDA with aspiration thrombectomy. He was then initiated on dual antiplatelet therapy (DAPT) and recovered appropriately. This case is presented with the goal of enlightening the academic community of a rare complication while presenting a judicious approach to management in an attempt to decrease the occurrence of "near misses" in the future.

1. Introduction

Blunt thoracic trauma commonly leads to blunt cardiac injury (BCI), i.e., injury of the myocardium and large vessels. BCI is reported to occur in as many as 20% of all blunt thoracic trauma cases [1]. However, amongst those cases, acute coronary artery occlusion is not common, especially occlusion of the RCA. We present the case of a young man without cardiac history or pertinent risk factors, who was found to have an acute myocardial infarction (AMI) in the setting of an RCA thrombosis secondary to blunt thoracic trauma via MVC.

2. Case Presentation

A 37-year-old male presented to the emergency department (ED) due to trauma sustained as the unrestrained driver in an MVC. He was without loss of consciousness, remained hemodynamically stable, but was combative with evidence of head trauma. He was sedated and intubated at the scene due to incipient airway compromise and was then transferred to the hospital by air ambulance.

In the ED, the patient was noted to be normotensive and tachycardic while sedated on ventilator support. Physical exam was notable for multiple areas of ecchymosis and lacerations. Workup revealed multiple fractures, a small right pneumothorax, and pelvic hematoma. ECG was concerning for AMI with ST elevations in the inferior and lateral leads (Figure 1). A bedside TTE demonstrated normal left ventricular ejection fraction, mild inferolateral hypokinesis, and absence of tamponade physiology. His initial Troponin-I was 0.56 ng/ml.

The patient was given aspirin 325 mg and subsequently observed without scheduled antiplatelet therapy due to incipient hemodynamic compromise in the setting of a hematoma and extensive trauma. In the interim, serial Troponin-I levels continued to rise sharply, peaking at 34.24 ng/ml, necessitating urgent coronary angiography via the right radial artery access, which revealed thrombosis in the pRCA, the rPL, and the distal PDA (Figure 2), at which point the patient underwent successful aspiration thrombectomy with the

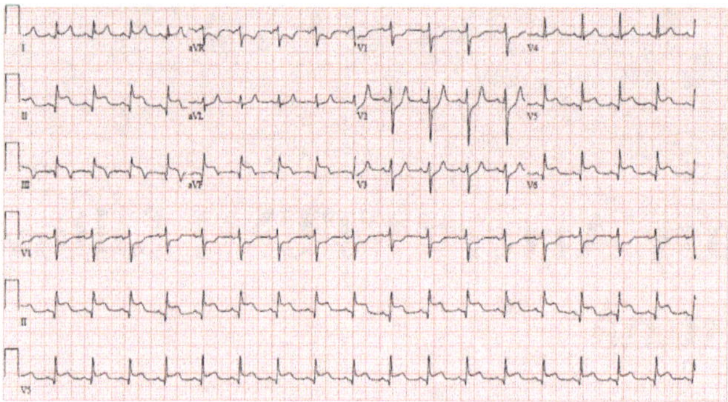

FIGURE 1: Inferolateral STEMI. ECG in the ED showing sinus tachycardia and ST-segment elevation in the inferolateral leads.

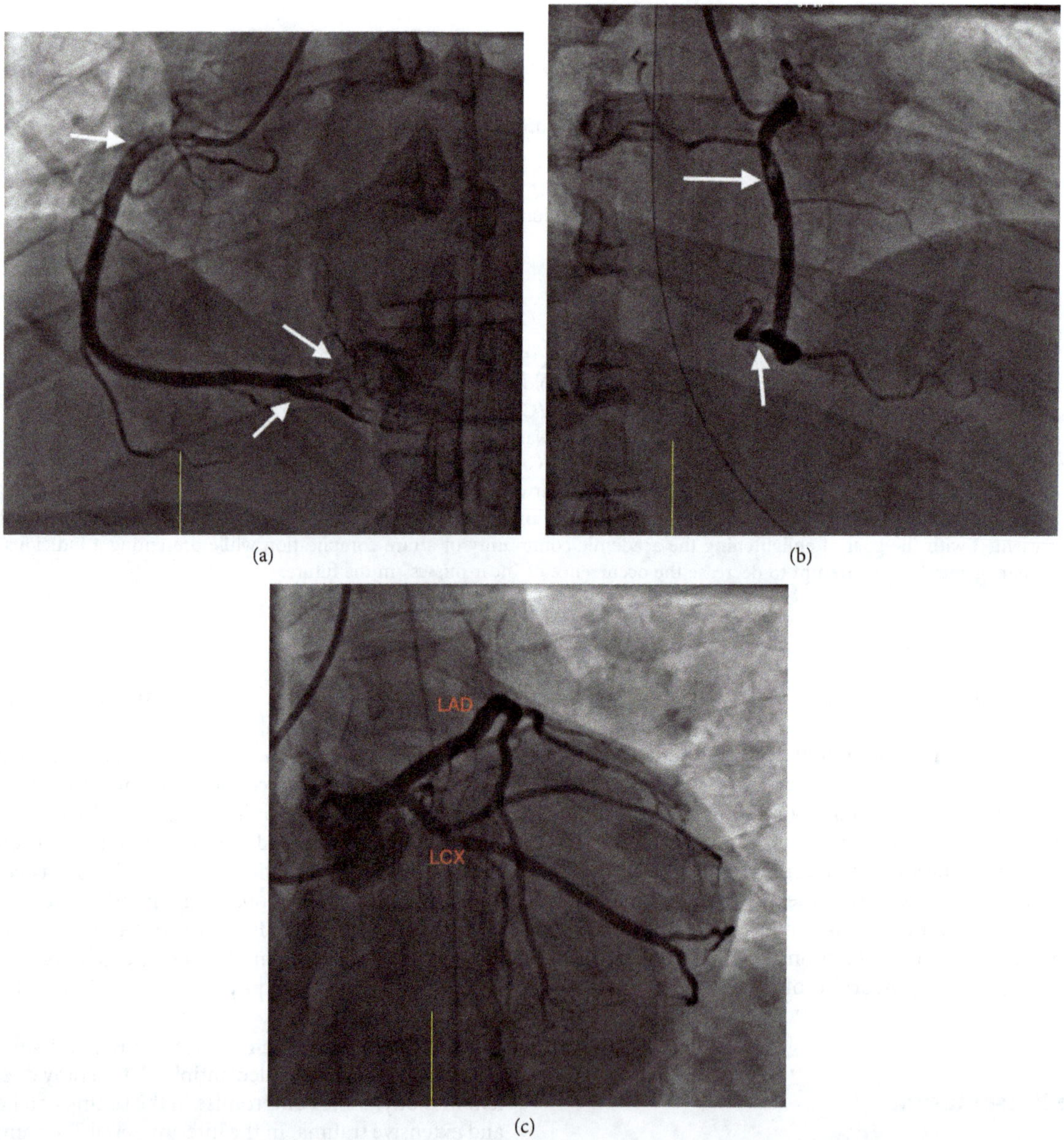

FIGURE 2: Coronary angiography prior to intervention. (a) pRCA, rPL, and PDA thrombus: coronary angiography (LAO view) showing thrombus in the proximal right coronary artery (pRCA), the right posterolateral (rPL), and the right posterior descending (PDA) branches (white arrows). (b) pRCA and rPL thrombus: coronary angiography (RAO view) showing thrombi in the pRCA and rPL branches (white arrows). (c) Normal left main, LAD, and LCX: coronary angiography (LAO cranial view) showing angiographically normal left main, left anterior descending (LAD), and left circumflex (LCX) arteries.

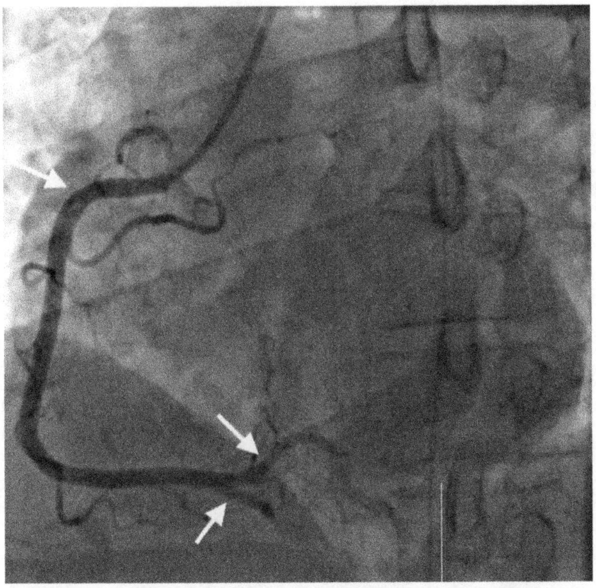

FIGURE 3: Coronary angiography after intervention. pRCA and rPL s/p aspiration thrombectomy: coronary angiography (LAO view) showing complete resolution of thrombi in the pRCA and rPL branches after aspiration thrombectomy (white arrows). However, the PDA remained occluded with microthrombi as a consequence of intervention in the proximal RCA (white arrow).

Pronto aspiration catheter system (Teleflex Medical OEM, Gurnee, IL, USA) without further evidence of underlying plaque or dissection. The distal PDA remained occluded in the aftermath of pRCA intervention, and attempts at aspiration thrombectomy were precluded by the small diameter of the vessel (<2 mm) (Figure 3). After the procedure, a glycoprotein IIb/IIa inhibitor infusion was administered for 12 hours. Intravenous Cangrelor, which had been initiated during the procedure, was changed to clopidogrel once additional orthopedic procedures were no longer anticipated. The patient recovered well after the procedure and was discharged home in a stable condition. He was prescribed DAPT for at least 12 months along with a high-intensity statin and beta-blocker.

3. Discussion

With extensive thoracic trauma, as in our case, a broader differential diagnosis needs to be considered to include cardiac contusion, large vessel dissection, external compression of the coronary artery, and stress-induced cardiomyopathy. These, along with valvular malfunction in the setting of a traumatic avulsion, pericardial effusion, and arrhythmias are known to be the most common cardiac complications resulting from blunt thoracic trauma [2]. AMI secondary to blunt thoracic trauma is rare, as direct injury to the coronary vessels is uncommon [3], occurring in only 3% of all BCIs [1]. However, this does occur with a proposed etiology due to the superficial anatomic location of the coronaries making the vessels susceptible to thrombosis formation in the setting of a traumatic event [4, 5]. Furthermore, since the left anterior descending artery is the most anterior vessel and hence in the most vulnerable position, it is also the most commonly injured [4, 6–13].

This case report of AMI with occlusion of the pRCA, rPL, and PDA represents an exceedingly rare complication of blunt thoracic trauma. Our patient had no cardiac history or risk factors for atherosclerotic coronary vascular disease, and no evidence of underlying coronary artery disease was found with angiography either. This suggests that blunt trauma-induced thrombosis was the most likely cause of the AMI. Fortunately, a complete cardiac workup upon presentation and early involvement of a cardiology team led to prompt diagnosis and treatment, which afforded the patient an excellent outcome. However, such is not always the case.

When a patient presents with blunt thoracic trauma, BCIs are often masked by precordial pain due to trauma to that area, making the diagnosis less clear [14]. For generalized cardiac complications, a workup including ECG and cardiac biomarkers is a must, as illustrated via a meta-analysis directly correlating abnormal values of such with patients requiring cardiac treatment [15]. Specifically for AMI as in our case, serial ECGs afforded the most useful diagnostic information, in addition to wall motion abnormalities noted on TTE, as well as elevated cardiac biomarkers [16]. Cardiac MRI with contrast and cardiac CT is also beneficial as has been shown useful in differentiating between cardiac contusion and acute MI [17, 18].

Although rare, providers should always maintain a high index of suspicion for BCI following blunt thoracic trauma. Workup should include, at a minimum, ECG, echocardiography, and trending of cardiac biomarkers to allow for early identification of AMI, i.e., need for coronary intervention, which is critical for improved outcomes [19–21].

Acknowledgments

This study was supported by the Continuing Medical Education fund for Internal Medicine Residents at UTCOM Chattanooga.

References

[1] J. M. Schultz and D. D. Trunkey, "Blunt cardiac injury," *Critical Care Clinics*, vol. 20, no. 1, pp. 57–70, 2004.

[2] Y. L. Lin and C. H. Yu, "Acute myocardial infarction caused by coronary artery dissection after a blunt chest trauma," *Internal medicine*, vol. 50, no. 18, pp. 1969–1971, 2011.

[3] M. D. Christensen, P. E. Nielsen, and P. Sleight, "Prior blunt chest trauma may be a cause of single vessel coronary disease; hypothesis and review," *International Journal of Cardiology*, vol. 108, no. 1, pp. 1–5, 2006.

[4] E. Atalar, T. Açil, K. Aytemir et al., "Acute anterior myocardial infarction following a mild nonpenetrating chest trauma–a case report," *Angiology*, vol. 52, no. 4, pp. 279–282, 2001.

[5] S. G. Foussas, G. D. Athanasopoulos, and D. V. Cokkinos, "Myocardial infarction caused by blunt chest injury: possible mechanisms involved–case reports," *Angiology*, vol. 40, no. 4, pp. 313–318, 1989.

[6] B. R. Fang and C. T. Li, "Acute myocardial infarction following blunt chest trauma," *European Heart Journal*, vol. 15, no. 5, pp. 705–707, 1994.

[7] O. Goktekin, A. Unalir, B. Gorenek et al., "Traumatic total occlusion of left main coronary artery caused by blunt chest trauma," *The Journal of Invasive Cardiology*, vol. 14, no. 8, pp. 463–465, 2002.

[8] M. Nikparvar, S. M. Asghari, and H. Farshidi, "Delayed diagnosis of myocardial infarction in a young man with a blunt chest trauma," *Journal of cardiovascular and thoracic research*, vol. 11, no. 3, pp. 251–253, 2019.

[9] A. Sinha, M. Sibel, P. Thomas et al., "Coronary thrombosis without dissection following blunt trauma," *Case Reports in Cardiology*, vol. 2016, Article ID 8671015, 2016.

[10] R. F. Al-Aqeedi, W. M. Ali, F. Al-Ani, Y. S. Abdulrahman, and A. Alnabti, "A blunt chest trauma causing left anterior descending artery dissection and acute myocardial infarction treated by deferred angioplasty," *Heart views: the official journal of the Gulf Heart Association*, vol. 12, no. 2, pp. 71–73, 2011.

[11] C. H. Li, T. F. Chiu, and J. C. Chen, "Extensive anterolateral myocardial infarction caused by left main coronary artery dissection after blunt chest trauma: a case report," *The American journal of emergency medicine*, vol. 25, no. 7, pp. 858.e3–858.e858005, 2007.

[12] M. J. Anto, S. G. Cokinos, and E. Jonas, "Acute anterior wall myocardial infarction secondary to blunt chest trauma," *Angiology*, vol. 35, no. 12, pp. 802–804, 1984.

[13] S. A. Abdolrahimi, H. R. Sanati, M. M. Ansari-Ramandi, S. O. Heris, and M. Maadani, "Acute myocardial infarction following blunt chest trauma and coronary artery dissection," *Journal of Clinical and Diagnostic Research: JCDR*, vol. 10, no. 6, pp. OD14–OD15, 2016.

[14] A. R. de Biasi, K. P. Seastedt, S. R. Eachempati, and A. Salemi, "Common cause of mortality in trauma but manageable nonetheless," *Circulation*, vol. 132, no. 6, pp. 537–545, 2015.

[15] R. L. Maenza, D. Seaberg, and F. D'Amico, "A meta-analysis of blunt cardiac trauma: ending myocardial confusion," *The American Journal of Emergency Medicine*, vol. 14, no. 3, pp. 237–241, 1996.

[16] G. Kotsovolis, Z. Aidoni, E. Geka, and M. Peftoulidou, "Occlusion of the right coronary artery after blunt thoracic trauma with fatal outcome: a case report and review of the literature," *Hippokratia*, vol. 17, no. 3, pp. 274–276, 2013.

[17] S. Southam, C. Jutila, and L. Ketai, "Contrast-enhanced cardiac MRI in blunt chest trauma: differentiating cardiac contusion from acute peri-traumatic myocardial infarction," *Journal of Thoracic Imaging*, vol. 21, no. 2, pp. 176–178, 2006.

[18] T. L. Lee, C. F. Hsuan, C. H. Shih et al., "Early detection of myocardial infarction following blunt chest trauma by computed tomography: a case report," *BMC Cardiovascular Disorders*, vol. 17, no. 1, p. 56, 2017.

[19] G. Oghlakian, P. Maldjian, E. Kaluski, and M. Saric, "Acute myocardial infarction due to left anterior descending coronary artery dissection after blunt chest trauma," *Emergency Radiology*, vol. 17, no. 2, pp. 149–151, 2010.

[20] L. T. Laubach, G. A. Burket, R. D. Barraco, D. Ramic, K. R. Weaver, and M. R. Greenberg, "Post-traumatic left anterior descending artery dissection," *The American journal of emergency medicine*, vol. 38, no. 6, pp. 1299.e3–1299.e5, 2020.

[21] M. D. Greenberg and C. L. Rosen, "Evaluation of the patient with blunt chest trauma: an evidence based approach," *Emergency medicine clinics of North America*, vol. 17, no. 1, p. 41, 1999.

32

Guide Extension Catheter-Facilitated Reverse Controlled Antegrade and Retrograde Tracking for Retrograde Recanalization of Chronic Total Occlusion

Rohit Mody,[1] **Debabrata Dash**,[2] **Bhavya Mody**,[3] **and Aditya Saholi**[4]

[1]*Department of Cardiology, MAX Super Specialty Hospital, Bathinda, Punjab, India*
[2]*Department of Cardiology, Zulekha Hospital, AL Zahra Street, Sharjah 457, UAE*
[3]*Department of Medicine, Kasturba Medical College, Manipal, Karnataka, India*
[4]*Department of Medicine, Irwin Hospital, Surja Ram Market, Malout, Punjab, India*

Correspondence should be addressed to Rohit Mody; drmody_2k@yahoo.com

Academic Editor: Yigit Canga

Background. In recent years, the retrograde approach has become a common practice in the treatment of chronic total occlusion (CTO) of coronary ostium which is arising abnormally and has an ambiguous proximal cap. In this case report, we report a case of retrograde percutaneous coronary intervention (PCI) done successfully on an abnormally originating artery which was guideliner assisted. *Case Presentation.* A 65-year-old gentleman with a history of hypertension, diabetes, and PCI presented to us with angina. Physical examination, electrocardiography (ECG), and echocardiography were done. Coronary angiography (CAG) revealed a normal left anterior descending artery (LAD), an anomalous circumflex (CX) artery arising from the right cusp. The abnormal CX had an implanted stent from which the abnormal right coronary artery (RCA) was arising and had a CTO. It also revealed the retrograde filling of distal RCA through grade 2 Werner collateral channels (CCs) from the LAD, a long CTO segment with a distal cap at the bifurcation. PCI of an RCA-CTO was scheduled utilizing a primary retrograde strategy, since antegrade ostium was abnormal in origin, and the patient was previously stented across the origin. The retrograde wire was externalized, and the procedure was completed with 3 overlapping drug-eluting stents (DESs). We used a guideliner which also assisted in the capture of retrograde corsair during the retrograde procedure of CTO [assisted reverse controlled antegrade and retrograde tracking (CART)]. These measures helped us to complete the CTO intervention successfully. *Conclusion.* The antegrade crossing is the most common approach to CTOs. However, it is sometimes difficult to penetrate the proximal hard ambiguous cap with guidewires, especially in the case of CTOs of anomalous coronary arteries because of a lack of support. Herein, we describe an iteration of reverse CART technique using a guide extensor catheter to facilitate externalizing the retrograde wire from false to true lumen.

1. Introduction

PCI of CTO has a lower success rate than PCI of nonoccluded coronary artery [1, 2]. In 1990, the first retrograde approach technique was applied for CTO via a degenerated saphenous vein graft. Over the next 2 decades, septal collateral branches were considered to be novel access for the retrograde approach [3]. With the emergence of new equipment and important iterations, this approach has become safer, faster, and more successful [4]. In this case report, we report a case of retrograde PCI done successfully on an abnormally originating artery which was guideliner assisted. Mozid et al. similarly described the utility of a guideliner catheter in retrograde PCI of a CTO with reverse CART—the "Capture" technique [5].

2. Case Presentation

2.1. History. A 65-year-old gentleman presented with Canadian Cardiovascular Society (CCS) Class III angina despite being on optimal medical therapy, including beta-blocker

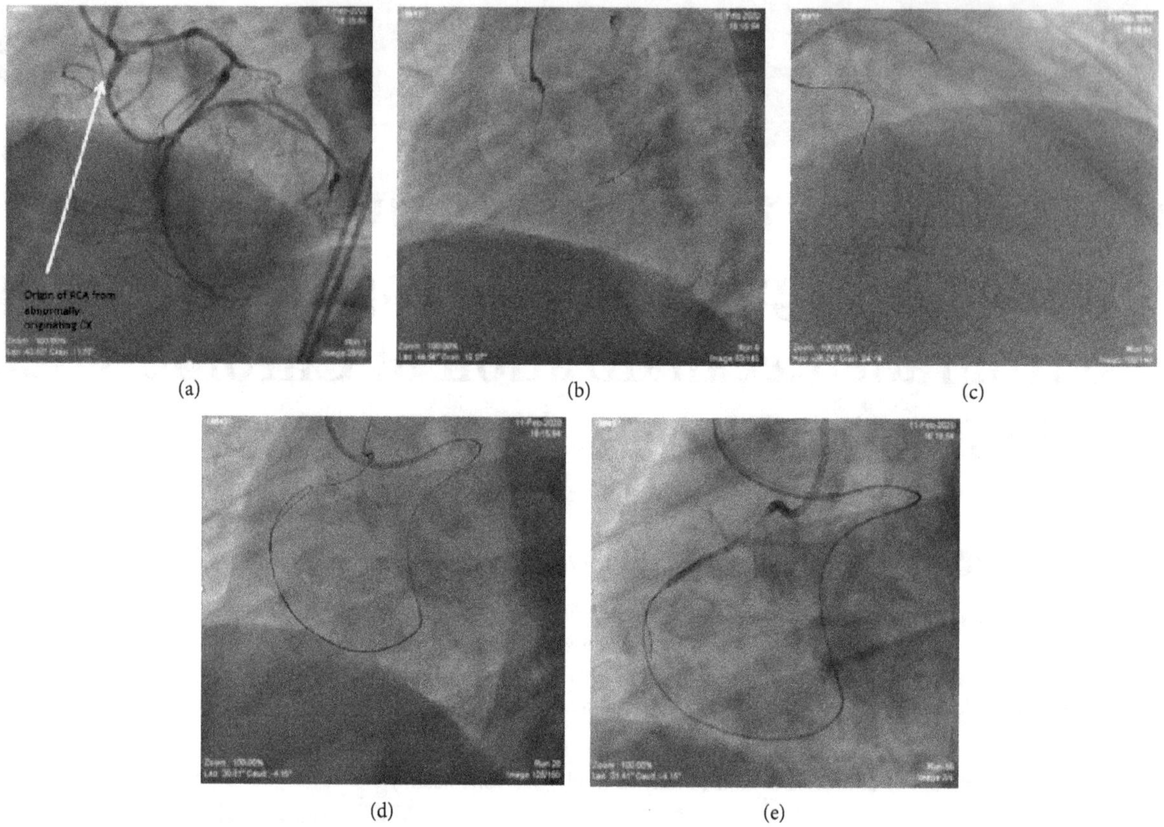

FIGURE 1: (a) Retrogradely filling abnormal RCA originating from abnormally originating CX. (b) POT done in CX stent. (c) Sion blue and Corsair crossed retrogradely. (d) Knuckle pilot wire reaching proximal RCA subintimaly. (e) Guideliner assisted creation of common space antegradely.

(Metocard XL 100 mg OD), long-acting nitrates (Nitrocontin 6.4 mg BD), calcium channel blocker (Dilzem SR 120 mg OD), and Ranolazine (Rancad 1 g OD). In addition to that, the patient used to take sublingual nitrates as and when required for angina. He was a known case of hypertension, diabetes, and a post-PCI of the proximal segment of an anomalous CX artery arising from the right cusp. The implanted stent was covering the abnormal origin of RCA from CX which had a CTO. He was also on dual antiplatelet therapy (DAPT) with aspirin 75 mg OD and Clopidogrel 75 mg OD as a post-PCI regimen. Also, the patient was on an oral hypoglycemic agent (Oxramet 5 mg/1000 mg OD) with poorly controlled diabetes (HbA1c: 8%).

2.2. Differential Diagnoses. In this patient, acute coronary syndrome was most suspected, followed by myocarditis, pericarditis, and stress cardiomyopathy.

2.3. Investigations. The patient's routine blood investigations were sent. An ECG revealed normal sinus rhythm at a rate of 62 beats/min without abnormal QS wave patterns. An echocardiogram revealed normal overall left ventricular function. Troponin I and CPK-MB were normal. The diagnostic CAG revealed a normal LAD and anomalous CX arising from the right coronary cusp along with a CTO in the proximal segment of the anomalous RCA. This RCA was arising from the proximal segment of abnormally originating CX artery. It also revealed the retrograde filling of distal RCA through grade 2 Werner CCs from the LAD, a long CTO segment with a distal cap at the bifurcation (Figure 1(a)). Therefore, the PCI of an RCA-CTO was scheduled utilizing a primary retrograde strategy.

2.4. Management. Vascular access was obtained using bilateral femoral 7-Fr long sheaths. Particularly, 7-Fr Hyperion AL 1 (Asahi Intecc, Aichi, Japan) and 7-Fr extra backup (EBU) 3.5 (Medtronic, USA) with side holes were utilized to engage the CX arising from the right cusp and the LAD, respectively. A workhorse wire was advanced into the distal abnormal CX. A 3.5×15 mm noncompliant (NC) balloon (Mozec™ NC PTCA Balloon) was used to postdilate the previously implanted stent for smooth navigation of gears (Figure 1(b)). A Sion wire (Asahi Intecc, Aichi, Japan) and 150 cm Corsair® microcatheter (Asahi Intecc, Aichi, Japan) were advanced through the septal CC into the posterior descending artery progressing easily until the distal cap of the occlusion (Figure 1(c)). Similarly, the escalation of the retrograde wire was done. The initial Sion blue was exchanged with Pilot 200 (Abbott Vascular International, Diegem, Belgium), and an attempt to navigate it through the distal cap was unsuccessful. Hence, the distal cap was crossed with a knuckle which could be advanced in subintimal space from distal to proximal RCA allowing delivery of the Corsair® (Figure 1(d)). Unable to progress further, a

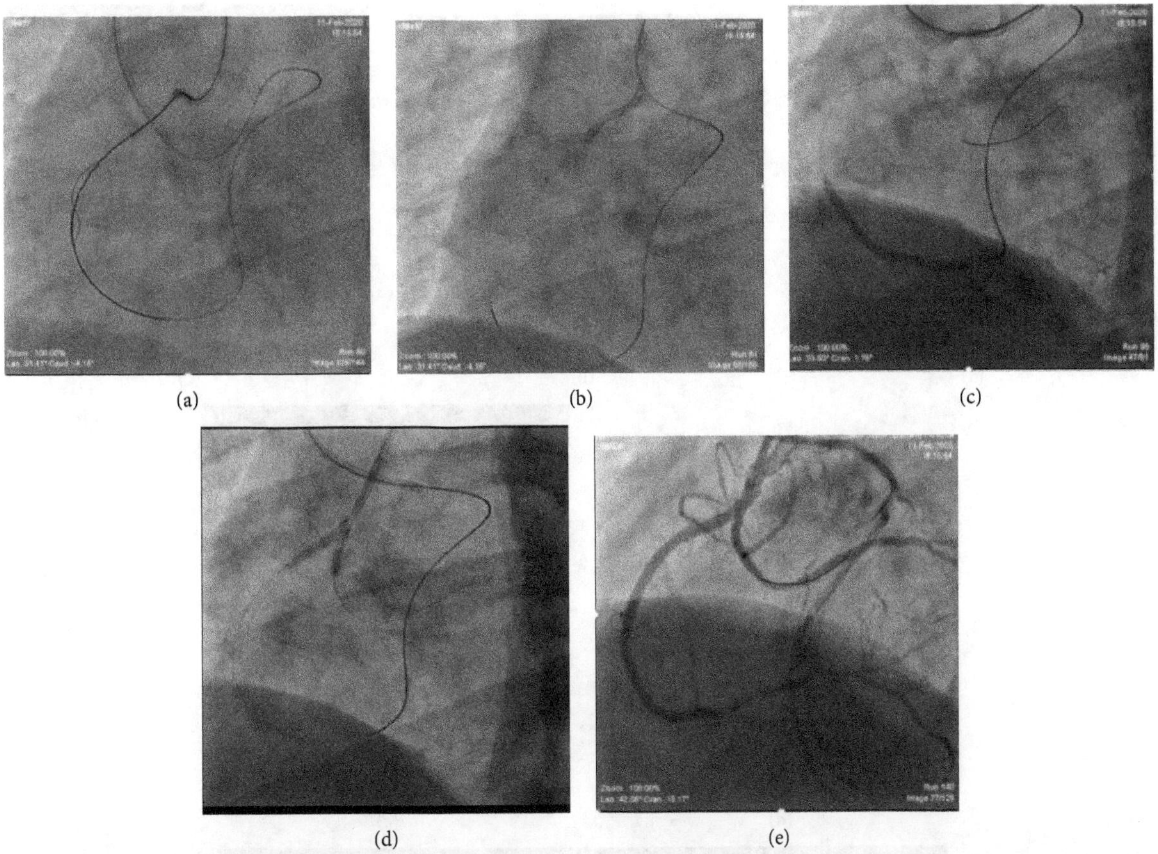

Figure 2: (a) RG3 wire externalized with the help of guideliner. (b) Corsair taken back. (c) 3 stents deployed sequentially. (d).Final proximal kissing. (e) Final result.

decision was made to introduce an anterograde subintimal track through the struts of an already deployed CX stent, from which abnormal RCA was arising, to meet the retrograde wire. A Gaia 2 (Asahi Intecc, Aichi, Japan) was taken through a Finecross microcatheter (Terumo Corp., Tokyo, Japan), escalated to Gaia 3, and finally Conquest Pro 12 (Asahi Intecc, Aichi, Japan). This entered the subintimal space anterogradely but was unable to meet the retrograde wire. To optimize the subintimal space, it was dilated with a 3×15 mm NC balloon. When this was also futile, a guide extension catheter (Guideliner [Vascular Solutions, Minneapolis, MN, USA]) was positioned in the antegrade subintimal space which created a target lumen enabling rapid reconnection with the true lumen from the retrograde wire (Figure 1(e)). Once the wire engaged the antegrade guide, the procedure became standard reverse CART with RG3 wire (Asahi Intecc, Aichi, Japan) externalized (Figure 2(a)). Following predilation with serial ballooning, 3 overlapping DESs were implanted (Figures 2(b) and 2(c)). The final proximal RCA stent, a 3.5×18 mm DES (cobalt-chromium everolimus-eluting stent; Xpedition; Abbott Vascular, Santa Clara, California), was deployed with T and protrusion (TAP) technique touching the CX stent. Final kissing was done with 3×15 mm NC balloon (Mozec™ NC PTCA Balloon) in the CX and withdrawn 3.5×18 mm stent balloon at 12 atm after the sequential dilatation of respective balloons to 18 atm (Figure 2(d)). The final angiographic result was excellent (Figure 2(e)). Finally, an optical coherence tomography (OCT) run was taken to see the final optimization which showed optimized stent deployment, no edge dissection, good bifurcation angle, and no major complication (Figure 3).

2.5. Follow-Up. The patient was followed up at 3-month intervals in the outpatient department. The patient is free of angina on minimal doses of beta-blocker (Metocard XL 50 mg OD) and long-acting nitrates (Imdur 30 mg OD), and there was no need for sublingual nitrates and calcium channel blockers. He had no symptoms pertaining to cardiovascular symptoms. His ECG was unremarkable, and ECHO showed EF of 60%. Blood sugar was better controlled with HbA1c of 7%.

3. Discussion

The most common cause of failure of PCI for CTO is the inability of wire to cross the occlusion [6, 7]. Recently, the retrograde approach through the CCs was introduced to overcome this problem, and several strategies and techniques for the retrograde approach have been developed to increase the efficacy and feasibility of this technique for CTO intervention [8–10]. Recently, Dash [4] described four iterations of reverse CART: (1) conventional reverse CART; (2) contemporary reverse CART involving the use

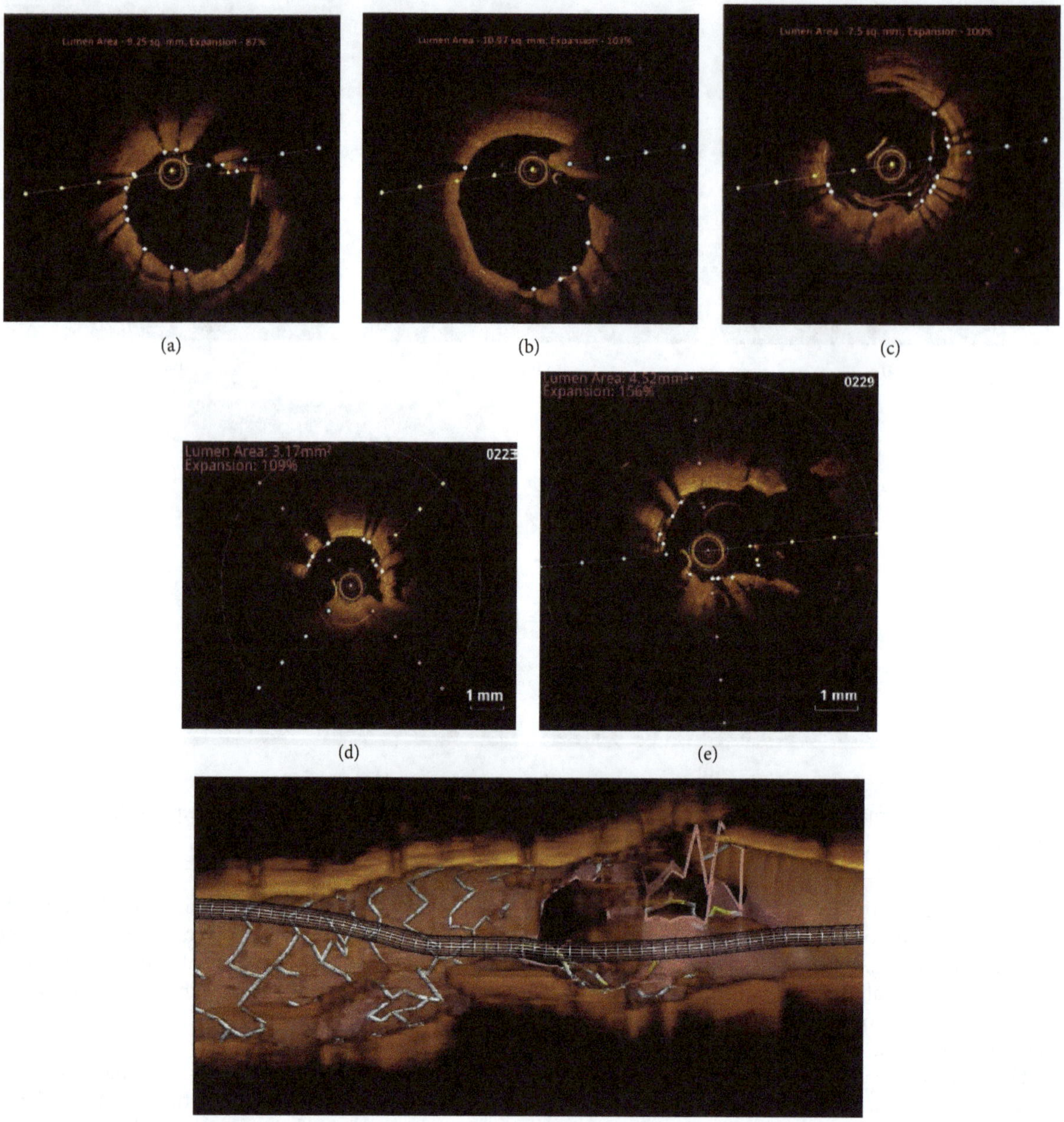

Figure 3: (a) RCA showing intimal tear within stented segment. (b) Proximal edge with no edge dissection. (c) RCA—distal edge. (d) CX—tissue prolapse. (e) CX bifurcation view—no pinching. (f). CX bifurcation view—longitudinal.

of small antegrade balloons and more active, intentional vessel tracking and penetration; (3) assisted reverse CART involving assistance from intravascular ultrasound (IVUS), stent, guide extension catheter, etc.; and (4) shifting reverse CART. Our case describes how the optimization of the reentry space can be escalated, with the advantage of the guide extensor catheter forming a clear open target, enabling rapid advancement of the retrograde wire into the proximal true lumen. This procedure could have been assisted by IVUS and stent. Stent-facilitated reverse CART is by nature an irreversible procedure as once the stent is deployed, it cannot be removed [4, 11, 12]. Unlike a stent, the guide extension device may be removed or repositioned once there is a failure of connection between the antegrade and retrograde true lumen [4, 11]. In our case, guideliner-assisted reverse CART was done. Firstly, in our case, the origin of the artery was abnormal; hence, good antegrade preparation was not possible with only AL1 support. Hence, guideliner was used. As the lesion was already stented previously so a good preparation with semicompliant balloon dilatation had to be made to advance guideliner through struts. As we know there may be compression or collapse of subintimal space after antegrade balloon inflation making wiring the true lumen more difficult even if common subintimal space does exist. We overcame this difficulty by the use of mother and child catheter. The advantage of this technique is that we can change the position of the guideliner to capture the retrograde microcatheter which otherwise cannot be done if the stent reverse CART technique is used [11]. Also, in our case, it was decided to go retrograde as an initial strategy as there was an abnormal origin and the segment had an overlying stent making antegrade entry ambiguous.

4. Conclusion

To conclude, retrograde PCI using reverse CART should be the first-line option for patients of CTO and abnormally originating artery. Also, during reverse CART in these lesions, guideliner can help support antegrade preparation as well as can help in the iteration of reverse CART.

Abbreviations

PCI: Percutaneous intervention
CTO: Chronic total occlusion
CX: Circumflex
CCS: Canadian Cardiovascular Society
LAD: Left anterior descending
RCA: Right coronary artery
CCs: Collateral channels
Fr: French
AL: Amplatz
NC: Noncompliant
CART: Controlled antegrade and retrograde tracking
CAG: Coronary angiography
ECG: Electrocardiogram
IVUS: Intravascular ultrasound
DAPT: Dual antiplatelet therapy
DES: Drug-eluting stent
TAP: T and protrusion
OCT: Optical coherence tomography.

Consent

Written consent has been obtained to publish the case report from the guardian. The consent copy is available with the authors and ready to be submitted if required.

Authors' Contributions

RM was involved in the collection of data, preparation of the first draft, and revision of the manuscript for important intellectual content. RM, DD, BM, and AS were involved in the collection of data and preparation of the first draft. RM, BM, and AS were involved in the conception of the study, revision of the manuscript for important intellectual content, and approval of the manuscript. All the authors have read and approved the manuscript.

References

[1] R. D. Safian, C. H. McCabe, M. E. Sipperly, R. G. McKay, and D. S. Baim, "Initial success and long-term follow-up of percutaneous transluminal coronary angioplasty in chronic total occlusions versus conventional stenoses," *The American Journal of Cardiology*, vol. 61, no. 14, pp. 23G–28G, 1988.

[2] C. W. Hamm, W. Kupper, K. H. Kuck, D. Hofmann, and W. Bleifeld, "Recanalization of chronic, totally occluded coronary arteries by new angioplasty systems," *The American Journal of Cardiology*, vol. 66, no. 20, pp. 1459–1463, 1990.

[3] Y.-H. Kim, S. H. Hwang, C. H. Lim et al., "Reverse controlled antegrade and retrograde subintimal tracking in chronic total occlusion of right coronary artery," *Korean Circulation Journal*, vol. 42, no. 9, pp. 625–628, 2012.

[4] D. Dash, "Iteration of reverse controlled antegrade and retrograde tracking for coronary chronic total occlusion intervention: a current appraisal," *Korean Circulation Journal*, vol. 50, no. 10, article e113, pp. 867–879, 2020.

[5] A. M. Mozid, J. R. Davies, and J. C. Spratt, "The utility of a guideliner™ catheter in retrograde percutaneous coronary intervention of a chronic total occlusion with reverse cart—the "capture" technique," *Catheterization and Cardiovascular Interventions*, vol. 83, no. 6, pp. 929–932, 2014.

[6] J. Y. Kim, J. Yoon, H. S. Jung et al., "The experience of transradial coronary intervention for chronic total occlusion," *Korean Circulation Journal*, vol. 33, pp. 805–812, 2003.

[7] T. Noguchi, M. D. Shunichi Miyazaki, I. Morii, S. Daikoku, Y. Goto, and H. Nonogi, "Percutaneous transluminal coronary angioplasty of chronic total occlusions: determinants of primary success and long-term clinical outcome," *Catheterization and Cardiovascular Interventions*, vol. 49, no. 3, pp. 258–264, 2000.

[8] J. F. Surmely, E. Tsuchikane, O. Katoh et al., "New concept for CTO recanalization using controlled antegrade and retrograde subintimal tracking," *The Journal of invasive Cardiology*, vol. 18, p. 3348, 2006.

[9] S. Saito, "Different strategies of retrograde approach in coronary angioplasty for chronic total occlusion," *Catheterization and Cardiovascular Interventions*, vol. 71, no. 1, pp. 8–19, 2008.

[10] N. Kukreja, P. W. Serruys, and G. Sianos, "Retrograde recanalization of chronically occluded coronary arteries: illustration and description of the technique," *Catheterization and Cardiovascular Interventions*, vol. 69, no. 6, pp. 833–841, 2007.

[11] D. Dash, "Retrograde coronary chronic total occlusion intervention using a novel reverse controlled antegrade and retrograde subintimal tracking," *Journal of interventional Cardiology.*, vol. 29, no. 1, pp. 70–74, 2016.

[12] R. Fung, E. B. Wu, and M. H. Jim, "Dislodged stent after stent reverse controlled antegrade and retrograde subintimal tracking (CART) - Is stent reverse CART a necessary tool or an unnecessary evil?," *J Cardiol Cases*, vol. 16, no. 6, pp. 205–209, 2017.

33

Retrograde Balloon Dilation outside the Main Branch Stent to Restore the Occlusion of Side Branch in Chronic Total Occlusion Bifurcation Lesions

Gao Hao-kao and Li Cheng-xiang

Department of Cardiology, The First Affiliated Hospital of Air Force Military Medical University, Xi'an 710032, China

Correspondence should be addressed to Li Cheng-xiang; 1256423656@qq.com

Academic Editor: Ming-Ren Chen

Percutaneous coronary intervention (PCI) of a chronic total occlusion (CTO) can be challenging when a bifurcation is present at the distal cap. We described a case of retrograde balloon outside the main branch stent to restore the occlusion of side branch in CTO bifurcation lesion through the jailed wire.

1. Introduction

Percutaneous coronary intervention for chronic total occlusion (CTO-PCI) remains one of the most challenging clinical scenarios in interventional cardiology and a lower success rate compared to non-CTO lesions [1, 2]. Although the antegrade approach is a general approach for CTO recanalization, a retrograde approach is currently widely used in complex CTO lesion and improves the success rate when antegrade techniques are unlikely to succeed [3]. The presence of a bifurcation lesion in the context of a CTO represents an additional difficulty. The jailed balloon technique (JBT) is now emerging for protection of the side branch (SB) acquiring high procedural success rate without SB occlusion [4].

But in this case, we described a retrograde small profile balloon outside the main branch stent to restore the occlusion of posterolateral vessel (PLV) in right coronary artery (RCA) CTO bifurcation lesion via a jailed wire.

2. Case Report

A 63-year-old man with 40 years smoking habit and known coronary artery disease presented with Canadian Cardiovascular Society (CCS) class II angina. Two weeks before, the patient had just successfully undergone CTO-PCI of the left circumflex artery (LCx) in our hospital, and at this time, he was referred for PCI to CTO in the RCA. Twelve-lead electrocardiography showed slight ST-segment depression in II/III/avF leads. Ultrasound echocardiography revealed the preserved left ventricular ejection fraction (LVEF = 52%) and hypokinesia of the inferior and posterior left ventricular wall. Three days after admission, we performed PCI for RCA CTO.

This time, we performed simultaneous left and right coronary angiography (CAG). PCI was performed with right femoral and radial arteries route. The RCA was engaged with a 7F SAL1.0 guide in the radial artery and the left coronary artery (LCA) with a 7F EBU 3.75 guide in the radial artery. CAG demonstrated severe stenosis of the proximal RCA and CTO of the RCA extending from the RCA middle to the posterior descending artery (PDA) and PLV bifurcation (Figure 1(a)). The LCA had a severe stenotic lesion in the distal of LCx, and two stents (Abbott Vascular, USA) were implanted there. The RCA distal bifurcation was well filled by CC2 septal collateral channels and CC3 epicardial collaterals from the left anterior descending artery (LAD) (Figure 1(b)).

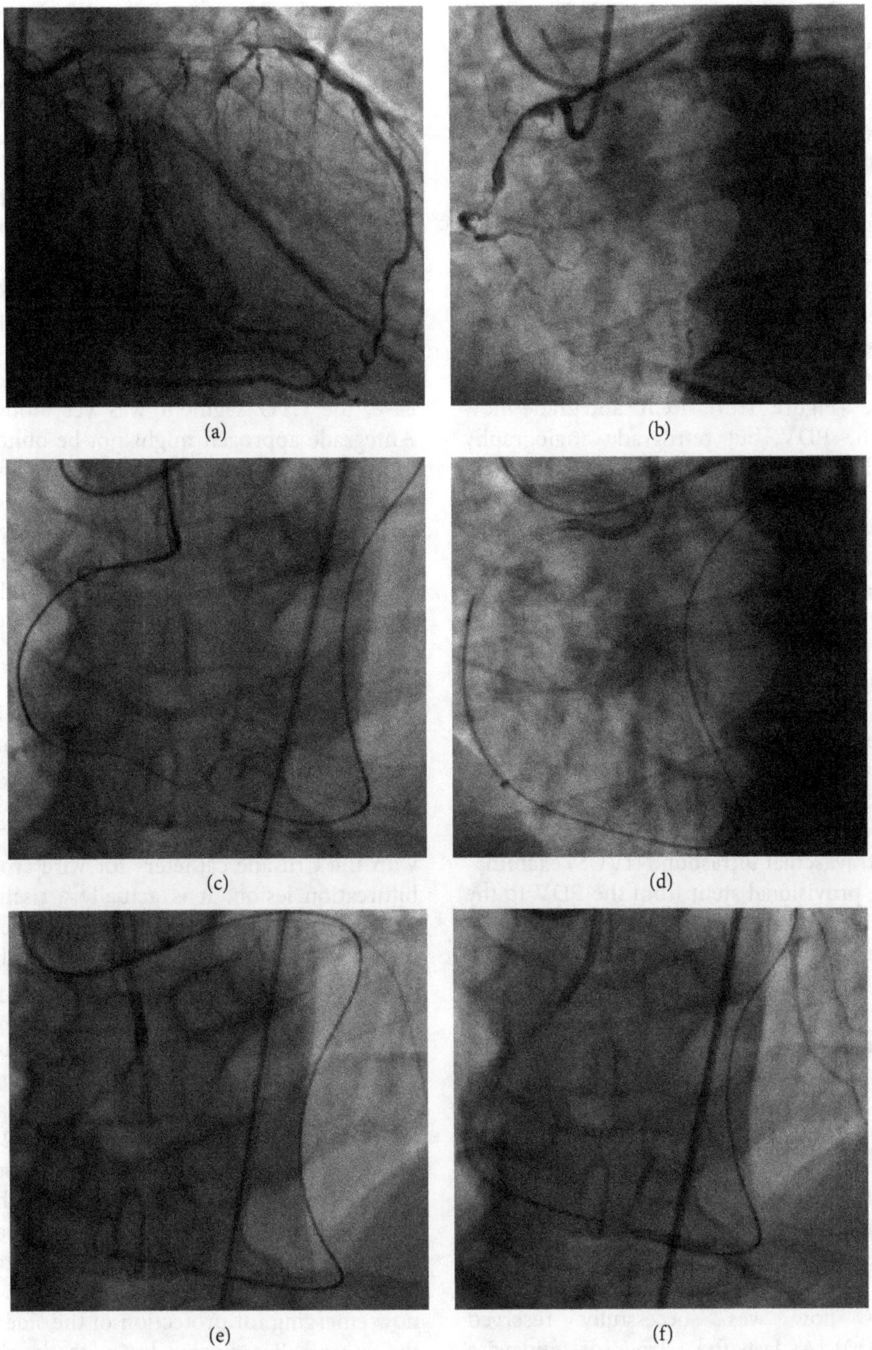

FIGURE 1: Recanalization of RCA CTO by a retrograde approach. (a) CAG showed LAD to RCA collaterals. (b) Simultaneous bilateral CAG showed long RCA CTO at bifurcation with large branches; (c) Corsair catheter in the right PDA placed retrograde via a epicardial collateral from the LAD, and tip injection showed antegrade wire in false lumen; (d) retrograde wire and Corsair into antegrade Guidezilla guide; (e) sequentially predilation RCA along antegrade RG3 wire; (f) retrograde angiography showed the severe disease in PLV.

2.1. One Retrograde Approach Successfully Opened RCA-PD CTO. The entrance of CTO was stumpless especially with big side branch and longer CTO segment. The J-CTO score for RCA CTO was 2. The lesion was initially approached antegradely with a Fielder XT-R wire (Asahi Intecc, Japan) supported by a Corsair microcatheter (Asahi Intecc, Japan), the Fielder XT-R could not be advanced, and composite core Gaia third wire (Asahi Intecc, Japan) was subsequently used but also failed to reenter into distal true lumen which was confirmed in false lumen by contralateral angiography (Figure 1(c)). Therefore, we switched to retrograde approach. The LAD provided larger and less tortuous epicardial collaterals, and a SION guide wire (Asahi Intecc, Japan) with a Corsair microcatheter was introduced into the epicardial branch. Selective tip injection through the Corsair revealed the occlusion site at the bifurcation with large branches (Figure 1(c)). A Fielder XT-R guide wire was advanced "knuckled" up into the RCA CTO segment and overlaps with the antegrade wire at the middle part of CTO. The retrograde and antegrade guiding wires were difficult to kiss, and next, we used the reverse controlled antegrade and retrograde subintimal tracking (CART) technique to enlarge subintimal space with a 2.0 mm × 20 mm balloon. The reverse CART technique facilitated Guidezilla (Boston Scientific, Natick, MA, USA) into CTO middle segment for picking up retrograde wire and manipulating the retrograde Pilot 200 wire (Abbott Vascular, USA) and Corsair into a Guidezilla guide (Figure 1(d)). The Pilot 200 wire was then exchanged with a 330 cm RG3 wire (Asahi Intecc, Japan) that was externalized. After sequentially predilation with a 1.5 × 20 mm/2.0 × 20 mm balloon along an antegrade RG3 wire (Figure 1(e)), RCA antegrade flow was restored into the PDV, but retrograde angiography showed the severe disease in the PLV (Figure 1(f)).

2.2. Another Retrograde Approach to Save PLV flow outside the Main Vessel Stent. Several attempts to wire PLV in the antegrade direction using several guide wires failed, and even "reverse bent wiring with the Crusade catheter" for a Field XT-R wire recrossing to the PLV still failed because of the retroflexed angle (Figure 2(a)). To preserve the PDA/PLV bifurcation, a Sion retrograde wire with a 150 cm long Corsair microcatheter was advanced into PLV distal via the second septal vessel. A 1.5 × 20 mm balloon mini-Trek (Abbott Vascular, USA) successfully predilated the PLV for Thrombolysis In Myocardial Infarction (TIMI) 3 grade flow (Figure 2(b)). The intravascular ultrasound (IVUS) examination showed that the provisional stent from the PDV to the RCA proximal segment was appropriate with a low rate of PLV occlusion (Figure 2(c)). Stenting of the RCA into the PDV was performed using four Xience Prime stents (Abbott Vascular, USA). But angiography showed that PLV flow was slower in TIMI 1 grade flow after stents (Figure 2(d)). A retrograde 1.5 × 20 mm balloon successfully advanced through outside the PDA stent into the PLV to dilate it, and the flow was rescued (Figure 2(e)). To avoid the plaque shift to the PDA and preserve PLV flow, an antegrade 3.0 × 15 mm balloon Trek (Abbott Vascular, USA) with retrograde 2.0 × 20 mm Trek balloon performed the final kissing technique (FKT) to dilate bifurcation lesion with 14 atm, respectively (Figure 2(f)). Angiography and IVUS showed that PLV flow was successfully reserved (Figures 2(g) and 2(h)). At last, the retrograde guidewire and microcatheter were withdrawn, and RCA angiography showed no collateral circulation damage and rupture.

The total fluoroscopy time of the procedure was 170 minutes, and the total contrast volume delivered was 380 ml. The patient was followed up six months without symptom.

3. Discussion

In this case report, we described a new kissing technique for bifurcation lesion where one balloon was antegradely advanced in the main vessel and the other retrogradely advanced outside the main vessel stent. This was the reasonable approach because one of the limbs of the bifurcation could not be wired via the antegrade route and not rewired via retrograde approach. Al Aloul et al. [5] reported a case where a bifurcation lesion was treated with antegrade and retrograde "Head-to-Toe" kissing balloon angioplasty. But our case was different with his case for our retrograde balloon through outside of the main vessel stent for performing the kissing technique. To our knowledge, this was the first case report using this technique to dilate a bifurcation lesion.

Treating CTOs with a bifurcation at the distal cap can be challenging and often result in recanalization of only one of the branches [6]. Although new technique and devices have been developed, restoration of antegrade flow into both branches with large caliber still can be challenging. For this case, the CTO segment was very long with side branch. Antegrade approach might not be quite effective and failed to enter into the true lumen at bifurcation. Then, we turned to retrograde approach, in which epicardial collateral wire advanced into CTO segment and overlapped antegrade wire at the middle of CTO. We performed reverse CART technique and Guidezilla picking up retrograde wire with a Corsair guide, and RG3 wire externalization to completed RCA CTO.

The distal occlusion was located at the bifurcation site which had a markedly angulated PLV. It is considered that access to SB is usually more difficult in the case with the carina angle of more than 70 degrees and can be particularly difficult when the carina angle exceeds 90 degrees. Nomura et al. [7] reported the application of a "reverse bent wiring with the Crusade catheter" for wire crossing to a SB at the bifurcation lesion. It is actually a useful technique in our PCI center. But unfortunately, we failed into PLV by this technique in this case. Finally, we used a septal retrograde approach to preserve PLV flow by small profile balloon dilating it. Although IVUS examination showed the ostial area of PLV was enough with a low rate to occlude and also we conventionally adopted a jailed wire technique, the PLV still occlude after main branch stent. Kotsia et al. [8] reported the use of a retrograde Confianza Pro 12 guide wire rewiring into the main vessel stent through side branch and put stents followed by wire externalization. His technique might be safe and effective, but in our case, the carina angle of nearly 90 degrees in PLV made it more difficult to rewire though the ostial plaque of the PLV had been modified. The JBT is now emerging for protection of the side branch by reducing the risk of SB occlusion but with the risk of jailed balloon entrapment. In our case, once the retrograde balloon entrapment would cause severe injury. To overcome the dilemma situation, we tried small profile balloon (1.5 × 20 mm) advanced through the outside space of the main vessel stent and restored the flow of the PLV. Finally, the balloon kissing technique provided PL better flow without the main branch stent deformation.

Our case demonstrated an effective use of a retrograde approach for preserving a bifurcation at the distal CTO cap especially retrograde balloon dilating side branch outside of the main vessel stent. The retrograde balloon was smaller comparing with a traditional kissing technique in case of retrograde access injury, and the most important thing to remember was not to hard push the retrograde balloon.

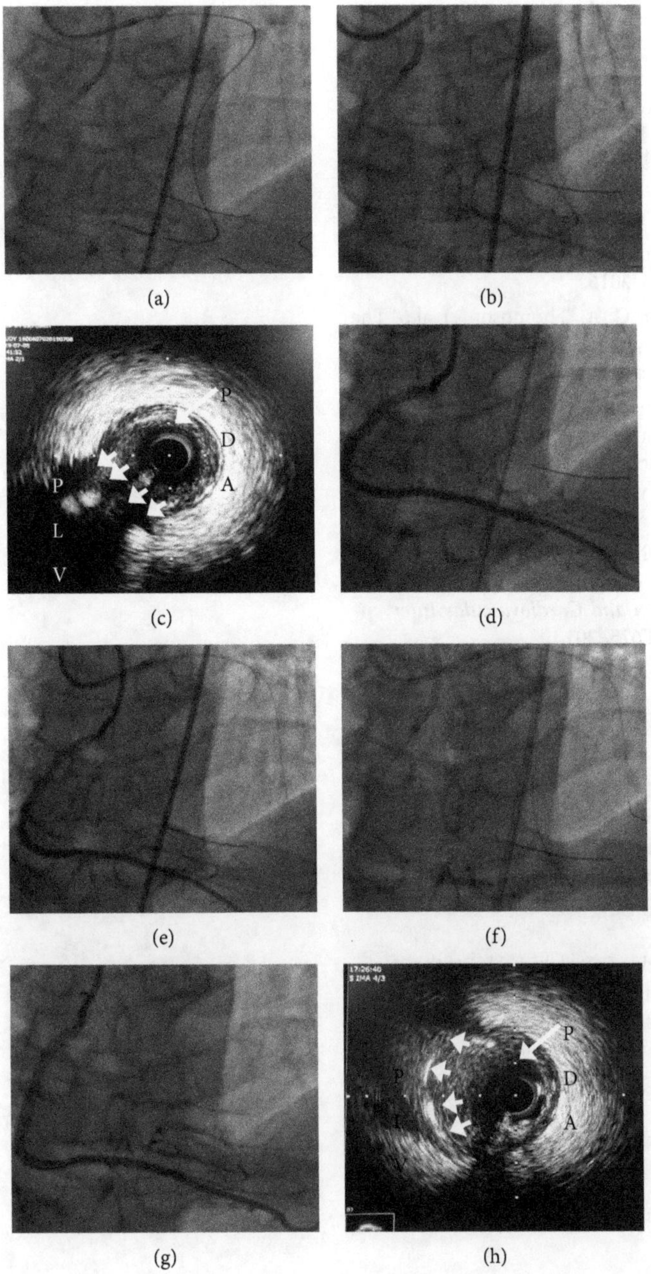

FIGURE 2: RCA bifurcation CTO PCI: (a) Corsair catheter in the right PLV placed retrograde via septal collaterals from the LAD and antegrade reverse bent wiring with the Crusade catheter failed into PLV; (b) recovery flow of PLV after retrograde balloon dilation; (c) IVUS showed PLV ostium had larger area before PDA stent; (d) angiography of RCA showing TIMI 1 grade flow in the right PLV after stent in the main vessel; (e) retrograde small profile balloon dilation to recovery PLV flow; (f) antegrade balloon and retrograde balloon outside the main branch stent final kissing technique; (g) the final result with flow in the right PDA and PLV; (h) IVUS showed the final PLV ostial area.

However, in similar cases, antegrade crossing was preferred if possible to keep side branch open, as it has a number of limitations. For example, it is difficult to cross or dilate small and tortuous septal channels and there exists the risk of septal injury. It is also easy to cause channel rupture, balloon trapping, and subintimal dissection.

However, given the technical difficulty and associated risks, the above technique of retrograde balloon dilating side branch outside of the main vessel stent should only be employed by experienced CTO operators. Additional cases are required to establish the success and reproducibility of this technique and to identify its limitations.

4. Conclusion

The technique of retrograde balloon dilating side branch outside the main vessel stent could be used to preserve both branches of a significant bifurcation at the CTO distal cap.

References

[1] E. S. Brilakis, S. Banerjee, D. Karmpaliotis et al., "Procedural outcomes of chronic total occlusion percutaneous coronary intervention: a report from the NCDR (National Cardiovascular Data Registry)," *JACC: Cardiovascular Interventions*, vol. 8, no. 2, pp. 245–253, 2015.

[2] W. M. Wilson, S. J. Walsh, A. T. Yan et al., "Hybrid approach improves success of chronic total occlusion angioplasty," *Heart*, vol. 102, no. 18, pp. 1486–1493, 2016.

[3] E. S. Brilakis, J. A. Grantham, C. A. Thompson et al., "The retrograde approach to coronary artery chronic total occlusions: a practical approach," *Catheterization and Cardiovascular Interventions*, vol. 79, no. 1, pp. 3–19, 2012.

[4] S. Saito, K. Shishido, N. Moriyama et al., "Modified jailed balloon technique for bifurcation lesions," *Catheterization and Cardiovascular Interventions*, vol. 92, no. 3, pp. E218–E226, 2018.

[5] B. Al Aloul, P. Guigari, and M. N. Burke, ""Head-to-toe" kissing balloon angioplasty during PCI of right coronary artery chronic total occlusion," *Catheterization and Cardiovascular Interventions*, vol. 82, no. 5, pp. E672–E675, 2013.

[6] E. S. Brilakis, J. A. Grantham, S. Rinfret et al., "A percutaneous treatment algorithm for crossing coronary chronic total occlusions," *JACC. Cardiovascular Interventions*, vol. 5, no. 4, pp. 367–379, 2012.

[7] T. Nomura, Y. Higuchi, and T. Kato, "Successful percutaneous coronary intervention for complex bifurcated lesions with combination of "reverse wire technique" and " reverse bent wiring with the crusade catheter" novel wire manipulation technique," *Catheterization and Cardiovascular Interventions*, vol. 87, no. 5, pp. 920–925, 2016.

[8] A. Kotsia, G. Christopoulos, and E. S. Brilakis, "Use of the retrograde approach for preserving the distal bifurcation after antegrade crossing of a right coronary artery chronic total occlusion," *The Journal of Invasive Cardiology*, vol. 26, no. 4, pp. E48–E49, 2014.

Polycythemia Vera Presenting as Cardiac Arrest: Novel Management Strategies

Mark I. Davis[1], **Brian K. Courtney**[1], **Gideon Cohen**[2], **Stephanie Poon**[1], **and Mina Madan**[1]

[1]*Division of Cardiology, Department of Medicine, Sunnybrook Health Sciences Centre, University of Toronto, Toronto, Canada*
[2]*Division of Cardiac Surgery, Department of Surgery, Sunnybrook Health Sciences Centre, University of Toronto, Toronto, Canada*

Correspondence should be addressed to Mina Madan; mina.madan@sunnybrook.ca

Academic Editor: Adam Torbicki

Acute coronary syndromes (ACS) usually occur in patients with multiple cardiac risk factors. In young adults, drug use and hypercoagulable states are common causes for ACS presentations. We report a case of a man in his early 30s who was diagnosed with polycythemia vera (PV) and had a cardiac arrest due to an anterolateral ST elevation myocardial infarction. We discuss his unique management and review the evidence on the management of arterial thromboembolism in PV patients.

1. Introduction

Acute coronary syndrome presentations in young adults are often unrelated to atherosclerosis and instead are commonly due to drug use (i.e., cocaine), underlying hypercoagulable states, and vascular abnormalities such as fibromuscular dysplasia. Additionally, myeloproliferative disorders such as polycythemia vera (PV) can lead to acute arterial thrombotic occlusions. Here, we present a case of a patient with PV, who had massive coronary artery thrombosis presenting with sudden cardiac arrest. Although there have been many similar case reports [1–6], none have described an ST elevation myocardial infarction with ventricular fibrillation arrest presentation nor the extent of arterial thrombosis observed in this patient and its unique management.

2. Case Report

A male in his early 30s had a witnessed cardiac arrest shortly after an emotionally stressful event. Bystander CPR was initiated immediately. When emergency medical services arrived, the presenting rhythm was ventricular fibrillation and 1 shock was delivered. He was intubated at the scene. Standard advanced cardiac life support was continued en route to the nearest emergency department. In total, four cycles of CPR, epinephrine, and defibrillation were given prior to the return of spontaneous circulation, obtained upon the patient's arrival at a community hospital. We were urgently contacted by the community hospital because his initial ECG was consistent with left bundle branch block morphology but then progressed on serial ECGs with significant ST elevations noted in leads I, AVL, and V4-V6 and ST depressions in leads III and aVF. The patient was transferred emergently to our institution for emergency coronary angiography in the setting of ST elevation myocardial infarction (STEMI). The patient's past medical history is significant for a stroke at age 7 without any residual deficits and hypertension. He was recently diagnosed with polycythemia vera (Janus kinase 2 (JAK2) positive) and was prescribed enteric-coated ASA 81 mg daily and hydroxyurea. The patient had previously been undergoing regular phlebotomy at our institution but had not attended these appointments over the last two months. It was unclear whether he was taking any medications at the time of presentation. Initial bloodwork showed the following: hemoglobin 184 g/L, hemotocrit 0.59, platelet count 1072×10^9/L, leukocytes 38.8×10^9/L, creatinine 142 μmol/L, hsTroponin 506 ng/L (peak 67322 ng/L) and CK 980 U/L (peak 9013 U/L), pH 7.12, and lactate was 9 mmol/L.

Upon arrival at our institution, he was in cardiogenic shock with a blood pressure (BP) of 95/80 mmHg and a heart rate (HR) of 110 bpm on 2.5 mcg/kg/min of intravenous (IV)

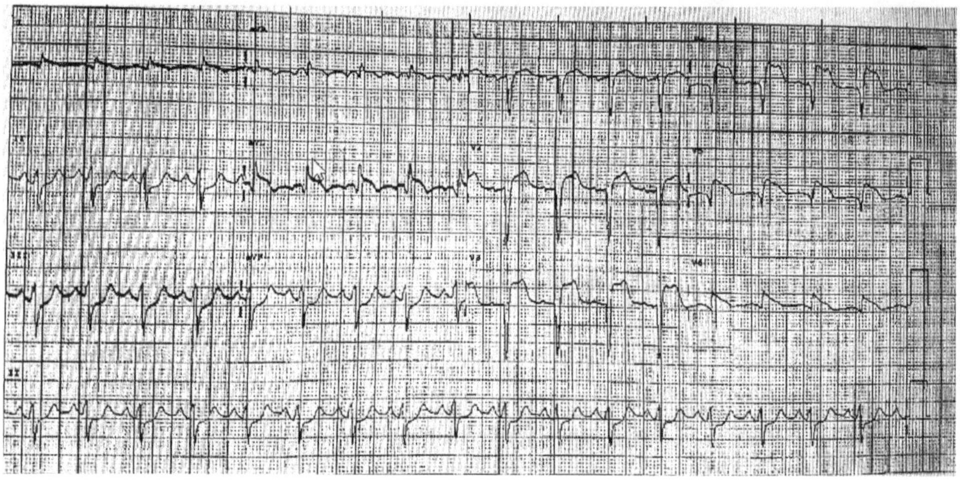

FIGURE 1: Presenting ECG at our institution: significant anterior and lateral ST elevations along with anterior and lateral Q waves. Based on this ECG as well as his extremis presentation, he was brought emergently to the cardiac catheterization lab.

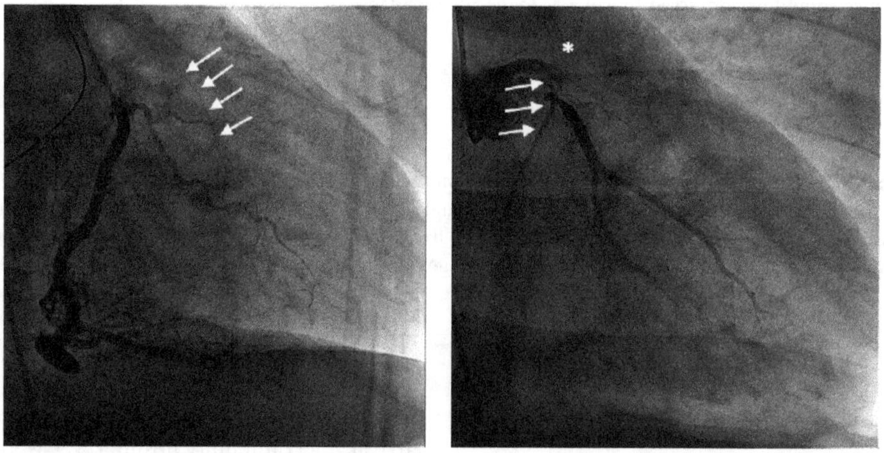

(a) (b)

FIGURE 2: (a). RAO projection demonstrating a normal and patent RCA and left-sided collaterals (white arrows). See Supplementary Video 1 for CINE. (b). RAO caudal projection of LCA. The LAD is occluded (*), and proximal LCX has a long 90% proximal stenosis (white arrows) and fills poorly after a large first obtuse marginal branch. See Supplementary Video 2 for CINE.

dopamine, 1 mg/min IV amiodarone, 20 mcg/kg/min IV propofol, and intermittent IV boluses of 50 mg rocuronium. He also received 120 mg of IV furosemide. IV norepinephrine was initiated at 10 mcg/min, and dopamine was discontinued. His ECG showed an anterolateral STEMI (Figure 1). ECASA 160 mg and ticagrelor 180 mg were given to the patient via the NG tube, and 4000 units of IV heparin was administered. He was brought urgently to the cardiac catheterization laboratory. Selective coronary angiography demonstrated a normal right coronary artery with collaterals to the left circumflex artery (LCX), complete occlusion of his left anterior descending artery (LAD), and a long 90% lesion of the proximal LCX (Figures 2(a) and 2(b), Supplementary Videos 1 and 2). The left ventricular end diastolic pressure was 30 mmHg. As he was on a significant amount of vasoactive medications for hemodynamic support, we did not believe it was appropriate to administer intra-arterial nitroglycerin at this time, nor did we feel this would lead to any change in his clinical management, as there was clear thrombus in the LM, LAD, and LCX. His oxygen saturation was 95% on 100% FiO_2, but his BP was 84/68 and HR 118 bpm, despite being on 15 mcg/min of IV norepinephrine. Based on the patient's clinical status and angiographic findings, an 8 French 40 cc intra-aortic balloon pump (IABP, Arrow® International, Teleflex Medical, Athlone, Ireland) was inserted into the right femoral artery followed by the administration of additional 7,000 IU (patient's weight was 110 kg and had already received 4000 units preprocedure) of intra-arterial heparin. We then proceeded with emergency percutaneous coronary intervention (PCI) on the LAD and LCX. There was a significant amount of thrombus in the LAD and LCX (Figure 3, Supplementary Video 3); and thus, 6 passes with a 6 French Export Advance™ Aspiration Catheter (Medtronic Inc., Minneapolis, MN) were performed. Soon after thrombectomy was completed, the patient experienced recurrent thrombosis of the left coronary system.

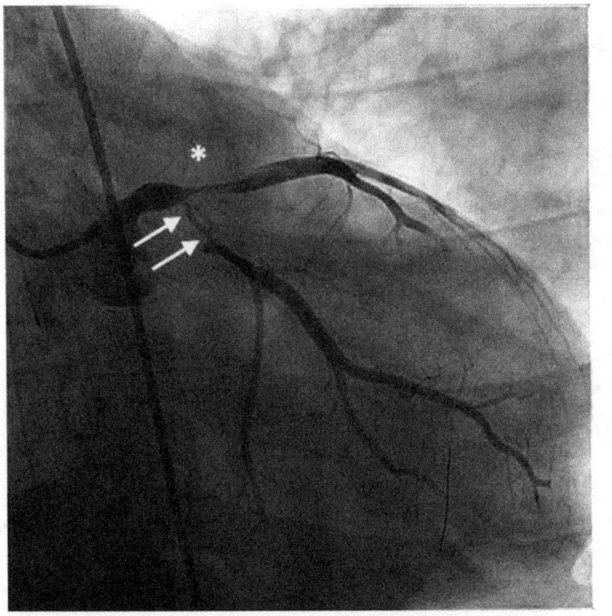

FIGURE 3: RAO caudal projection after initial ballooning of the LAD and LCX: extensive thrombus burden is noted in the LAD (*) and a 90% proximal LCX lesion (white arrows). See Supplementary Video 3 for CINE.

Repeat thrombectomy was performed; however, the thrombectomy catheter itself became clotted.

To combat the extensive thrombus formation in the setting of PV, we performed intraprocedural phlebotomy. A total of 550 mL of blood was phlebotomized, and two boluses of intracoronary eptifibatide were given. Despite this fact, there was a significant amount of recurrent thrombus formation and a second dose of intra-arterial heparin at 100 IU/kg was given for a total of 21,000 IU of IV unfractionated heparin which was administered for the procedure. Although an ACT was not drawn during the case, at the end of the case, it was 250 seconds. Eventually, the de novo coronary thrombosis stopped, and complex bifurcation stenting of the LAD, left main artery, and LCX could be performed using 2 drug-eluting stents and a bifurcation minicrush technique (Figure 4, Supplementary Videos 4 and 5). Despite these efforts, he remained in cardiogenic shock (BP 101/57 mmHg, HR 107 bpm) while on significant hemodynamic support (IABP at 1 : 1 cycle, IV norepinephrine 20 mcg/min, IV vasopressin 0.04 units/min, and IV epinephrine 20 mcg/min). The advanced heart failure and cardiac surgical teams were consulted, and the decision was made to bring the patient directly to the operating room for an emergency left ventricular assist device (LVAD-CentriMag, Thoratec Corporation, Pleasanton, CA), which the teams felt to be more appropriate than an extracorporeal membrane oxygenation circuit. Additionally, 1 g of hydroxyurea was given at the end of the procedure via an oral gastric tube following consultation with hematology for the acute treatment of PV.

His postoperative course was complicated by left-sided weakness and radiologic evidence of a new stroke (right occipital parietal subacute infarct with hemorrhagic transformation along with multiple small subacute infarcts in the right frontal, left frontal, and left parietal occipital regions), pneumonia, and a slow wean from the LVAD-CentriMag. Postprocedure imaging demonstrated evidence of significant mitral regurgitation secondary to complete flail of the anterior mitral valve leaflet with chordal rupture, which may have occurred following the emergency insertion of the CentriMag device. The patient underwent an Alfieri stitch procedure on LVAD removal, to reduce the degree of mitral regurgitation from severe to moderate. The patient eventually made significant neurological recovery and was discharged from the hospital to an inpatient cardiac rehabilitation facility, 38 days after admission to our institution. His ejection fraction at discharge was 25-35% with moderate mitral regurgitation.

After discharge, the patient had a single chamber ICD inserted due to the persistence of severe LV dysfunction with a left ventricular ejection fraction of 20-25% as well as moderate-to-severe RV dysfunction. The distal half of his LV, as well as the septum, was thinned and akinetic. Within 3 months after discharge, he was readmitted to the hospital with right-sided heart failure symptoms and weight gain. Investigations revealed portal vein thrombosis and right-sided heart failure as the causes. He has required multiple dose adjustments of his cardiac medications due to development of cardiorenal syndrome. At 1 year post MI, his ejection fraction remained <30% with anterior wall akinesis, aneurysmal apex, and moderate to severe mitral regurgitation. He continues to be followed by cardiology, a dedicated heart failure clinic, respirology, neurology, haematology, and nephrology.

3. Discussion

Polycythemia vera is a type of chronic myeloproliferative neoplasm. The diagnosis is based on the World Health Organization criteria [7], requiring all three majors or the first major and 1 minor criterion (major criteria: (1) hemoglobin > 165 g/L in men and >160 g/L in women or hematocrit > 49% in men and >48% in women or increased red cell mass, (2) hypercellular bone marrow with trilineage growth, and (3) presence of a JAK2 mutation; minor criteria: hypercellular bone marrow with trilineage growth, low serum erythropoietin levels, and endogenous erythroid colony formation). Clinical symptoms include pruritus, splenomegaly, vasomotor symptoms, and arterial and venous thrombosis. The JAK2 mutation is 95 to 100% sensitive in the diagnosis of PV. Our patient had both the major criteria at the time of diagnosis and has had evidence of arterial thromboembolism both on this current presentation (coronary and cerebrovascular) as well as when he was a child (cerebrovascular). We learned from the patient's hematologist that he was noncompliant with therapy, despite being prescribed cytoreductive therapy (hydroxyurea). Hydroxyurea has been shown to significantly reduce recurrent thrombotic complications such as stroke and myocardial infarction [8]. The incidence of thrombotic complications in PV patients ranges from 13 to 60%. The presence of traditional cardiac risk factors further increases the risk of thrombosis,

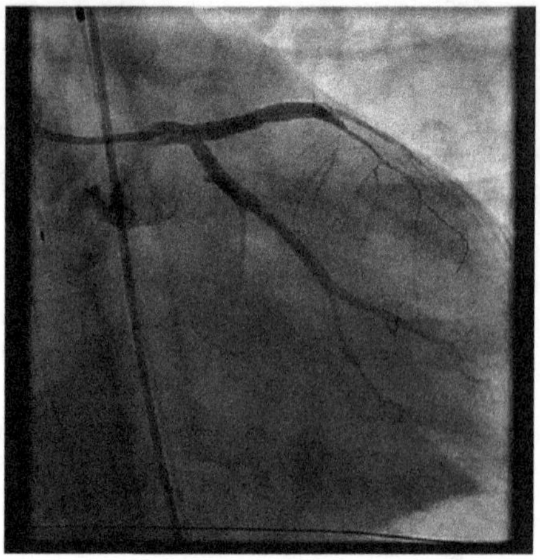

(a)

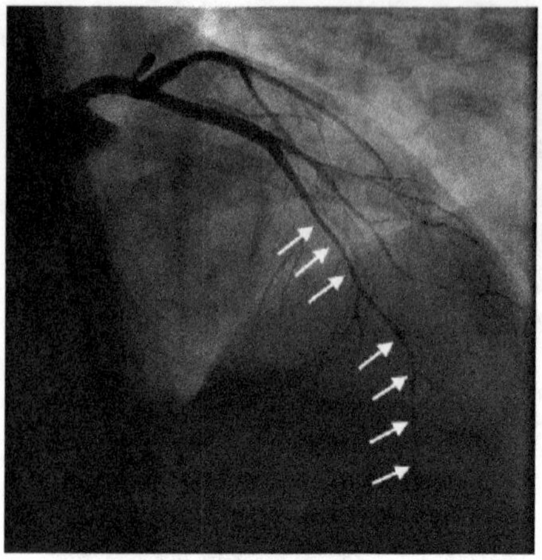

(b)

FIGURE 4: (a). RAO caudal projection. After PCI, the left main artery, LAD, and LCX are patent. See Supplementary Video 4 for CINE. (b). Diffuse distant vasoconstriction of the coronary arteries (white arrows) following PCI due to high doses of IV norepinephrine, epinephrine, and vasopressin. See Supplementary Video 5 for CINE.

especially coronary artery thrombosis [9]. Our patient had hypertension and was an active smoker, satisfying the above criteria.

In patients with PV, arterial thrombi form due to platelet activation, adhesion, and aggregation [10]. Proposed mechanisms of thrombogenesis are multifactorial but involve increased shear stress due to high hematocrit leading to vessel wall inflammation and closer contact of platelets to the endothelium leading to platelet activation. The use of intracoronary eptifibatide or abciximab inhibits platelet aggregation by reversibly blocking the GP IIb/IIIa receptor, decreasing fibrinogen and von Willebrand factor-mediated platelet activation [11]. Intracoronary eptifibatide doses can be up to 1000 times that delivered intravenously and can disaggregate the thrombus itself [12]. In the case of our patient, initially, there was recurrent thrombosis and the use of intracoronary eptifibatide may have decreased further thrombus formation, allowing the visualization of the coronary anatomy and PCI to be performed. Previously, a meta-analysis comparing the use of intracoronary to intravenous abciximab demonstrated a mortality benefit of intracoronary abciximab in primary PCI patients, although more recent data suggest no difference in myocardial damage with intracoronary or intravenous GP IIb/IIIa inhibitors [13, 14]. The subsequent INFUSE-AMI trial showed that among early presenting anterior STEMI patients, infarct size is decreased with the use of intracoronary abciximab but not manual aspiration thrombectomy [11]. In our patient, high-dose heparin was used synergistically with eptifibatide to block the coagulation cascade and prevent further intracoronary thrombus formation. To our knowledge, no other case reports have reported double bolus IV unfractionated heparin during primary PCI when there is such extensive thrombus burden. Although our ACT was therapeutic, we believed that in this young male, the benefit of extra heparin outweighed the risk of a potential bleed, and without preventing further thrombus formation, he likely would have died intraprocedurally. As the heparin and eptifibatide took effect, de novo thrombus formation decreased and PCI to the LAD and the LCX was possible. We do not feel that the intraprocedural heparin contributed to the hemorrhagic conversion of his thrombotic stroke, as the procedure and stoke were separated by multiple days and the heparin would have already been cleared from his system. He still would have had to have some heparin on board due to the CentriMag, and this could have increased the risk of hemorrhagic conversion.

In situations where the pathology is unclear, both IVUS and OCT can be helpful to determine pathology and possibly change management [15, 16]. It was clear that the LAD and LCX were occluded with thrombus, which is known to occur in patients with polycythemia vera without underlying atherosclerosis. As seen in the RCA injections, there was some collateral flow to the left system, although collaterals can form quite acutely and do not suggest chronic atherosclerotic disease in this patient [17]. Since this patient was hemodynamically unstable, the goal was to reestablish blood flow, irrespective of the underlying pathology; thus, no adjunctive imaging modalities were used. Furthermore, as we were unable to establish any significant flow down the coronary arteries until stent deployment, there would not have been enough opacification with contrast for OCT to be beneficial.

Prior publications have reported intraprocedural phlebotomy to combat thrombus formation, although they were not known to us at the time [3]. There are no guidelines addressing the acute management of arterial thromboembolism in patients with PV, especially in those with extremis presentations like our patient. The decision for phlebotomy as well as NG hydroxyurea was made empirically by the treatment team to try all means possible to preserve cardiac function and life. Our goal was to acutely reduce the hematocrit to <45%. Indeed, a prior study of non-PV patients which stratified STEMI patients based on hematocrit levels (anemia with hematocrit < 36% for women and <39% for men, normal hematocrit, or erythrocytosis with hematocrit > 46% for women and >47% for men) showed that although the one-month mortality was highest in patients with anemia, the odds ratio for mortality in patients with erythrocytosis was 4.3 [18]. Furthermore, PV treatment guidelines suggest targeting a hematocrit < 45% in PV patients to prevent arterial thromboembolism through phlebotomy and the use of cytoreductive therapy such as hydroxyurea [19, 20]. Although we used these measures to treat his PV acutely, these measures were maintained throughout his subsequent hospital stay. It is unlikely that randomized controlled trials would be able to be conducted with a sufficient number of patients to determine the optimal treatment method for PV patients with massive arterial thromboembolism presenting in an extremis fashion as the patient in our case, and we are acknowledging there is no evidence to support our treatment method.

The management of high intracoronary thrombus burden is difficult, and there are no guidelines regarding this management. Strategies to deal with high intracoronary thrombus burden include the use of adjunctive thrombectomy, intracoronary GP IIb/IIIa inhibitors, and/or intracoronary thrombolysis with PCI if immediate intervention is required, usually due to poor flow or an occluded vessel. But if there is TIMI 3 flow, another approach includes IV heparin and the use of IV GP IIb/IIIa inhibitors to allow for clot dissolution and then PCI later. Although the most recent ACC/AHA STEMI guidelines [21] have decreased the use of mechanical thrombus aspiration to Class 2b, for selective use, we do believe our patient was appropriate for aspiration thrombectomy. The ESC STEMI guidelines, [22] also recommended against routine thrombus aspiration, do suggest that thrombus aspiration may be considered in patients with large residual thrombus after wire and balloon attempts to open the vessel (which our patient would fall under) [23]. Although we agree that thrombectomy should not be used in all situations, for this patient, both his LAD and LCX were completely occluded by thrombus and he was in cardiogenic shock. These patients were not included in most of the thrombectomy trials [11, 24], or the number of cardiogenic shock patients was not identified for subgroup analysis [25, 26].

There are no large-scale trials that look at the use of intracoronary thrombolytics but only small single-centre trials that have shown positive results for thrombus dissolution after the use of thrombectomy and/or intracoronary GP IIb/IIIa inhibitors. The DISSOLUTION trial [27], which included approximately 100 patients, with 50 in each arm, showed decreased thrombus burden but no measurable change in MACE. The same was the case for the even smaller ICE T TIMI 49 study, which had 10 patients in each arm and once again showed that there was a decrease in thrombus burden but was not powered for a difference in MACE. Both studies demonstrated safety of IC thrombolytics with minimal to no bleeding events. The dosage used was between 1/5 and 1/3 of the systemic dose. At this dosage, there were no significant bleeding events. In these two small studies and a few other case reports, there seemed to be successful establishment of TIMI 3 flow after other standard PCI techniques failed without significant morbidity or mortality. The best approach in this situation would be the use of a microcatheter to allow for directed thrombolytic injection and not injection through the guide catheter which would result in significant "spillage" and a more systemic effect.

PV patients who undergo PCI are left with having a higher than normal risk of stent thrombosis, although the true risk is unknown, nor do any guidelines exist on the antiplatelet regimen that should be followed. Logically, using more potent P2Y12 inhibitors such as ticagrelor or prasugrel in combination with ASA would lead to a lower stent thrombosis risk than that of clopidogrel. No data exists on the use of anticoagulants in this scenario. Given the propensity for stent thrombosis in these patients, we agree that if the patient can be adequately treated without stent insertion, this would be preferable, but if unavoidable, dual antiplatelet therapy with aspirin and ticagrelor/prasugrel, in addition to hydroxyurea and phlebotomy, would likely result in the least long-term morbidity/mortality and the lowest risk of stent thrombosis.

4. Conclusion

Here, we presented a case of a young male with polycythemia vera who was noncompliant with treatment and who presented with sudden cardiac arrest due to massive and recurrent coronary thrombosis. Our unique treatment included a multipronged approach employing thrombectomy, acute phlebotomy, double-bolus intracoronary eptifibatide, and double-dose IV unfractionated heparin, allowing thrombus removal and prevention of recurrent coronary thrombosis. The patient eventually required temporary LVAD placement until his cardiac status improved and he made a relatively complete neurological recovery over 5 weeks from his initial presentation. This case highlights the importance of maintenance therapy among patients with polycythemia vera and the extremis presentation they can have with arterial thrombosis.

Supplementary Materials

Supplementary 1. Supplementary Video 1: RAO projection of the RCA demonstrating collaterals to the left system. Cinepak Codec.

Supplementary 2. Supplementary Video 2: RAO caudal projection of the LCA demonstrating an occluded LAD and significant stenosis of the proximal LCX. Cinepak Codec.

Supplementary 3. Supplementary Video 3: RAO caudal projection of the LAD and LCX post initial balloon dilation of the LAD. Extensive thrombus burden is seen. Cinepak Codec.

Supplementary 4. Supplementary Video 4: RAO caudal projection of the LAD and LCX post bifurcation stenting of the LAD, LM and LCX. The proximal vessels are patent with distal vessel constriction due to high doses of vasoconstrictors. Cinepak Codec.

Supplementary 5. Supplementary Video 5: RAO cranial projection of the LAD demonstrating a patent vessel with distal vessel vasoconstriction from high doses of norepinephrine, vasopressin, and epinephrine. Cinepak Codec.

References

[1] E. Rattarittamrong, L. Norasetthada, A. Tantiworawit et al., "Acute non-atherosclerotic ST-segment elevation myocardial infarction in an adolescent with concurrent hemoglobin H-constant spring disease and polycythemia vera," *Hematology Reports*, vol. 7, no. 3, p. 5941, 2015.

[2] A. Fujino, H. Hao, N. Kajimoto et al., "Restenosis after drug-eluting stent implantation in a patient with polycythemia vera: optical coherence tomography and pathological findings," *JACC: Cardiovascular Interventions*, vol. 8, no. 7, pp. e111–e112, 2015.

[3] C. F. Wu, G. P. Armstrong, R. A. Henderson, and P. N. Ruygrok, "Polycythaemia vera presenting as ST-elevation myocardial infarction," *Heart, Lung & Circulation*, vol. 14, no. 1, pp. 51–53, 2005.

[4] P. Venegoni and G. Cyprus, "Polycythemia and the heart. A review," *Texas Heart Institute Journal*, vol. 21, no. 3, pp. 198–201, 1994.

[5] T. Inami, M. Okabe, M. Matsushita et al., "JAK2 mutation and acute coronary syndrome complicated with stent thrombosis," *Heart and Vessels*, vol. 31, no. 10, pp. 1714–1716, 2016.

[6] H. Bahbahani, K. Aljenaee, and A. Bella, "Polycythemia vera presenting as acute myocardial infarction: an unusual presentation," *Journal of the Saudi Heart Association*, vol. 27, no. 1, pp. 57–60, 2015.

[7] D. A. Arber, A. Orazi, R. Hasserjian et al., "The 2016 revision to the World Health Organization classification of myeloid neoplasms and acute leukemia," *Blood*, vol. 127, no. 20, pp. 2391–2405, 2016.

[8] A. Tefferi, A. M. Vannucchi, and T. Barbui, "Polycythemia vera treatment algorithm 2018," *Blood Cancer Journal*, vol. 8, no. 1, p. 3, 2018.

[9] R. Landolfi, M. C. Cipriani, and L. Novarese, "Thrombosis and bleeding in polycythemia vera and essential thrombocythemia: pathogenetic mechanisms and prevention," *Best Practice & Research Clinical Haematology*, vol. 19, no. 3, pp. 617–633, 2006.

[10] M. H. Kroll, L. C. Michaelis, and S. Verstovsek, "Mechanisms of thrombogenesis in polycythemia vera," *Blood Reviews*, vol. 29, no. 4, pp. 215–221, 2015.

[11] G. W. Stone, A. Maehara, B. Witzenbichler et al., "Intracoronary abciximab and aspiration thrombectomy in patients with large anterior myocardial infarction: the infuse-ami randomized trial," *JAMA*, vol. 307, no. 17, pp. 1817–1826, 2012.

[12] H. E. Speich, R. R. Furman, L. T. Lands, G. D. Moodie, and L. K. Jennings, "Elevating local concentrations of GPIIb-IIIa antagonists counteracts platelet thrombus stability," *Journal of Thrombosis and Thrombolysis*, vol. 36, no. 1, pp. 31–41, 2013.

[13] Y. J. Shimada, N. C. Nakra, J. T. Fox, and Y. Kanei, "Meta-analysis of prospective randomized controlled trials comparing intracoronary versus intravenous abciximab in patients with ST-elevation myocardial infarction undergoing primary percutaneous coronary intervention," *The American Journal of Cardiology*, vol. 109, no. 5, pp. 624–628, 2012.

[14] I. Eitel, J. Wöhrle, H. Suenkel et al., "Intracoronary compared with intravenous bolus abciximab application during primary percutaneous coronary intervention in ST-segment elevation myocardial infarction: cardiac magnetic resonance substudy of the AIDA STEMI Trial," *Journal of the American College of Cardiology*, vol. 61, no. 13, pp. 1447–1454, 2013.

[15] T. Ma, B. Zhou, T. K. Hsiai, and K. K. Shung, "A review of intravascular ultrasound-based multimodal intravascular imaging: the synergistic approach to characterizing vulnerable plaques," *Ultrasonic Imaging*, vol. 38, no. 5, pp. 314–331, 2016.

[16] M. J. Suter, S. K. Nadkarni, G. Weisz et al., "Intravascular optical imaging technology for investigating the coronary artery," *JACC: Cardiovascular Imaging*, vol. 4, no. 9, pp. 1022–1039, 2011.

[17] C. Seiler, M. Stoller, B. Pitt, and P. Meier, "The human coronary collateral circulation: development and clinical importance," *European Heart Journal*, vol. 34, no. 34, pp. 2674–2682, 2013.

[18] G. Greenberg, A. Assali, H. Vaknin-Assa et al., "Hematocrit level as a marker of outcome in ST-segment elevation myocardial infarction," *The American Journal of Cardiology*, vol. 105, no. 4, pp. 435–440, 2010.

[19] R. Marchioli, G. Finazzi, G. Specchia et al., "Cardiovascular events and intensity of treatment in polycythemia vera," *New England Journal of Medicine*, vol. 368, no. 1, pp. 22–33, 2013.

[20] A. Tefferi and J. L. Spivak, "Polycythemia vera: scientific advances and current practice," *Seminars in Hematology*, vol. 42, no. 4, pp. 206–220, 2005.

[21] G. N. Levine, E. R. Bates, J. C. Blankenship et al., "2015 ACC/AHA/SCAI focused update on primary percutaneous coronary intervention for patients with ST-elevation myocardial infarction: an update of the 2011 ACCF/AHA/SCAI guideline for percutaneous coronary intervention and the 2013 ACCF/AHA guideline for the management of ST-elevation myocardial infarction," *Journal of the American College of Cardiology*, vol. 67, no. 10, pp. 1235–1250, 2016.

[22] B. Ibanez, S. James, S. Agewall et al., "2017 ESC guidelines for the management of acute myocardial infarction in patients presenting with ST-segment elevation the task force for the management of acute myocardial infarction in patients presenting with ST-segment elevation of the European Society of Cardiology (ESC)," *European Heart Journal*, vol. 39, no. 2, pp. 119–177, 2018.

[23] S. S. Jolly, S. James, V. Džavík et al., "Thrombus aspiration in ST-segment–elevation myocardial infarction," *Circulation*, vol. 135, no. 2, pp. 143–152, 2017.

[24] G. Sardella, M. Mancone, C. Bucciarelli-Ducci et al., "Thrombus aspiration during primary percutaneous coronary intervention improves myocardial reperfusion and reduces infarct size: the EXPIRA (thrombectomy with export catheter in infarct-related artery during primary percutaneous coronary intervention) prospective, randomized trial," *Journal of the American College of Cardiology*, vol. 53, no. 4, pp. 309–315, 2009.

[25] S. S. Jolly, J. A. Cairns, S. Yusuf et al., "Randomized trial of primary PCI with or without routine manual thrombectomy," *New England Journal of Medicine*, vol. 372, no. 15, pp. 1389–1398, 2015.

[26] T. Svilaas, P. J. Vlaar, I. C. van der Horst et al., "Thrombus aspiration during primary percutaneous coronary intervention," *New England Journal of Medicine*, vol. 358, no. 6, pp. 557–567, 2008.

[27] C. Greco, F. Pelliccia, G. Tanzilli et al., "Usefulness of local delivery of thrombolytics before thrombectomy in patients with ST-segment elevation myocardial infarction undergoing primary percutaneous coronary intervention (the delivery of thrombolytics before thrombectomy in patients with ST-segment elevation myocardial infarction undergoing primary percutaneous coronary intervention [DISSOLUTION] randomized trial)," *The American Journal of Cardiology*, vol. 112, no. 5, pp. 630–635, 2013.

Deep Vein Thrombosis after Femoral Arterial Access: Pathophysiologic and Therapeutic Challenges

Evan Harmon, Yoo Jin Lee, Sula Mazimba, Kanwar Singh, Aditya Sharma, and Younghoon Kwon

University of Virginia Health System, Charlottesville, VA, USA

Correspondence should be addressed to Evan Harmon; eharmon@virginia.edu

Academic Editor: Manabu Shirotani

Deep vein thrombosis (DVT) after femoral arterial access is a rare complication of left heart catheterization (LHC). The reasons for paradoxical venous clot formation after arterial access are identifiable in some cases but less clear in others. Here, we present one case of provoked DVT after femoral access followed by a second case in which clot formation appears to be spontaneous. Additionally, though each of the patients presented here demonstrated thrombus resolution, only one received anticoagulation. These cases highlight the complex pathophysiology of DVT following femoral arterial access and the challenges of management strategy selection.

1. Introduction

Femoral access site complications following left heart catheterization (LHC) or coronary angiography are well described and include arterial thrombosis, hematoma (both femoral and retroperitoneal), pseudoaneurysm, and arteriovenous fistula. Another vascular femoral access site complication that is less often encountered is deep vein thrombosis (DVT). The few reports of DVT after femoral arterial access in the published literature have also cited one or more other provoking factors which could explain venous thrombus formation. However, a subset of patients without overt DVT risk factors appear to suffer DVT after femoral arterial access for reasons that remain unclear.

2. Case Descriptions

2.1. Case 1. An 83-year-old man with a history of rheumatic mitral stenosis (MS) and atrial fibrillation underwent preoperative cardiac catheterization with the artery and venous access obtained under direct ultrasound visualization without difficulty using a 6 Fr sheath and 7 Fr sheath, respectively, for concurrent left and right heart catheterization. Femoral access was chosen given recent computed tomography (CT) angiogram of the chest, abdomen, and pelvis demonstrating extremely tortuous supra-aortic vessels, complicating radial access. Upon completion of his catheterization procedure, the arterial sheath was removed once ACT was below 180 seconds. Per standard catheterization laboratory protocol, firm manual compression with full pressure was applied for five minutes, followed by gentler pressure for five minutes until hemostasis was visually ascertained. An intermittent pedal pulse check confirmed distal perfusion during this time. In the immediate postcatheterization period, the patient was noted to have a small right groin hematoma which resolved with an additional few minutes of direct compression.

Five days later, the patient presented to the emergency department with progressive right thigh pain, ecchymoses, swelling, and difficulty ambulating. CT scan demonstrated a 14 cm right-sided femoral hematoma, and follow-up CT angiogram revealed a $2.3 \times 2.0 \times 3.5$ cm right profunda femoris proximal branch pseudoaneurysm associated with the hematoma. This study also demonstrated severe stenosis of the right superficial femoral vein secondary to extrinsic compression with nonocclusive wall adherent thrombus in the right midpopliteal vein (Figure 1).

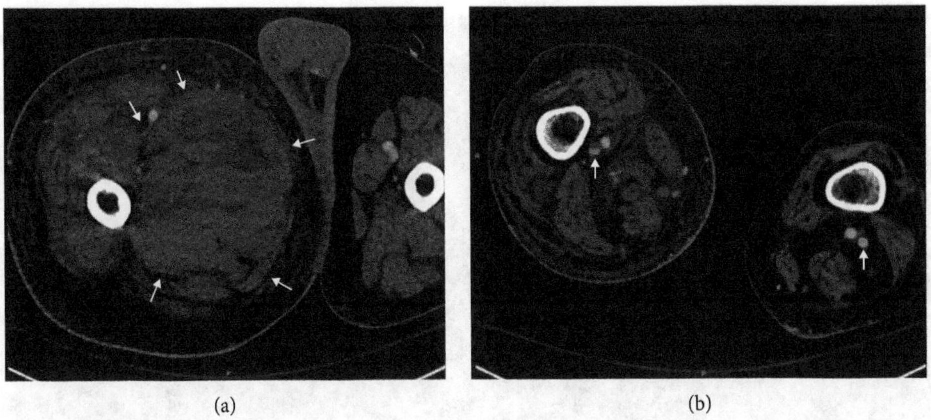

FIGURE 1: (a) Collapsed right-sided common femoral vein (white arrow) due to massive hematoma (yellow arrows). (b) Nonocclusive thrombus in right-sided midpopliteal vein, compared to patient left-sided midpopliteal vein (white arrows).

Coil embolization of his pseudoaneurysm was attempted, but two hours post procedure, the patient demonstrated severe motor and sensory deficits in the right lower extremity with associated hemoglobin drop from 8.1 g/dL to 6.0 g/dL. He was taken for emergent surgical evacuation of his right thigh hematoma.

Though his course was further complicated by additional mild, transfusion-responsive bleeding events, his bleeding ultimately stabilized and the patient was successfully transitioned back to his home warfarin dose by the day of discharge to be continued indefinitely in the setting of his known atrial fibrillation. A follow-up ultrasound obtained two weeks after initial identification of the patient's midpopliteal DVT demonstrated thrombus resolution.

2.2. Case 2. A 40-year-old man with a history of hypertension and hyperlipidemia was referred for a one-month history of exertional chest pain consistent with typical angina. Cardiac CT demonstrated multivessel disease, and LHC was pursued.

The right femoral artery was accessed using a 6 Fr sheath under direct ultrasound visualization. Following the procedure, an Angio-Seal™ closure device (St. Jude Medical, Minnetonka, Minnesota) was used to achieve hemostasis. Manual compression was still applied for about three minutes. Access site examination was unremarkable, without bruit auscultation or evidence of hematoma.

One week after PCI, the patient reported new, worsening groin pain radiating to the abdomen. Ultrasound was ordered for suspected pseudoaneurysm but instead demonstrated nonocclusive thrombus within the right common femoral vein without evidence of hematoma or arterial pathology (Figure 2). Hypercoagulability testing was unrevealing: antithrombin-III function, Protein C activity, Protein S activity, anti-cardiolipin IgM/IgG, and anti-beta-2-glycoprotein-1 IgM/IgG were all within normal limits. Factor V Leiden and prothrombin assays were unremarkable. Serum homocysteine was only mildly elevated at 14 μmol/L (reference range 5-12 μmol/L). Given these findings, three months of oral anticoagulation in addition to the patient's dual antiplatelet regimen was planned, but it was later found that the patient had not taken his oral anticoagulation as instructed. Interestingly, he did report resolution of his groin pain and ipsilateral edema, and follow-up CT venogram one month later revealed thrombus resolution (Figure 3).

3. Discussion

DVT following femoral arterial access is considered to be a relatively rare vascular complication of LHC with an estimated incidence of 0.05% [1]. Though radial rather than femoral access is becoming more common for routine LHC, the latter remains critical for procedures requiring larger vascular sheath sizes (and longer compression times) such as intra-aortic balloon pump or percutaneous left ventricular assist device placement. It is also the preferable access modality for patients with coronary artery bypass grafts and hemodialysis arteriovenous fistula [2, 3]. DVT incidence following LHC may therefore be underestimated, though prospective investigations with systematic screening are necessary to objectively confirm.

The majority of published DVT cases following femoral arterial access demonstrate a clear provocation in the form of mechanical deep venous compression by a known hematoma, or by concurrent arterial and venous access, such as in Case 1 [4]. Additionally, the age and relative immobility of the patient described in Case 1 represent at least two additional nonmechanical risk factors for DVT formation. In contrast, Case 2 represents only the second reported case of seemingly unprovoked DVT formation following LHC utilizing femoral arterial access [5]. In such "unprovoked" cases, we suspect a likely inadvertent venous compression during femoral arterial hemostasis as the mechanism for DVT formation. Supporting this hypothesis is the evidence that DVTs in this setting arise almost universally in the proximal rather than distal lower extremity venous system, which is reflected in our two cases. Literature review demonstrates only one other case of distal DVT following LHC [5], suggesting a strong anatomical relationship between the sites of access, hemostasis, and subsequent thrombus formation.

An important question to consider is whether and to what degree the use of a vascular closure device (VCD) in Case 2 may have contributed to DVT formation. To date,

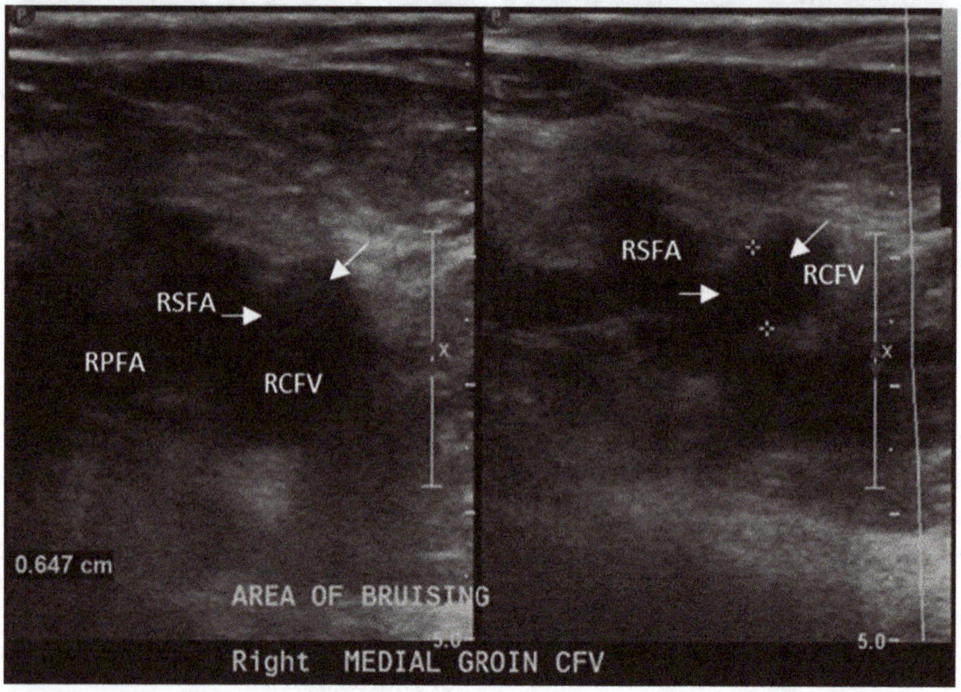

(a) (b)

Figure 2: Partially thrombosed (white arrows) right common femoral vein. (a) is without compression; (b) is with compression, which demonstrates incomplete collapse of the RCFV.

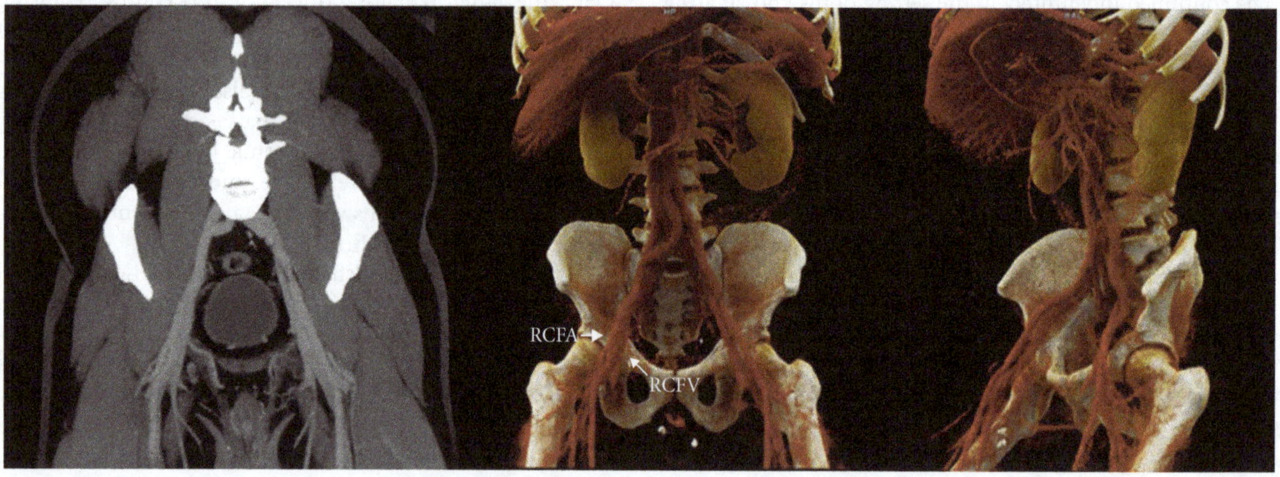

Figure 3: MIP (maximal intensity projection) and 3D cinematic rendering images of the CT venogram performed 1 month after the ultrasound exam were normal, with no evidence of residual venous thrombus or traumatic pseudoaneurysm.

large meta-analyses comparing outcomes between manual compression and VCDs have yielded conflicting results. However, the ISAR-CLOSURE trial, which randomized over four thousand patients undergoing coronary angiography to the hemostasis strategies of manual compression, intravascular closure device, or extravascular closure device in a 1 : 1 : 1 fashion, demonstrated that VCDs overall have similar rates of vascular complications compared to manual compression while achieving hemostasis quicker [6]. Among the VCD group, intravascular closure devices such as Angio-Seal™ trended toward significantly fewer access site complications while achieving hemostasis significantly quicker than extravascular devices. These findings would suggest that the use of the Angio-Seal™ closure device in Case 2 is unlikely to explain DVT formation, though an important limitation of the ISAR-CLOSURE trial and others is the lack of inclusion of DVT formation as part of the primary endpoint. One prospective study of over six hundred patients found no difference in minor complications (including DVT) between Angio-Seal™, StarClose™ (extravascular closure device), and manual compression, but additional studies with specific focus on DVT formation following femoral arterial access are needed [7].

Additionally, hypercoagulable workup may be reasonable in select patients in whom the factors contributing to DVT formation following femoral arterial access are not immediately clear. For example, our patient in Case 2 was found to have mild hyperhomocysteinemia, a well-described risk factor for inherent endothelial dysfunction [8]. This finding supports the notion that it is likely the combination of inadvertent arterial compression during hemostasis *and* underlying patient susceptibility which results in seemingly "unprovoked" DVT formation in a subset of cases.

Finally, DVT formation following a percutaneous coronary intervention (PCI) may be therapeutically challenging. In these cases, "triple therapy," i.e., the addition of oral anticoagulation to dual antiplatelet therapy (DAPT), in the post-PCI setting markedly increases bleeding risk [9]. Nonetheless, current European Society of Cardiology (ESC) guidelines recommend that among most patients with a baseline anticoagulation indication (e.g., atrial fibrillation and mechanical heart valve) undergoing PCI, triple therapy should be continued through at least one month postprocedurally [10]. The most recent CHEST guidelines recommend OAC for three-month duration in the setting of an acute provoked proximal DVT [11]. This regimen was recommended to the patient in Case 2, though he ultimately demonstrated spontaneous resolution of his DVT without anticoagulation. This raises the interesting question of whether less aggressive antithrombotic regimens may be reasonable in select patients found to have DVT following femoral arterial access. Overall, however, these challenges in management should highlight the importance of emphasizing DVT prophylaxis strategies in standard post-LHC management protocols.

In summary, DVT formation is an important potential complication of femoral access LHC. A subset of patients suffer seemingly unprovoked DVT, the pathophysiology of which is unclear but may be attributable to inadvertent venous compression during hemostasis in combination with patient-specific susceptibility factors. Additional research is necessary to guide therapeutic decision-making, particularly in patients requiring DAPT.

4. Conclusion

DVT formation is a rare but increasingly reported complication of femoral arterial access LHC. Clot formation in some cases is easily attributable to mechanical venous compression due to arterial complications such as hematoma formation. However, there appears to be a subset of patients in whom DVT formation is unprovoked. The pathophysiology of unprovoked DVT in this setting is unclear but may be attributable to inadvertent venous compression during arterial hemostasis in combination with patient-specific susceptibility factors. Additional research is necessary to not only clearly delineate the mechanism responsible for unprovoked DVT after femoral arterial access but also guide therapeutic decision-making, particularly in patients on DAPT.

References

[1] K. Filis, F. Arhontovasilis, D. Theodorou et al., "Management of early and late detected vascular complications following femoral arterial puncture for cardiac catheterization," *Hellenic Journal of Cardiology*, vol. 48, no. 3, pp. 134–142, 2007.

[2] T. T. Michael, M. Alomar, A. Papayannis et al., "A randomized comparison of the transradial and transfemoral approaches for coronary artery bypass graft angiography and intervention: the RADIAL-CABG trial (RADIAL versus femoral access for coronary artery bypass graft angiography and intervention)," *JACC: Cardiovascular Interventions*, vol. 6, no. 11, pp. 1138–1144, 2013.

[3] National Kidney Foundation, "Clinical Practice Guidelines for Vascular Access," *American Journal of Kidney Diseases*, vol. 48, Supplement 1, pp. S248–S273, 2006.

[4] M. Kim, J. Y. Lee, C. W. Lee et al., "Deep vein thrombosis due to hematoma as a rare complication after femoral arterial catheterization," *Yeungnam University Journal of Medicine*, vol. 30, no. 1, pp. 31–35, 2013.

[5] S. Y. Min, J. H. Shin, S. W. Lee et al., "A case of deep vein thrombosis after coronary angiography in a patient using antidepressants and anxiolytics," *Korean Circulation Journal*, vol. 43, no. 2, pp. 132–134, 2013.

[6] S. Schulz-Schüpke, S. Helde, S. Gewalt et al., "Comparison of vascular closure devices vs manual compression after femoral artery puncture: the ISAR-CLOSURE randomized clinical trial," *JAMA*, vol. 312, no. 19, pp. 1981–1987, 2014.

[7] H. Yeni, M. Axel, A. Ornek, T. Butz, P. Maagh, and G. Plehn, "Clinical and subclinical femoral vascular complications after deployment of two different vascular closure devices or manual compression in the setting of coronary intervention," *International Journal of Medical Sciences*, vol. 13, no. 4, pp. 255–259, 2016.

[8] M. M. Eldibany and J. A. Caprini, "Hyperhomocysteinemia and thrombosis: an overview," *Archives of Pathology & Laboratory Medicine*, vol. 131, no. 6, pp. 872–884, 2007.

[9] D. L. Staudacher, M. Kaiser, C. Hehrlein, C. Bode, and I. Ahrens, "Triple antithrombotic therapy after percutaneous coronary intervention (PCI) in patients with indication for oral anticoagulation: data from a single center registry," *PLoS One*, vol. 10, no. 10, article e0140101, 2015.

[10] M. Valgimigli, H. Bueno, R. A. Byrne et al., "2017 ESC focused update on dual antiplatelet therapy in coronary artery disease developed in collaboration with EACTS: the Task Force for dual antiplatelet therapy in coronary artery disease of the European Society of Cardiology (ESC) and of the European Association for Cardio-Thoracic Surgery (EACTS)," *European Heart Journal*, vol. 39, no. 3, pp. 213–260, 2018.

[11] C. Kearon, E. A. Akl, J. Ornelas et al., "Antithrombotic therapy for VTE disease: CHEST guideline and expert panel report," *Chest*, vol. 149, no. 2, pp. 315–352, 2016.

36

Achalasia as an Unusual Cause of Acute Cellular Rejection of a Transplanted Heart

Amanda Fernandes,[1] Crystal Lihong Yan,[1] Phillip Ruiz,[2] and Nina Thakkar Rivera[3]

[1]*Division of Internal Medicine, University of Miami/Jackson Memorial Hospital, Miami, FL, USA*
[2]*Departments of Surgery and Pathology, University of Miami/Jackson Memorial Hospital, Miami, FL, USA*
[3]*Division of Cardiology, Miami Transplant Institute, University of Miami/Jackson Memorial Hospital, Miami, FL, USA*

Correspondence should be addressed to Crystal Lihong Yan; crystaly@med.miami.edu

Academic Editor: Gopal Chandra Ghosh

A 68-year-old female with end-stage heart failure presented to the hospital for heart transplant. She was diagnosed with achalasia 14 months prior and treated with frequent botulinum toxin injections. She underwent orthotopic heart transplant on the day of admission and was extubated a few days later. She developed intractable nausea and vomiting. Her first endomyocardial biopsy revealed moderate, approaching severe rejection. She was treated with high-dose intravenous pulse steroids. Fluoroscopy at the time of follow-up biopsy showed undigested pills in her esophagus with narrowing at the distal end and thus failure to deliver immunosuppressive therapy. This case highlights achalasia as an etiology for acute rejection and its potential management.

1. Introduction

Acute allograft rejection is the most feared complication following heart transplantation. There are several types of rejection of which the classification and appropriate treatment are based on the type (cellular or humoral), timing posttransplant (hyperacute, acute, and chronic), and grade (mild, moderate, and severe) [1]. The most common type of heart transplant rejection is acute cellular rejection. It is a T-cell-mediated process that often happens in the first 3 to 6 months posttransplant. However, it may occur any time and can be prevented with adequate doses of maintenance immunosuppressive therapy. Hyperacute rejection is rare given the ABO matching between donor and recipient prior to transplant and the prospective cross-matching for HLA. In high-risk cases, higher doses of immunosuppression are given perioperatively (called induction therapy) to avoid the donor antigen expression and subsequent immune response by the recipient [1, 2].

While rejection is mostly commonly thought of as having an immunologic etiology, the etiology can also be mechanical. Esophageal dysmotility and subsequent failure to deliver immunosuppressive therapy are a rare etiology of allograft rejection posttransplant. Prompt identification of a mechanical etiology is crucial to treat rejection. In the following case, we report an unusual cause of transplant rejection due to a preexisting anatomic abnormality from achalasia resulting in the inability to achieve proper immunosuppression.

2. Case Presentation

A 68-year-old female with a past medical history of end-stage heart failure with reduced ejection fraction secondary to nonischemic cardiomyopathy on chronic milrinone infusion for the past 13 months, presented to the hospital at the instruction of her transplant team after being matched with a donor. She was originally listed as UNOS status 1B and later converted to UNOS status 4 with the new allocation system. She had also been diagnosed with achalasia 14 months prior with biopsies negative for eosinophilic esophagitis and serologies negative for Chagas disease. Due to high surgical risk, her achalasia was managed with frequent botulinum toxin (Botox) injections, resulting in improvement of her dysphagia. The last injection was one month prior to heart transplant.

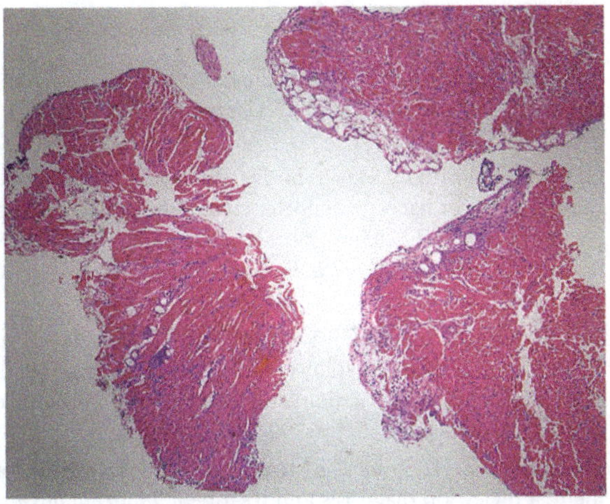

FIGURE 1: First endomyocardial biopsy posttransplant demonstrating moderate acute cellular rejection with mildly diffuse lymphocytic infiltrates and focal myocardial ischemic injury.

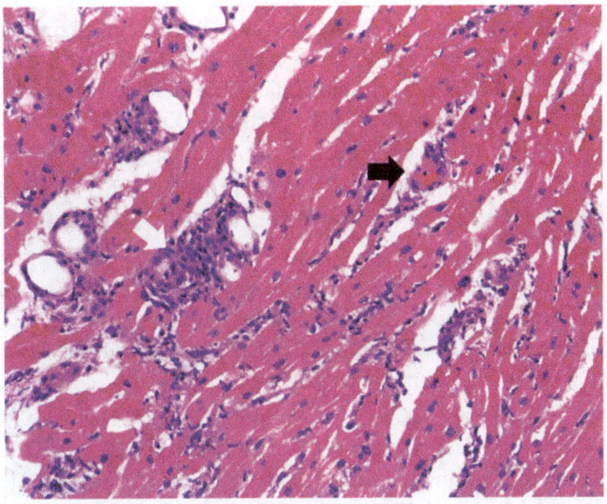

FIGURE 2: Close up image showing cardiac myocytes surrounded by dense collections of inflammatory cells (white arrow) and focal capillaritis (black arrow), consistent with grade 2R (borderline 3R) rejection.

She underwent orthotopic heart transplant on the day of admission and was successfully extubated on postoperative day 4 (POD). However, over the following days, she developed intractable nausea and vomiting. Her first endomyocardial biopsy on POD 12 revealed grade 2R approaching 3R rejection (Figures 1 and 2). She remained hemodynamically stable and was treated with high-dose intravenous pulse steroids. Fluoroscopy at the time of follow-up biopsy revealed undigested pills in her esophagus and narrowing at the distal end (Figure 3). This led to a barium swallow series (Figure 4), which confirmed the diagnosis of achalasia as the etiology for her acute rejection.

To address the cause of her rejection, she underwent percutaneous endoscopic gastrostomy (PEG) tube placement within three weeks of transplantation for the sole purpose of immunosuppression delivery. Furthermore, she received a

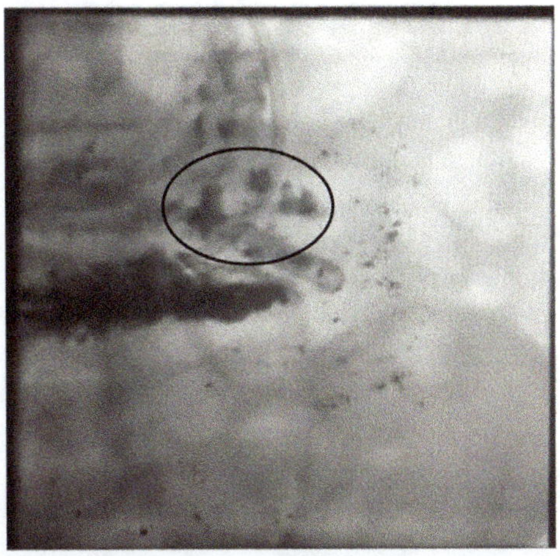

FIGURE 3: Fluoroscopy images at the time of endomyocardial biopsy demonstrating residual medications at the distal end of the esophagus (circle).

temporizing injection of Botox to her lower esophageal sphincter with relief of her refractory nausea and vomiting. She was discharged after a 5-week hospital course in stable condition and with control of her acute rejection down to grade 1R. Unfortunately, her disease course was further complicated by multiple admissions for a clogged PEG tube, compromising her immunosuppression delivery. In addition, she continued to receive multiple Botox injections for dysphagia and severe acid reflux until it no longer worked. Given her history of multiple PEG tube malfunctions and inability to take her transplant antirejection medications orally, she underwent a laparoscopic Heller myotomy procedure 7 months posttransplant. Since then, she has remained without rejection and on stable doses of immunosuppression.

3. Discussion

Achalasia is rare type of neurodegenerative dysmotility disorder with an estimated incidence of around 1.5 to 2 per 100,000 person-years [3]. It affects the lower portion of the esophagus causing dysphagia, weight loss, chest pain, acid reflux, and food regurgitation [4]. The most definitive therapy for achalasia is surgical myotomy, followed by graded pneumatic dilation [5]. However, posttransplant, surgery is ideally avoided for up to 1 year.

In our case, we kept the patient stable without rejection for as long as we could and ultimately opted for surgical myotomy sooner than 1 year because of her risk for rejection without adequate delivery of her immunosuppressive medications. Botox can be a temporary treatment in patients with high surgical risk, as was our patient, although its efficacy is debatable. Studies have shown minimal improvement in symptoms for a limited time [4] or no improvement [6].

Solid organ transplant recipients are commonly affected by gastrointestinal complications, which can be related to the surgical procedure itself, opportunistic infections, or side effects from immunosuppressive medications [7]. In a retrospective cohort study, the presence of esophagogastric outflow obstruction, gastroesophageal reflux, and incomplete transit of

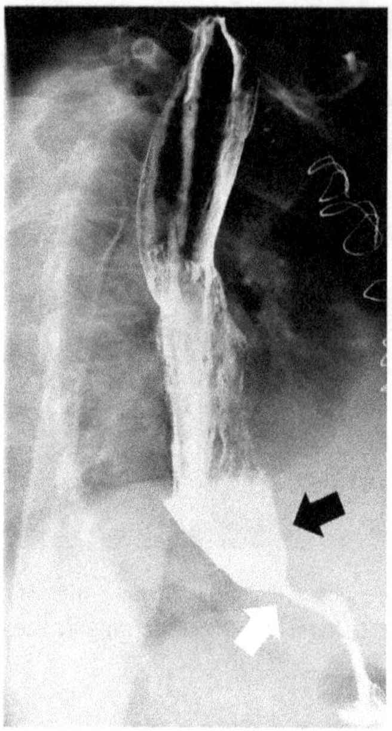

Figure 4: Barium swallow study demonstrating achalasia. There is significant narrowing at the lower esophageal sphincter (white arrow) with pooling of contrast in the distal esophagus (black arrow) and markedly delayed transit of contrast into the stomach.

food bolus were independently associated with obstructive chronic lung allograft dysfunction [8], but there is no data on those factors being related to heart transplant rejection.

To the best of our knowledge, this is the first reported case describing a patient with a pretransplant diagnosis of achalasia who was managed initially with Botox injections due to her high surgical risk and developed acute heart transplant rejection because of failure to deliver an immunosuppressive regimen at the absorbing portion of her gastrointestinal tract. Fluoroscopy performed during follow-up endomyocardial biopsy revealed the undigested pills in her distal esophagus and was key in allowing prompt recognition of the true etiology behind her acute rejection.

The current indications for PEG tube placement are for long-term enteral feeding in patients with functional gastrointestinal systems or for gastric decompression [9]. But here, we report another feasible and life-saving indication, which is to avoid transplant rejection in patients with esophageal dysmotility. In our case, the PEG tube was a temporary measure until her recovery post-heart transplant in order to receive the appropriate long-term solution.

4. Conclusion

We described a case of achalasia causing acute allograft rejection due to the anatomic inability to deliver immunosuppressive therapy after heart transplantation. In patients undergoing evaluation for solid organ transplant and with clinical concern for esophageal dysmotility, it is important to rule out achalasia on barium swallow and manometry studies. If confirmed, a multidisciplinary plan should be created prior to transplantation given the heightened risk of acute allograft failure.

References

[1] J. Lindenfeld, G. G. Miller, S. F. Shakar et al., "Drug therapy in the heart transplant recipient," *Circulation*, vol. 110, no. 24, pp. 3734–3740, 2004.

[2] C. Sánchez-Enrique, U. P. Jorde, and J. González-Costello, "Trasplante cardiaco y soporte circulatorio mecanico para pacientes con insuficiencia cardiaca avanzada," *Revista Española de Cardiología (English Edition)*, vol. 70, no. 5, pp. 371–381, 2017.

[3] P. R. Harvey, T. Thomas, J. S. Chandan et al., "Incidence, morbidity and mortality of patients with achalasia in England: findings from a study of nationwide hospital and primary care data," *Gut*, vol. 68, no. 5, pp. 790–795, 2019.

[4] J. Tuason and H. Inoue, "Current status of achalasia management: a review on diagnosis and treatment," *Journal of Gastroenterology*, vol. 52, no. 4, pp. 401–406, 2017.

[5] C. E. Weber, C. S. Davis, H. J. Kramer, J. T. Gibbs, L. Robles, and P. M. Fisichella, "Medium and long-term outcomes after pneumatic dilation or laparoscopic Heller myotomy for achalasia," *Surgical Laparoscopy, Endoscopy & Percutaneous Techniques*, vol. 22, no. 4, pp. 289–296, 2012.

[6] F. Mion, S. Marjoux, F. Subtil et al., "Botulinum toxin for the treatment of hypercontractile esophagus: results of a double-blind randomized sham-controlled study," *Neurogastroenterology and Motility*, vol. 31, no. 5, article e13587, 2019.

[7] B. Díaz, F. González Vilchez, L. Almenar et al., "Gastrointestinal complications in heart transplant patients: MITOS study," *Transplantation Proceedings*, vol. 39, no. 7, pp. 2397–2400, 2007.

[8] A. Tangaroonsanti, A. S. Lee, M. D. Crowell et al., "Impaired esophageal motility and clearance post-lung transplant: risk for chronic allograft failure," *Clinical and Translational Gastroenterology*, vol. 8, no. 6, article e102, 2017.

[9] A. A. Rahnemai-Azar, A. A. Rahnemaiazar, R. Naghshizadian, A. Kurtz, and D. T. Farkas, "Percutaneous endoscopic gastrostomy: indications, technique, complications and management," *World Journal of Gastroenterology*, vol. 20, no. 24, pp. 7739–7751, 2014.

37

Acute Limb Ischemia Caused by Dissection following Percutaneous Coronary Intervention using Right Radial Approach

Haris Ahmed,[1] Jonathan Brown,[1] Brooke Walterscheid,[1] Phebe Abraham,[1] Junaid Alam,[1] Nabeel Ahmad,[1] and Syed Arman Raza[2]

[1]*Department of Internal Medicine, HCA Houston Kingwood/University of Houston College of Medicine, USA*
[2]*Department of Cardiology, HCA Houston Kingwood/University of Houston College of Medicine, USA*

Correspondence should be addressed to Haris Ahmed; haris.ahmed@hcahealthcare.com

Academic Editor: Muhammad Zia-Ul-Haq

Iatrogenic aortic dissection is a rare but potentially fatal complication of percutaneous coronary intervention (PCI). Iatrogenic aortic dissection following PCI is rare with most cases reporting dissection originating within the coronary vessels with propagation into the ascending aorta. In this specific case, dissection was without coronary involvement, with dissection extending from the ascending aorta into the descending aorta and iliac vessels. Although PCI via radial approach is associated with fewer vascular complications than with femoral approach, significant adverse outcomes may still occur and require prompt intervention. This case highlights the highly atypical presentation of iatrogenic aortic dissection following cardiac catheterization presenting as acute limb ischemia. In such patients as with ours, immediate surgical intervention is necessary with overall poor prognosis.

1. Introduction

Iatrogenic aortic dissection (IAD) secondary to PCI may present variably and without prompt diagnosis and intervention, while outcomes may be unfavorable. Percutaneous coronary intervention via radial approach has been associated with reduced complications and bleeding rates when compared with femoral approach; however, features associated with radial approach may predispose patients to aortic dissection with coronary involvement. We present the rare case of extensive type A aortic dissection extending into the descending aorta causing limb ischemia following right radial heart catheterization.

2. Case Presentation

We present a 56-year-old male with past medical history of coronary artery disease status post-PCI ×2 presenting with chest pain and dyspnea. Labs were remarkable for elevated troponin (1.24 ng/mL), and EKG findings were consistent with NSTE-ACS with ST depression more so within inferior leads. He was medically optimized with ACS directed therapy while troponins continued to uptrend (3.04 ng/mL) overnight. Transthoracic echocardiogram demonstrated normal systolic function (EF: 50-54%) with normal aortic root diameter (3.4 cm) and aortic valve function. Right radial arterial area was prepared, and a 5-French Tiger catheter was used to perform the right coronary angiography. Catheter was unsuccessful in engaging the left coronary artery despite multiple attempts and therefore was replaced with a 6-French JL4 diagnostic catheter, and left coronary angiography was performed. Left heart catheterization was remarkable for significant 80% stenosis of the mid left anterior descending artery (LAD). For the PCI part of the procedure, the EBU 4, 6-French guide catheter was used to support and engage the left coronary artery, and the 0.014 runthrough wire was used to cross the lesion and parked distally. The target lesion at the mid LAD was predilated using the 3.0

× 20 mm Emerge compliant balloon with sequential inflation followed by the placement of a Boston Scientific Synergy 3.5 × 48 mm drug-eluting stent from proximal to mid LAD. Post-PCI results were satisfactory with TIMI grade 3 flow and without dissection of left main and other coronary arteries (Figure 1). Within a few hours after the procedure, the patient developed left lower extremity paresthesia with complete loss of pulses and severe left flank pain. Arterial Doppler showed occlusion/stenosis of the left common femoral artery with near absent distal flow. Heparin drip was initiated due to concern for embolic occlusion with subsequent return of pulses, and vascular surgery was consulted. CTA chest and abdominal aorta demonstrated an ascending and descending aortic dissection (Figure 2(a)) extending into (1) left main renal artery with left kidney infarction (Figure 2(b)), (2) inferior mesenteric artery with possible right colon ischemia, and (3) >70% narrowing in the left common iliac artery. CTA chest further reviewed the extensive type A dissection involving the aortic root which had increased in size to 4.6 cm with extension into the right brachiocephalic and right common carotid artery (Figure 3). Upon return from CT, patient was unarousable and was intubated by the ICU team. CT head without contrast did not show intracranial hemorrhage or any acute abnormality. Heparin drip was discontinued, and patient was managed in the intensive care unit with goal of maintaining systolic blood pressure of <120 mmHg. Patient was transferred to a tertiary medical center for an elephant trunk aortic replacement; unfortunately, the patient expired after the intervention.

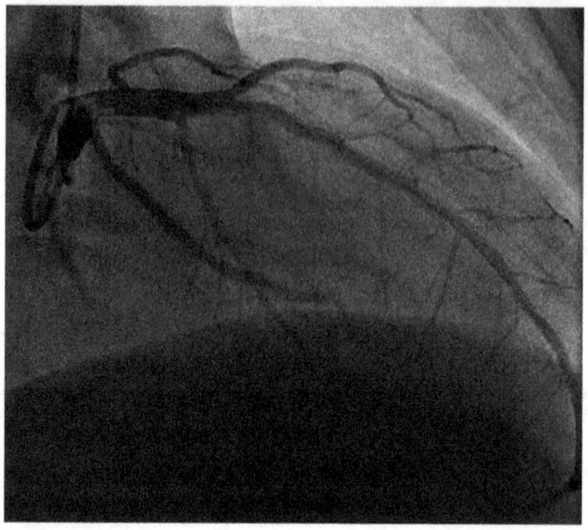

Figure 1: Coronary angiography showing no dissection of the left main coronary artery.

3. Discussion

Radial approach has gained significant interest and usage within interventional cardiology. One of the more significant aims of this approach includes decreasing bleeding and postoperative complications. Comparisons between percutaneous angioplasty using radial and femoral approach showed similar clinical outcomes with decreased access site complications using radial approach [1]. Despite data supporting radial approach, proficiency and experience with this technique plays a pivotal role [2]. Ball et al. showed that success with transradial PCI, comparable to an experienced operator, is dependent on reaching a minimum case volume of ≥50 cases [2]. A lower case volume was associated with increased PCI failure, increased contrast use, and longer fluoroscopy time [2]. Certain limitations with radial approach such as anatomic variation and tortuosity can lead to significant complications [3]. Overall intraoperative aortic dissection (IAD) following PCI is exceedingly rare, as evidenced in a review of 139,262 patients who underwent cardiac catheterization in which the incidence of IAD was 0.06% [4]. Most cases in literature highlight IAD following PCI as a result of retrograde propagation of coronary artery dissection [5]. Interestingly, few cases have reported aortic dissection following heart catheterization without dissection originating within the coronary vessels. In our case, the coronary angiogram postprocedure revealed normal coronary vessels without dissection, pointing to a supracoronary entry point. Upon review of other similar cases, most occurred via right radial access with entry point of dissection occurring around the junction of the right subclavian and brachiocephalic artery. Anatomic anomalies of the subclavian-brachiocephalic axis and tortuosity of the upper limb arteries may predispose such vessels to catheter-induced trauma [6]. The causative factor in the reviewed cases appears multifactorial (calcified vessels, cystic media degeneration, severe atherosclerosis); however, catheter-induced trauma appears to be the focal causative factor. In similar cases, Khan et al. attributed their case to aggressive manipulation of the guide wire into the subclavian loop [3], whereas Noguchi et al. postulated aggressive manipulation of the guiding catheter through the radial artery approach causing intimal tear around the brachiocephalic artery [6]. Similarly, in our case, catheter-induced trauma using right radial approach was the likely inciting factor due to difficulty in engaging the left coronary artery despite multiple attempts.

What makes our patient's case incredibly unique is the extent of dissection from the ascending aorta into the abdominal aorta and run-off vessels affecting the relative organ systems. In this case, the patient's symptoms of severe flank pain and lower extremity paresthesia soon after PCI were the only emergent signs of the underlying complication. Imaging confirmed extensive dissection of the abdominal aorta with dissection extending into the left renal, inferior mesenteric, and left iliac arteries causing the relative symptoms in this case. Such cases involving the ascending and descending aorta have high mortality rates and require extensive surgery known as the "elephant trunk" procedure. Our patient was sent to a tertiary medical center where replacement of the supracoronary ascending aorta with arch repair was followed by treatment of the distal aortic aneurysm. Unfortunately, due to this patient's critical condition and extensive dissection, he expired soon after the initial procedure. To the best of our knowledge, this is the first case reporting ascending aortic dissection involving the abdominal aorta and vessels causing limb ischemia using right radial approach. In conclusion, although radial access may hold certain advantages, rare but fatal complications exist which

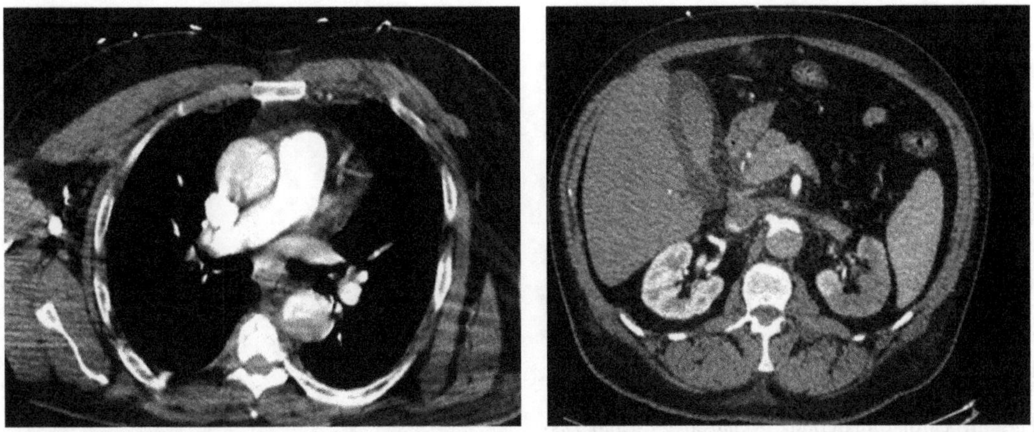

(a) (b)

FIGURE 2: (a) Ascending aortic, descending aortic, and aortic arch aneurysm. (b) L renal infarct and descending aortic aneurysm.

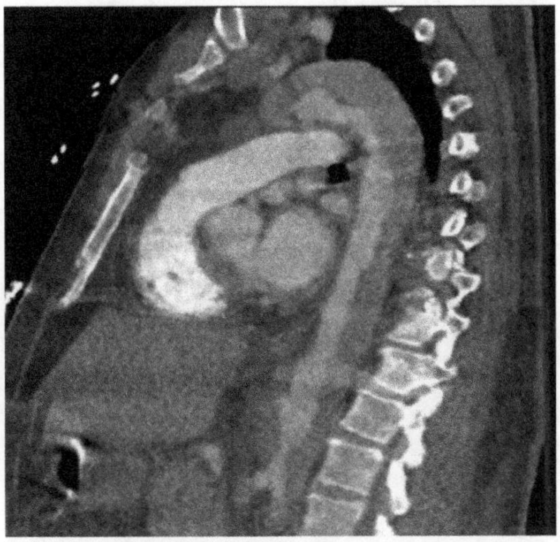

FIGURE 3: Extensive aortic dissection.

may be more frequent using radial approach. Such complications may be secondary to complex anatomy of the upper extremity vasculature predisposing these patients to catheter-induced trauma and subsequent dissection with supracoronary entry [3]. In such cases, immediate recognition and medical management is crucial in avoiding extensive dissection, thereby reducing mortality.

4. Conclusion

In conclusion, although radial access may have certain advantages, rare however significant complications may exist likely secondary to the complex anatomy of the upper extremity vasculature predisposing such patients to catheter-induced trauma. In such cases, immediate recognition and medical management is crucial in avoiding extensive dissection, thereby reducing mortality. To the best of our knowledge, this is the first case reporting extensive aortic dissection involving the abdominal aorta and run-off vessels causing limb ischemia using right radial approach.

Abbreviations

PCI: Percutaneous coronary intervention
NSTE-ACS: Non-ST segment elevation-acute coronary syndrome
GDMT: Guideline directed medical therapy
CTA: Computed tomography angiography
ACS: Acute coronary syndrome
LAD: Left anterior descending artery
IAD: Intraoperative aortic dissection
EKG: Electrocardiogram.

Additional Points

Learning Objectives. (i) Recognizing aortic dissection following cardiac catheterization as a complication. (ii) To understand the potential complications of PCI via radial approach. (iii) Immediate recognition and medical management of aortic dissection is crucial in avoiding extensive aortic dissection.

Consent

Written consent has been obtained from the patient and is available on request.

References

[1] M. Megaly, A. Karatasakis, B. Abraham et al., "Radial versus femoral access in chronic total occlusion percutaneous coronary intervention," *Circulation. Cardiovascular Interventions*, vol. 12, no. 6, article e007778, 2019.

[2] W. T. Ball, W. Sharieff, S. S. Jolly et al., "Characterization of operator learning curve for transradial coronary interventions," *Circulation. Cardiovascular Interventions*, vol. 4, no. 4, pp. 336–341, 2011.

[3] M. Z. Khan, L. Guzman, L. R. Gharai, and J. E. Exaire, "Dissection of ascending aorta: a complication of transradial artery access of coronary procedure," *Heart Views.*, vol. 19, no. 2, pp. 63–66, 2018.

[4] S. Leontyev, M. A. Borger, J. F. Legare et al., "Iatrogenic type a aortic dissection during cardiac procedures: early and late outcome in 48 patients," *European Journal of Cardio-Thoracic Surgery*, vol. 41, no. 3, pp. 641–646, 2012.

[5] M. Lambelin, L. Janssens, and L. Haenen, "Iatrogenic ascending aorta dissection during diagnostic coronary angiography: rare but life-threatening," *Case Reports in Cardiology*, vol. 2014, Article ID 809398, 2014.

[6] K. Noguchi, D. Hori, Y. Nomura, and H. Tanaka, "Iatrogenic acute aortic dissection during percutaneous coronary intervention for acute myocardial infarction," *Annals of Vascular Diseases*, vol. 5, no. 1, pp. 78–81, 2012, PMID:23555491.

38

A Cardiac Pseudoaneurysm as a Thromboembolic Source: Acute Visual Loss due to Cardiac Emboli

Fernando Montenegro Sá, Sara I. L. Fernandes, Rita J. R. Carvalho, Luís M. G. Santos, José A. S. Antunes, Joana M. Guardado, and João C. A. Morais

Cardiology Department, Leiria Hospital Center, Portugal

Correspondence should be addressed to Fernando Montenegro Sá; fernando.m.sa@gmail.com

Academic Editor: Ertugrul Ercan

Acute visual loss is rarely caused by a heart condition. This manuscript transcribes a case report of a 36-year-old patient with a 2-year history of aortic valve replacement due to bicuspid aortic valve endocarditis that presents to the emergency department with an acute right eye visual loss. After ophthalmologic investigation identified a central retinal artery occlusion, a transthoracic echocardiography was performed to search for a possible cardiac embolus, despite the patient presenting INR values of 2-2.5 for the last year. A mitral-aortic intervalvular fibrosa pseudoaneurysm was identified. A transoesophageal echocardiography was then performed, identifying a small clot logged inside the pseudoaneurysm that protruded to the left ventricle outflow tract. After INR-adjusted warfarin treatment to levels between 3 and 4, the pseudoaneurysm was surgically closed. This is a rare case since the likely source of embolism to the central retinal artery was the thrombus logged inside the pseudoaneurysm despite a standardly accepted therapeutic INR.

1. Introduction

The mitral-aortic fibrosa (MAF) consists of a thin layer of fibrous avascular tissue that separates the anterior mitral leaflet from the posterior portion of the aortic root [1]. It is limited by the left atrium (posterolaterally), the left ventricular outflow tract (LVOT, inferiorly), and the pericardium (superiorly). It is prone to infection, and, as a result, a pseudoaneurysm (PMAF) may develop—an uncommon condition that typically consists in a pulsatile cavity in the mitral-aortic junction communicating with the left ventricular outflow tract (LVOT) [1–3]. It is most frequently caused by aortic valve endocarditis, particularly in prosthetic valves [1, 4]. It may be identified by transthoracic echocardiography (TTE) and transoesophageal echocardiography (TOE) in postcardiac surgery asymptomatic patients or may present itself with many unspecific symptoms: the current literature describes fever and active signs of endocarditis in nearly 40% of PMAF patients and heart failure signs in 16%. Only 12% presents with cerebrovascular or embolic events [2]. It may be a severe condition if complete rupture occurs [5], but treatment is available through surgical or percutaneous closure [2, 4, 6].

2. Case Presentation

2.1. History of Presentation. A 36-year-old male presented to the emergency department with complaints of acute (approximately 1-hour evolution) and painless visual loss of the right eye. He was promptly observed by ophthalmology that determined a fully preserved (6/6) visual acuity of the left eye but near blindness of the right eye (6/60). The patient was agitated but had no other complaints. At inspection, the eye had no signs of infection or trauma. Neurological exam did not identify any change: sensory and motor examinations were normal and there was no facial asymmetry, aphasia, dysarthria, or dysmetria. Oculomotor movements and pupillary reflexes were preserved.

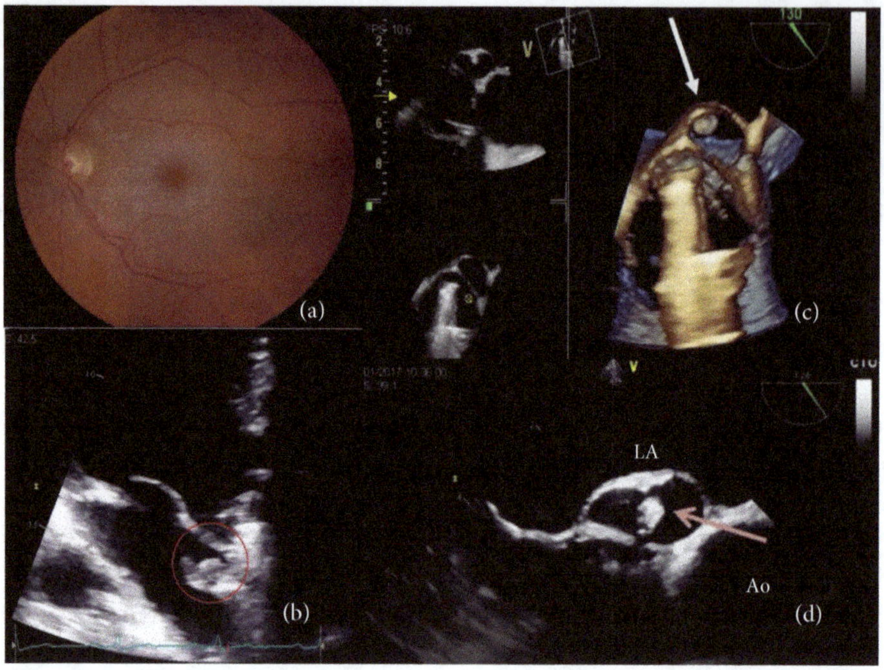

FIGURE 1: (a) Cherry red spot at the center of the fundoscopy. (b) Echolucent area in the mitral-aortic fibrosa with a hyperechogenic structure inside (red circle). (c) Reconstruction through transoesophageal echocardiography showing the mitral-aortic intervalvular fibrosa with a pseudoaneurysm (arrow) communicating with the left ventricle outflow tract and a free thrombus inside. (d) Transoesophageal echocardiography at 126° showing a free hyperechogenic highly mobile structure inside a pseudoaneurysm in the mitral-aortic intervalvular fibrosa, protruding into the LVOT through a small orifice. LA: left atrium; LV: left ventricle; Ao: ascending aorta.

2.2. Past Medical History. Previous medical history included a known bicuspid aortic valve disease. 2 years later, and after a dental procedure, the patient developed an aortic valve endocarditis due to an infection from *Streptococcus sanguinis*. This led to an ischemic stroke, from which the patient recovered completely. He was under antibiogram-directed antibiotic therapy for 1 month when a second stroke happened, and he was then submitted to an urgent surgical replacement of the aortic valve for a mechanical prosthesis that went well. He was discharged with a transthoracic echo referring a normofunctional prosthesis with no other significant alterations and an indication for warfarin therapy for INR target between 2 and 3. At the time of presentation of this case, the patient had medical records available that confirmed INR values between 2 and 2.5 for the last year.

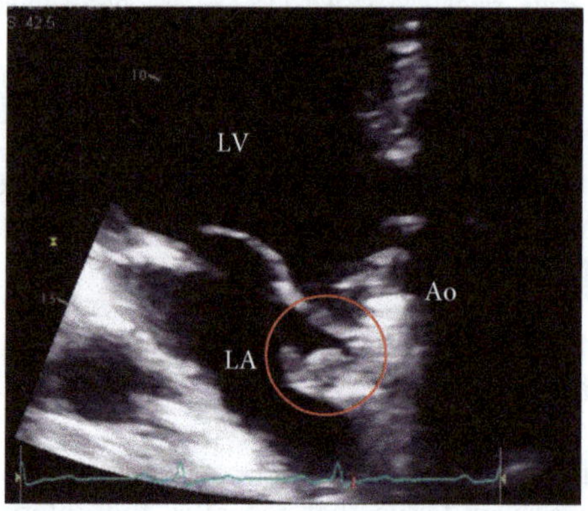

FIGURE 2: Echolucent area in the mitral-aortic fibrosa with a hyperechogenic structure inside (red circle). LA: left atrium; LV: left ventricle; Ao: ascending aorta.

2.3. Differential Diagnosis. Differential diagnosis for single eye acute visual loss includes an acute stroke/transient ischemic accident, compressive lesion, trauma, infection, Purtscher retinopathy and occlusion of the central retinal artery due to either atherosclerotic disease, embolism, arteritis or the presence of a hypercoagulable state (due to neoplastic disease or inherited pro-coagulative diseases, for example) [7].

2.4. Investigations. A fundoscopic exam was immediately performed and identified the foveola assuming a cherry red spot-like image with retinal whitening, which suggested that the visual loss had been caused by a central retinal artery occlusion (Figure 1(a)). Due to the patient's previous medical history, cardiology observation was required to search for a cardiac source of embolism. The patient's physical exam was normal, with cardiac auscultation identifying a clear metallic click as the second cardiac sound and a slight nonradiating systolic murmur (I/VI). A TTE was performed, showing a nonobstructive aortic prosthesis and a periprosthetic echolucent pulsatile region with a hyperechogenic mobile round structure inside (Figures 1(b) and 2). To better characterize these findings, a TOE was performed (Figures 1(c), 1(d), 3, and 4) revealing a free hyperechogenic highly mobile structure suggestive of a free thrombus inside a pseudoaneurysm in the mitral-aortic intervalvular fibrosa, protruding into the left ventricular outflow tract through a small communication orifice (supplementary material video 1 and 2).

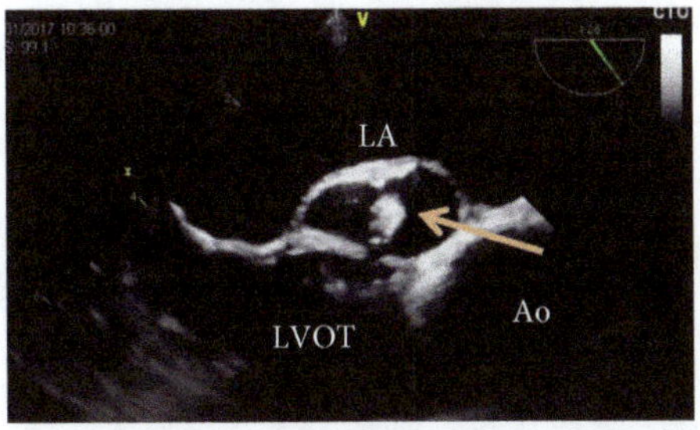

FIGURE 3: Transoesophageal echocardiography at 126° showing a free hyperechogenic highly mobile structure inside a pseudoaneurysm in the mitral-aortic intervalvular fibrosa, protruding into the LVOT through a small orifice. LA: left atrium; LVOT: left ventricle outflow tract; Ao: ascending aorta.

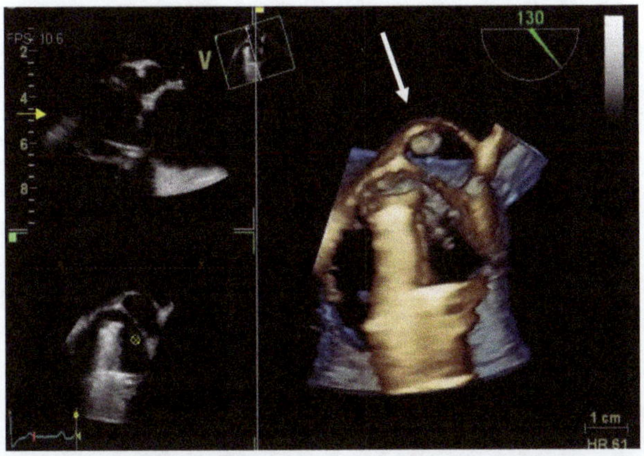

FIGURE 4: 3D reconstruction through transoesophageal echocardiography showing the mitral-aortic intervalvular fibrosa with a pseudoaneurysm (arrow) communicating with the left ventricle outflow tract and a free thrombus inside.

2.5. Treatment. In the acute setting in the emergency department, treatment consisted of the intermittent digital massage of the affected eye and the use of ocular hypotensive drugs and intravenous acetazolamide. The patient had a partial recovery of right eye visual acuity to 6/12. After 3 months of INR-adjusted warfarin treatment for target 3.0–3.5, the patient was submitted to a surgical pseudoaneurysm closure with a synthetic patch.

2.6. Outcomes. Since surgical pseudoaneurysm closure, and after the 1-year follow-up, the patient had no other embolic event. Visual acuity had no further improvements.

3. Discussion

This case represents a scenario of a postcardiac surgery complication with a very rare clinical presentation. In our understanding, the PMAF created a low-flow condition that, despite an INR between 2 and 2.5, still allowed a thrombus formation. The embolization of this small thrombus was the highly probable cause for the central retinal artery occlusion that caused the patient's symptoms. Regarding ophthalmological investigation, and after fundoscopy identification of retinal whitening with a macular cherry red spot, no further tests are indicated [7].

A review of all relevant English language articles published until 2010 identified 88 PMAF cases in the literature: only 11 patients presented with a cerebrovascular or an embolic complication. Of these, a clot was identified inside the pseudoaneurysm in only 5 cases [2]. Stroke due to a thrombus inside the PMAF was previously described, but to our knowledge, this is the first described case of central retinal artery occlusion.

Acute visual loss is rarely due to a cardiac cause, but in patients with high embolic risk conditions, it should be systematically thought of, since diagnosis may be difficult [5] but specific adequate treatment is available [6]. In this case, the final diagnosis was a cardioembolic central retinal artery occlusion, and most patients continue to experience severe vision loss during follow-up despite the current standard therapy [8].

This case highlights that in patients with a high embolic risk, the search for a cardiac embolism after any possible embolic event must be thorough. According to guidelines and recommendations, TTE is the first tool, and sometimes a TOE is also required [3]. This report represents a clinical scenario where a rare extracardiac manifestation (visual loss) was the event that prompted an exhaustive investigation that allowed surgical correction for the underlying problem.

Supplementary Materials

Supplementary 1. Video 1: transoesophageal echocardiography at 126° showing the mitral-aortic intervalvular fibrosa with a pseudoaneurysm and a highly mobile hyperechogenic mass suggestive of a small thrombus.

Supplementary 2. Video 2: transoesophageal echocardiography with 3D reconstruction showing a highly mobile mass (the thrombus) protruding through the ostium of the pseudoaneurysm to the left ventricular outflow tract.

References

[1] I. Afridi, M. A. Apostolidou, R. M. Saad, and W. A. Zoghbi, "Pseudoaneurysms of the mitral-aortic intervalvular fibrosa: dynamic characterization using transesophageal echocardiographic and Doppler techniques," *Journal of the American College of Cardiology*, vol. 25, no. 1, pp. 137–145, 1995.

[2] S. Sudhakar, A. Sewani, M. Agrawal, and B. F. Uretsky, "Pseudoaneurysm of the mitral-aortic intervalvular fibrosa (MAIVF): a comprehensive review," *Journal of the American Society of Echocardiography.*, vol. 23, no. 10, pp. 1009–1018, 2010.

[3] G. Habib, P. Lancellotti, M. J. Antunes et al., "2015 ESC guidelines for the management of infective endocarditis: the Task Force for the Management of Infective Endocarditis of the European Society of Cardiology (ESC). Endorsed by: European Association for Cardio-Thoracic Surgery (EACTS), the European Association of Nuclear Medicine (EANM)," *European Heart Journal*, vol. 36, no. 44, pp. 3075–3128, 2015.

[4] S. Jiménez Valero, E. García, Á. González Pinto, and J. L. Delcán, "Percutaneous closure of pseudoaneurysm of the mitral-aortic

intervalvular fibrosa," *Revista Española de Cardiología*, vol. 58, no. 12, pp. 1473–1475, 2005.

[5] C. Frances, A. Romero, and D. Grady, "Left ventricular pseudoaneurysm," *Journal of the American College of Cardiology*, vol. 32, no. 3, pp. 557–561, 1998.

[6] E. Apostolidou, C. Beale, A. Poppas, and P. Stockwell, "Pseudoaneurysm of the mitral-aortic intervalvular fibrosa: a case series with literature review," *CASE*, vol. 1, no. 6, pp. 221–226, 2017.

[7] R. G. Jones and A. Peall, "Sudden unilateral visual field loss," *Journal of Emergencies, Trauma, and Shock*, vol. 2, no. 3, pp. 211-212, 2009.

[8] A. K. Rudkin, A. W. Lee, E. Aldrich, N. R. Miller, and C. S. Chen, "Clinical characteristics and outcome of current standard management of central retinal artery occlusion," *Clinical & Experimental Ophthalmology*, vol. 38, no. 5, pp. 496–501, 2010.

39

Persistent Left Superior Vena Cava and Absent Right Superior Vena Cava with Left Subclavian Vein Stenosis: Technical Challenges with Pacemaker Implantation

Khalil Kanjwal, Michael Soos, Daniel Gonzalez-Morales, Ibrahim Shah, Mohan Madala, Majid Mughal, and Muhammad Awais Kang

McLaren Greater Lansing Hospital, Lansing, MI, USA

Correspondence should be addressed to Khalil Kanjwal; khalilkanjwal@yahoo.com

Academic Editor: Kathleen Ngu

We present a challenging case of a 75-year-old female with a history of paroxysmal atrial fibrillation (PAF) and symptomatic sick sinus syndrome (SSS) who presented for a dual chamber pacemaker implantation and was found to have persistent left superior vena cava and absent right superior vena cava with stenosis of the left subclavian vein. In this report, we discuss the implant technique in this group of patients.

1. Introduction

Persistent left superior vena cava (PLSVC) along with absent right SVC is a rare occurrence. It has been reported in 0.1% of the general population [1–3]. There have been only less than 15 cases reported in the literature. Pacemaker implantation can be very challenging in such patients, and there has not been much reported on various techniques of implanting pacemaker in such patients. To our knowledge, this is a second report of pacemaker implantation in a patient with persistent left SVC and absent right SVC. In addition, our patient also had left subclavian vein stenosis and thus complicating the implant procedure further.

2. Case

A 75-year-old female with symptomatic paroxysmal atrial fibrillation (PAF), statuspost atrial fibrillation ablation, and prior history of breast cancer, statuspost bilateral mastectomy and left lymphadenectomy, presented with diziness and near syncope and was found to have sinus bradycardia. Given her symptomatic sick sinus syndrome (SSS), she was planned for a dual chamber pacemaker implantation.

The placement of a dual chamber pacemaker insertion was attempted from the right side as the patient previously underwent left-sided lymphadenectomy. The right subclavian vein access was obtained and cannulated under fluoroscopy. The right ventricular (RV) lead was advanced attempting to access the right superior vena cava (SVC). While attempting to advance the lead, resistance was encountered and the lead was withdrawn. A venogram was performed revealing the absence of a right SVC with the presence of a persistent left superior vena cava draining into a massively dilated coronary sinus (Figures 1 and 2).

The lead could not be advanced into the right ventricle, and as a result, the procedure was aborted and cardiothoracic surgery was consulted for possible epicardial lead placement.

After discussing the potential need for cardiothoracic surgery with the patient, she considered another attempt at transvenous placement of a dual chamber pacemaker with us. After repeated attempts, left subclavian vein access could not be obtained. The venogram revealed stenosis of the left subclavian vein. The decision was made to make an additional attempt from the right subclavian vein utilizing the previous pocket. After successful cannulation of the right subclavian vein, an active fixation lead was advanced through the subclavian vein into the PLSVC through the coronary

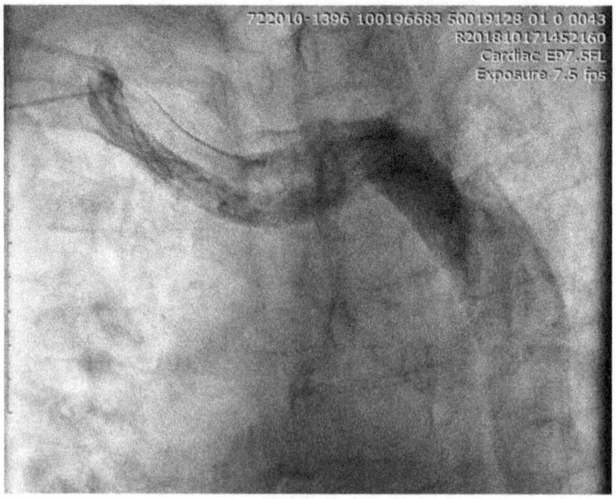

FIGURE 1

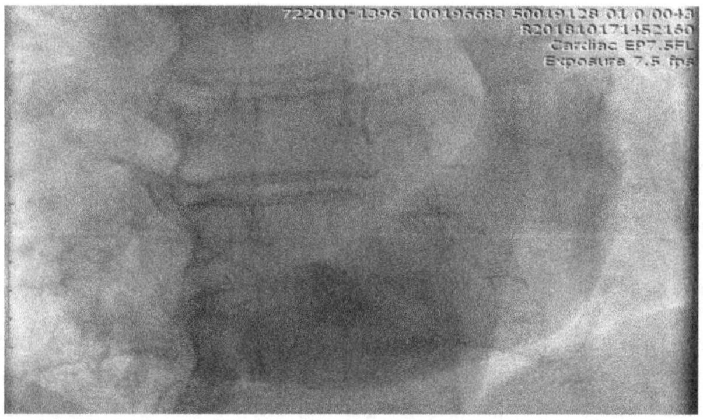

FIGURE 2

sinus and then through the tricuspid valve into the right ventricular septum. Following successful right ventricular lead placement, an active fixation bipolar pacing lead was advanced into the right atrium using a straight stylet and secured to the right atrial wall.

Stimulation and sensing thresholds were determined to be satisfactory in both leads. A St. Jude Medical generator was connected to the leads, and the pocket was closed.

3. Discussion

PLSVC is a rare congenital anomaly found in approximately 0.3-0.5% of the general population [1–3], and its occurrence along with absent right-sided SVC is reported in 0.1% of the general population. It results from the failure of the vessel to involute during embryologic development.

This anomaly usually exists with the presence of a right superior vena cava (SVC) and is usually found incidentally during cardiac device implantation. In patient with PLSVC, the cardiac devices are implanted from the right subclavian approach as the lead manipulation and deployment can be challenging from the left side. Absent right SVC with PLSVC occurs extremely rarely in less than 0.1% of the general population [1, 2]. In this report, we outline the technical approach to the placement of dual chamber pacemaker leads in a patient with solitary PLSVC. Our case was further complicated by subclavian stenosis on the left side. The right subclavian access was obtained using a micropuncture needle under fluoroscopy. The venography demonstrated the absence of right-sided SVC, and the wire could easily pass over the left SVC. The sheath was advanced over the wire, and a 65 cm active fixation lead could be easily advanced through the right subclavian into the left SVC and the coronary sinus and through the coronary sinus os into the right atrium in the right anterior oblique (RAO) fluoroscopic view. As the lead came out of the coronary sinus, it is directed in a direction opposite to that of the RV inlet, thus making the implantation and manipulation of the RV lead challenging. The most critical part of the procedure is crossing the tricuspid valve, and inability to do that will result in failure of the lead placement. In our patient, when the lead came out of the coronary sinus, it was further advanced without the stylet towards the right atrial wall. The forward movement against the RA free wall formed a loop, and subsequently, the part of the lead was prolapsed into the right ventricle. The stylet with a spiral curve made at the end of the stylet was introduced and advanced, and when it reached the coronary sinus os, the pull and push maneuver on the stylet and the lead was performed. The lead tip crossed the RV inlet and was further advanced into the RV towards RV septum. The septal location was confirmed in the left anterior oblique (LAO) fluoroscopic position, and subsequently, the helix was deployed (Figure 3).

There are few technical considerations the implanting physicians need to be aware of while implanting cardiac devices in patients with PLSVC and absent right SVC.

The course of the right subclavian to PLSVC is long. A longer sheath may be considered while navigating the lead through anomalous course of the vein. In addition, a longer lead (65 cm) would be a preferred length lead given the long course of right subclavian, PLSVC, and coronary sinus. The prolapse technique with a spiral curve of the stylet should be considered during such implants.

Other potential alternatives may be included using a coronary sinus deliver system. A 0.35″ wire may be advanced through the subclavian/left SVC venous system through coronary sinus os and through the RV inlet into the right ventricle followed by advancing the delivery system over the wire into the right ventricle.

The right atrial lead does not pose a technical challenge in such patients. When it comes out of the CS OS, it is directed towards the right free wall; however, it could be challenging sometimes to direct the lead into the right atrial appendage. A clockwise torque with a J-shaped stylet may help in such situation.

To the best of our knowledge, there has been only one report of pacemaker implantation in a patient with persistent left SVC with absent right SVC from the right subclavian vein [4]. The use of a fixed-shaped sheath and a lumen less bipolar pacing lead from Medtronic has been

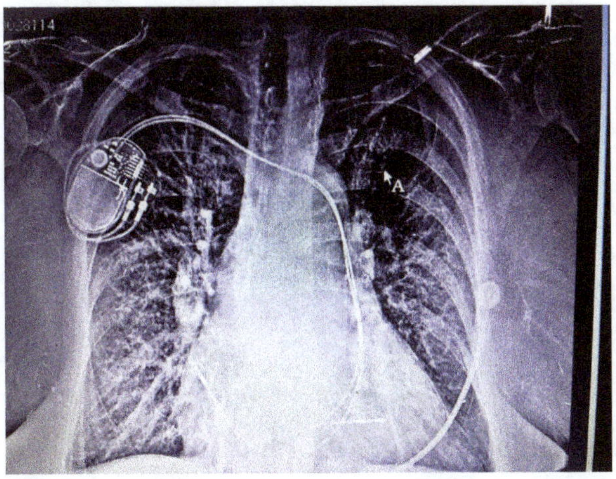

Figure 3

recently reported for implantation of a pacemaker from the left brachiocephalic system through the left persistent SVC [5].

4. Conclusion

Venous anomalies can be encountered during cardiac device implantations. Preprocedure venography may help identify such anomalies, and the physicians can plan on the techniques and need for special equipment ahead of time to have a better patient outcome.

Additional Points

Teaching Points. (1) Preimplant venograms provide crucial information about venous anatomy. (2) Implanting physicians should be aware of venous anomalies encountered during device implants. (3) A clear concept of venous anomalies and trouble shooting skills may improve patient outcomes.

References

[1] T. C. Demos, H. V. Posniak, K. L. Pierce, M. C. Olson, and M. Muscato, "Venous anomalies of the thorax," *American Journal of Roentgenology*, vol. 182, no. 5, pp. 1139–1150, 2004.

[2] Ö. Uçar, H. Çiçekçioğlu, I. Kocaoğlu, S. Aydoğdu, L. Paşaoğlu, and M. Vural, "Persistent left superior vena cava with absent right superior vena cava: a case report and review of the literature," *Cardiovascular Journal of Africa*, vol. 21, no. 3, pp. 164–166, 2010.

[3] S. T. MacDonald, Y. Emmanuel, S. Myerson, B. Prendergast, S. Neubauer, and P. Leeson, "Absent right superior vena cava: multimodality imaging of upper venous drainage via left-sided superior vena cava and azygos venous system," *Circulation: Cardiovascular Imaging*, vol. 2, no. 5, pp. e34–e36, 2009.

[4] J. Rizkallah, J. Burgess, and V. Kuriachan, "Absent right and persistent left superior vena cava: troubleshooting during a challenging pacemaker implant: a case report," *BMC Research Notes*, vol. 7, no. 1, p. 462, 2014.

[5] K. Sasaki, S. Tateishi, and C. Sawada, "Usefulness of a lead delivery system consisting of a fixed-shaped sheath and a lumenless bipolar lead in a patient with absent right and persistent left superior vena cava: a case report," *Indian Pacing and Electrophysiology Journal*, vol. 18, no. 6, pp. 234–236, 2018.

40

Blood Cyst of the Mitral Valve Diagnosed in an Adult after Systemic Thrombolysis

Diana C. Ramírez-Mesías,[1,2] Juan F. Contreras-Valero,[3,4] Gabriel D. Pinilla-Monsalve,[3,4] and Carlos E. Vesga-Reyes[3,4]

[1]*Hospital Universitario San Ignacio, Bogotá 110231, Colombia*
[2]*Pontificia Universidad Javeriana, Bogotá 110231, Colombia*
[3]*Fundación Valle del Lili, Cali 760032, Colombia*
[4]*Universidad Icesi, Cali 760031, Colombia*

Correspondence should be addressed to Carlos E. Vesga-Reyes; carlos.vesga@fvl.org.co

Academic Editor: Assad Movahed

Blood cysts in valves are very rare entities in adults, which can be distinguished through their echocardiographic features. A 57-year-old woman developed sudden dyspnea while hospitalized in the context of urinary sepsis; high-risk pulmonary embolism was diagnosed and she was prescribed systemic thrombolysis. She persisted with fever raising the suspicion of bacterial endocarditis. Transthoracic echocardiography did not report any masses, but later transesophageal imaging revealed a vegetation that was finally characterized as a blood cyst of the mitral valve based on ultrasound features. The patient evolved satisfactorily and did not require surgery.

1. Introduction

As detailed by Khan et al., intracardiac hematic cysts are benign "thin-walled structures lined by cobblestone-shaped epithelium, filled with non-organized blood" [1]. They were first defined by Elässer and are usually seen on atrioventricular valves in infants younger than six months but rarely in adults [2]. In 1983, Hausser et al. presented the first echocardiographic description of a hypoechogenic structure showing a synchronic movement with the tendinous cords towards the left ventricle outflow tract. Surgical and histological observations confirmed that this mass was consistent with a blood cyst [3]. Within the cardiac structure, they are mainly detected on valves with few cases of cysts attached to atria or ventricles [1]. Additionally, content echogenicity and intracystic microbubbles suggesting ventricle-to-cyst lumen connections [4] seem to be signs compatible with blood cysts.

Here, we report the case of a 57-year-old woman with a blood mitral valve cyst diagnosed after systemic thrombolysis for pulmonary embolism.

2. Case Presentation

This is the case of a 57-year-old Colombian obese woman who was admitted to the emergency department complaining of abdominal pain, urinary symptoms, and fever. Her medical history was positive for systemic arterial hypertension, type 2 diabetes mellitus, and nephrolithiasis. Ten days before the symptoms' onset, she underwent a dental procedure for tooth decay. In the beginning, she was treated in another facility for ketoacidosis, renal failure, and bacterial urinary tract infection, developing pneumonia as well. She required renal replacement therapy and received a course of antibiotics including amino-penicillins, carbapenems, and glycopeptides.

During hospitalization, the patient suddenly presented right calf pain; a duplex ultrasound was requested evidencing deep venous thrombosis of soleal and peroneal veins. She complained as well of dyspnea, chest pain, and palpitations, raising the suspicion of pulmonary embolism (Wells' criteria: 4.5 points). Thoracic CT angiography showed thrombosis of the pulmonary trunk and both main branches, and the initial transthoracic echocardiography (4 days after admission) reported left ventricle diastolic dysfunction with impaired relaxation, trivial mitral regurgitation, mild right ventricle dilation, mild tricuspid regurgitation, and an intermediate probability of pulmonary hypertension (PSAP 40 mmHg) with no other findings. Systemic thrombolysis with streptokinase was the chosen treatment for the high-risk pulmonary embolism; subsequently, she was started on enoxaparin with bridge therapy to warfarin.

After thrombolysis, the patient remained febrile with chest discomfort despite antibiotic treatment suggesting dialysis catheter-related infection or bacterial endocarditis. A transesophageal echocardiogram was carried out, revealing a mitral valve mass considered as a bacterial vegetation, and therefore, she continued receiving vancomycin. For exploring therapeutic alternatives, she was transferred to our hospital and stayed in the intensive care unit for one month. Her vital signs were normal (36.8°C, 95 beats per min, 20 breaths per min, 132/55 mmHg, SpO_2 94% on room air), but she was pale and cardiopulmonary auscultation was positive for S3 sound. No heart murmurs, abnormal breath sounds, or jugular ingurgitation was detected.

Laboratory analysis demonstrated leukocytosis (13.010 cells/μL), moderate anemia (7.4 g/dL), mild thrombocytopenia (146.000/μL), and increased C-reactive protein levels (17 mg/L, normal concentrations up to 5 mg/L). Moreover, renal function was severely compromised (creatinine 5.3 mg/dL and blood uremic nitrogen 42 mg/dL) and arterial blood gases showed metabolic acidosis (pH of 7.37, HCO_3 13.9 mmol/L, PCO_2 24 mmHg, SaO_2 87%, and base excess -10.6). Urine cultures were positive for IRT-resistant *Escherichia coli* and azole-sensitive *Candida albicans*, while no germs could be isolated on blood cultures. Consequently, fluconazole was added to the antibiotic regimen.

Transesophageal echocardiogram (16 days after admission) demonstrated preserved left ventricular dimensions and ejection fraction. Mitral valve exhibited a rounded image of 10 × 10 mm with hyperrefringent edges and hypoechogenic content within the anterior ring, corresponding to A1 and A2 segments (Figure 1). This lesion did not compromise the valve function nor obstructed the left ventricle outflow tract. The rest of the valves, cavities, and vessels were normal, except for a small left pleural effusion. The density of the mass and the absence of any other imaging features compatible with endocarditis (i.e., highly and asynchronously mobile pedicled mass) supported the diagnosis of a blood cyst. Contrast echocardiogram with sulfur hexafluoride microbubbles was not available in our institution.

Aside from the mass, she did not fulfill any other Duke's criteria and blood cultures were negative. Besides, there was no valvular regurgitation that supported the diagnosis of a leaflet aneurysm and the cyst remained the same size in transesophageal echocardiogram despite anticoagulation, being less likely that it corresponded to a thrombus adhered to the valve in a patient with no predisposing factors. Researchers have highlighted elsewhere that echogenicity is the key to differentiate other entities (infections, neoplasms, and thrombi) from blood cysts as the last exhibit a homogenous hypoechogenic content [1]. Unfortunately, we could not obtain the initial transthoracic echocardiogram for reviewing and confirming that the mass was not present at that point.

After 10 days of antifungals, the inflammatory response completely resolved and the antibiotic course was not extended as bacterial endocarditis was disregarded. The patient did not present any bleeding or embolic events and was discharged without any disability. Unfortunately, she did not attend to the Outpatient Clinic but, in a telephone follow-up, no recurrence of cardiovascular symptoms was reported.

3. Discussion

Valvular blood cysts may be present in approximately 50% of random fetal and infant autopsies with diameters reaching up to 3 mm and a slight, but not significant, predominance in males ($p = 0.103$) [5]. In adults, cysts can be the consequence of blunt trauma and valvular surgery [6]. Until 2009, eleven cases of blood cysts on the mitral valve had been reported (54.54% were women, median age was 44 years, IQR 32-48) with the anterior leaflet (81.8%) as the most commonly affected structure [6]. Intracardiac cysts have been related to a variety of symptoms including dyspnea, chest pain at rest and on exertion [7, 8], or even syncope [9]; neurological deficits are less prevalent and associated with embolic stroke [1] or transient ischemic attack [3] after cyst rupture.

According to Dencker et al. and other authors, there are five hypotheses for explaining the occurrence of blood cysts: entrapment of blood during valve development; vascular occlusion in the setting of inflammatory, autonomic, metabolic, or hemorrhagic conditions generating subvalvular hematomas; presence of heteroplastic tissue from the embryonic pericardium; valvular blood vessel ectasia; and tumor proliferation in the form of angiomas [6]. We believe that in this patient there is a considerable probability that septic status due to urinary infection and systemic thrombolysis could have produced a hematoma in the shape of a cyst as proposed by the second hypothesis. Although the improbable non-regression of a congenital cyst cannot be excluded, these tend to be smaller [5] than those found in adults [6]. Furthermore, the lesion was not seen in the initial transthoracic echocardiogram and the patient's condition significantly improved without interventions other than stated, while no pathological sample could be obtained to favor different explanations. Histologically, cysts are delimited by homogeneous and dense connective tissue with layers of endothelial cells [5, 7] and occasional lymphocytic infiltrate [10].

Echocardiography is considered the method of choice for diagnosis [8] due to its accessibility and live assessment of valve function. However, cysts could be misdiagnosed as

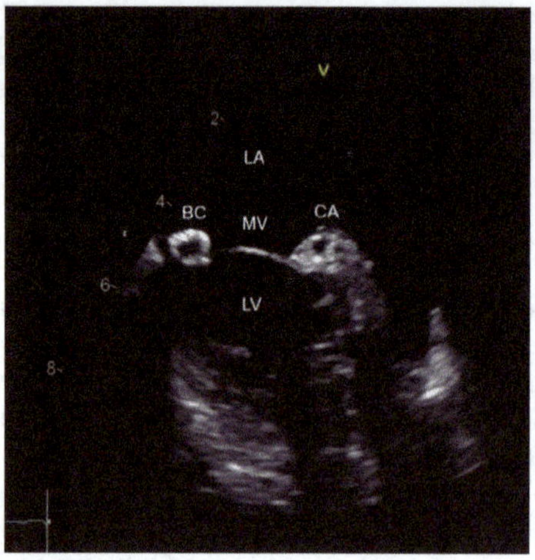

(a)

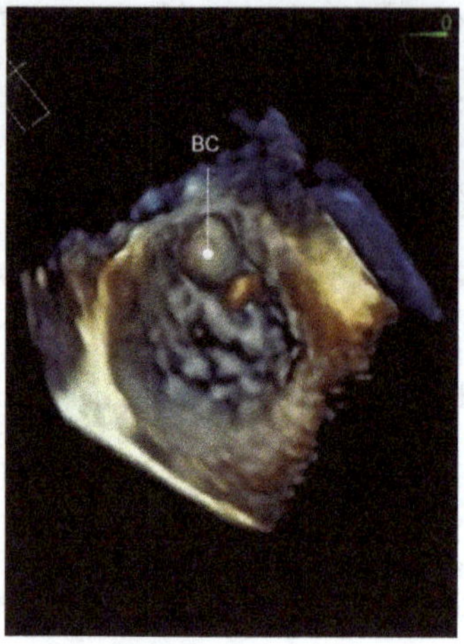

(b)

FIGURE 1: Transesophageal echocardiogram (a) with 3D reconstruction (b), exhibiting a blood cyst attached to the anterior leaflet of the mitral valve. LA: left atrium; LV: left ventricle; MV: mitral valve; BC: blood cyst; CA: circumflex artery.

adherent thrombus [7] or bacterial vegetation such as in this case. Contrast echocardiography might be of help as stated before [4]. Related to other imaging modalities, cysts can be isodense in CT scans [8]; cardiac magnetic resonance (CMR) is usually obtained to clarify tissue characteristics, but blood cysts are variably observed as hyperintense in T2W [11], isointense in turbo spin echo [8], and/or with a prolonged T1 relaxation time in special breath-held inversion-recovery sequences [12]. Early gadolinium enhancement is not common [8].

For this patient, the blood cyst could have been overlooked in the initial transthoracic echocardiogram. In fact, limited sensitivity and negative likelihood ratio of 71% (95% CI 0.56-0.82) and 0.37 (95% CI 0.20-0.68), respectively, have been reported for detecting vegetations through this modality [13]. Furthermore, no diagnostic accuracy studies have been published comparing CMR with transesophageal echocardiography for identifying intracardiac blood cysts, but the last (with or without 3D reconstruction) has a discriminative capacity higher than 90% for thrombus or myxoma diagnosis. Transesophageal echocardiogram seems more accurate than CT scan, but false negatives can occur when masses are located in the left ventricle due to difficulty for visualizing the ventricular apex [14]. In the compilation of cases by Dencker, only 2 out of 11 cases had a cardiac MRI for supporting the diagnosis [6]; nevertheless, this modality has been relevant for confirming (rather than discarding) the echocardiographic finding [1, 8, 15]. Lamentably, there are still administrative barriers that impede access to advance image modalities in developing countries.

Currently, there are no treatment guidelines for blood cysts because of the low incidence, but the majority of symptomatic patients have undergone surgery for ruling out malignancy and preventing stroke [16]. β-blocking, antiaggregation, or anticoagulation remain controversial [15]. The prognosis is benign as congenital cysts tend to resolve spontaneously, but in fewer cases, valvular disease or obstruction of the ventricular outflow tracts can be present [9].

4. Conclusion

Intracardiac blood cysts are infrequent in adults and can be congenital or acquired after trauma or surgery. We presented the rare case of a blood cyst of the mitral valve in the context of severe infection and bleeding diathesis precipitated by thrombolysis. Echocardiographic assessment is useful for differential diagnosis based on functional and structural features. Treatment should be individualized according to clinical status and complications.

References

[1] T. Khan, S. El-Sharkawy, and F. Schafer, "A heart within the heart - A rare congenital cause of an embolic stroke," *BMJ Case Reports*, vol. 2012, 2012.

[2] G. J. Liese, S. C. Brainard, and U. Goto, "Giant blood cyst of the pulmonary valve. Report of a case," *The New England Journal of Medicine*, vol. 269, no. 9, pp. 465–467, 1963.

[3] A. M. Hauser, K. Rathod, J. McGill, B. F. Rosenberg, S. Gordon, and G. C. Timmis, "Blood cyst of the papillary muscle: Clinical, echocardiographic and anatomic observations," *The American Journal of Cardiology*, vol. 51, no. 3, pp. 612-613, 1983.

[4] F. Migliore, V. Scarabeo, A. Corfini, and P. Piovesana, "Microbubbles contrast inside the cyst: a pathognomonic sign of mitral valve blood cyst," *Journal of Cardiovascular Medicine*, vol. 11, no. 4, pp. 294–296, 2010.

[5] K. G. Zimmerman, S. H. Paplanus, S. Dong, and R. B. Nagle, "Congenital blood cysts of the heart valves," *Human Pathology*, vol. 14, no. 8, pp. 699–703, 1983.

[6] M. Dencker, T. Jexmark, F. Hansen, P. Tydén, A. Roijer, and C. Lührs, "Bileaflet blood cysts on the mitral valve in an adult," *Journal of the American Society of Echocardiography*, vol. 22, no. 9, pp. 1085.e5–1085.e8, 2009.

[7] S. W. Xie, O. L. Lu, and M. H. Picard, "Blood cyst of the mitral valve: detection by transthoracic and transesophageal echocardiography," *Journal of the American Society of Echocardiography*, vol. 5, no. 5, pp. 547–550, 1992.

[8] F. Bonenfant, B. Essadiqi, G. Gahide, H. Jeanmart, and P. Farand, "Mitral valve blood cyst detected by multimodality imaging," *Canadian Journal of Cardiology*, vol. 30, no. 9, pp. 1109.e5–1109.e6, 2014.

[9] X. Ma, X. Zeng, Y. Wu et al., "Mitral valve blood cyst occlusion of the aortic valve leading to syncope: detection by transthoracic and contrast echocardiography," *The Journal of International Medical Research*, vol. 47, no. 8, pp. 3487–3490, 2019.

[10] J. Kuvin, P. Saha, H. Rastegar, R. N. Salomon, N. Pandian, and D. DeNofrio, "Blood cyst of the mitral valve apparatus in a woman with a history of orthotopic liver transplantation," *Journal of the American Society of Echocardiography*, vol. 17, no. 5, pp. 480–482, 2004.

[11] A. Reichelt and N. Khaladj, "MRI of a blood cyst of the mitral valve," *RöFo - Fortschritte auf dem Gebiet der Röntgenstrahlen und der bildgebenden Verfahren*, vol. 185, no. 1, pp. 68-69, 2013.

[12] S. Romano, K. Krishnasamy, N. Jariwala, J. Chung, and A. Farzaneh-Far, "Giant mitral blood cyst: cardiovascular magnetic resonance imaging features," *International Journal of Cardiology*, vol. 203, pp. 17-18, 2016.

[13] M. Bonzi, G. Cernuschi, M. Solbiati, G. Giusti, N. Montano, and E. Ceriani, "Diagnostic accuracy of transthoracic echocardiography to identify native valve infective endocarditis: a systematic review and meta-analysis," *Internal and Emergency Medicine*, vol. 13, no. 6, pp. 937–946, 2018.

[14] S. Turhan, O. Ulas Ozcan, and C. Erol, "Imaging of intracardiac thrombus," *Cor et Vasa*, vol. 55, no. 2, pp. e176–e183, 2013.

[15] D. Ludhwani, B. Sheikh, and Y. Sheikh, "Evaluation of mitral apparatus blood cyst: a case report and review of literature," *Cureus*, vol. 11, no. 10, article e5812, 2019.

[16] S. Yilmaz, M. Gül, S. Unal, U. Canpolat, and Z. Gölbasi, "Blood cyst of the mitral valve in an adult," *Herz*, vol. 40, no. 2, pp. 329–331, 2015.

41

An Unusual Cause of Dyspnea and Thoracic Pressure

Claire Chakkalakal, Rezo Jorbenadze, and Meinrad Gawaz

University Hospital, Department of Cardiology and Cardiovascular Medicine, University of Tübingen, 72076 Tübingen, Germany

Correspondence should be addressed to Meinrad Gawaz; meinrad.gawaz@med.uni-tuebingen.de

Academic Editor: Magnus Baumhäkel

There is a high prevalence of hepatic cysts in the general population. Simple cysts are most of the times asymptomatic and are usually detected incidentally on ultrasonography, computed tomography, or magnetic resonance imaging. Symptoms may range from abdominal discomfort and pain, early satiety, dyspepsia, nausea, and vomiting to jaundice and portal hypertension due to obstruction of adjacent structures. Complications include spontaneous hemorrhage, infection, thrombosis, and atrophy of surrounding hepatic tissue. We present a unique case of a middle-aged patient with acute onset of dyspnea and thoracic pressure due to compression of the right ventricle by a large hepatic cyst.

1. Introduction

Nonparasitic hepatic cysts occur in approximately 5% of the global population [1]. Since most hepatic cysts remain asymptomatic, the exact number is unknown. Liver cysts are fluid-filled cavities and normally require no treatment. The symptoms are strongly variable and usually depend on the cysts' size, location, type, and number. Most commonly described symptoms are abdominal pain or discomfort, early satiety, and nausea. In some cases, obstructive jaundice or portal hypertension may occur due to compression of adjacent structures. Hypotension and thrombosis due to atypical vena cava-compression syndrome are rare. Complications include spontaneous cyst rupture, hemorrhage into the abdominal cavity, and infections. Besides symptomatic treatment, therapeutic options range from percutaneous drainage and open or laparoscopic deroofing to hepatic resection [1]. We present a rare case of a middle-aged female patient with sudden onset of cardiopulmonary symptoms due to a large simple cyst of the liver.

2. Case Presentation

A 51-year-old woman presented herself in our emergency room (ER) with dyspnea and retrosternal thoracic pressure. The symptoms had started 2 years earlier, with a distinct deterioration over the course of the 4 weeks preceding her admission. According to the patient, the symptoms had culminated in acute shortness of breath and tightness of the chest, accompanied by nocturnal panic attacks, dyspepsia, and general weakness 2 nights before. The symptoms primarily occurred when lying down. There were no cardiovascular risk factors except for a positive family history for aortic aneurysms. Except for a hysterectomy many years earlier, her medical history was empty. The electrocardiograms (ECGs) recorded at her general practitioner (GP) during the past few years and, in particular, during the weeks prior to her admission, were all normal. A physical stress test had been performed at a local cardiologist with no conclusive results regarding exercise-induced alteration in repolarization or arrhythmias. Two weeks before, she had been referred to a local radiological center for computed tomography (CT) of the chest in order to detect potential lung embolism or aortic aneurysms. In regard to her family history, this seemed to be a relevant differential diagnosis, but the scan remained without noticeable mediastinal findings.

Upon admission to our ER, the initial ECG showed no abnormalities, blood pressure was 130/70 mmHg, oxygen saturation was between 97 and 100%. Her lab results were all normal. With troponin, CK, and D-dimers within physiological range, there were again no indicators for lung embolism, aortic aneurysm, or myocardial infarction. Furthermore, no infection or other pathological findings like elevated liver or kidney values were detected in the blood test results.

Echocardiography showed a good left-ventricular function and no valve dysfunctions. However, in the four- and five-chamber view, the right ventricle appeared to be compressed from the outside. The subxiphoid view confirmed this. The structure compressing the right side of the heart proved to be a large cystic lesion of the liver. In the consecutive ultrasound of the abdomen, the cyst measured 9 × 7 cm. Its size and subdiaphragmatic location left no doubt that it caused the symptoms described by the patient, in the absence of any other pathological findings.

She was referred to abdominal surgery and after negative echinococcus test results, a laparoscopic unroofing was scheduled. Several days before the appointment, the patient was readmitted due to increasing shortness of breath. The ultrasound showed that the cyst's total dimensions were 10.7 × 8.3 cm now and thus had grown over 1 cm per side in only 3 weeks. This fast progress explains why the affection appeared as a sudden onset, although the symptoms had started 2 years earlier.

Laparoscopic cystectomy was performed without complications. The symptoms previously described ceased abruptly afterwards. The histopathological findings gave no evidence of infection or inflammatory processes (Figure 1).

3. Discussion

Simple cysts account for the majority of hepatic cysts. Less frequent and more complicative cystic lesions include echinococcosis, cystadenoma, and cystadenocarcinoma [2]. In regard to the relatively high prevalence of hepatic cysts in general, symptoms or complications are rare. The most frequent ones are abdominal discomfort, nausea, and other gastrointestinal symptoms [1].

Cyst rupture and hemorrhage as well as infections account for the most common complications. Cardiopulmonary symptoms or complications are an exception and usually manifest themselves in form of hypotension and thrombosis. Acute severe retrosternal pressure or thoracic tightness and respiratory symptoms, such as dyspnea, are rather typical for cardiac or cardiopulmonary conditions, the most common ones being myocardial infarction, heart failure, aortic aneurysms, and lung embolism. Similar symptoms have been described to occur in pericardial cysts [3, 4] due to hemodynamic alterations and compression of the right ventricle as was also presented in this case (Figures 2 and 3). Isolated compression of the right heart chambers has also occurred in a few cases of patients with pectus excavatum, who showed comparable symptoms, such as dyspnea and thoracic pain or tightness [5–7].

This is the first reported case in which an abdominal cyst was compromising organs of the adjacent cavity to such an extent that it manifested itself as acute cardiopulmonary condition.

Since simple hepatic cysts are usually asymptomatic, the diagnosis is mostly incidental. They range from a few millimeters to enormous sizes, and the predominant location is the right hepatic lobe [2]. Laboratory results are usually

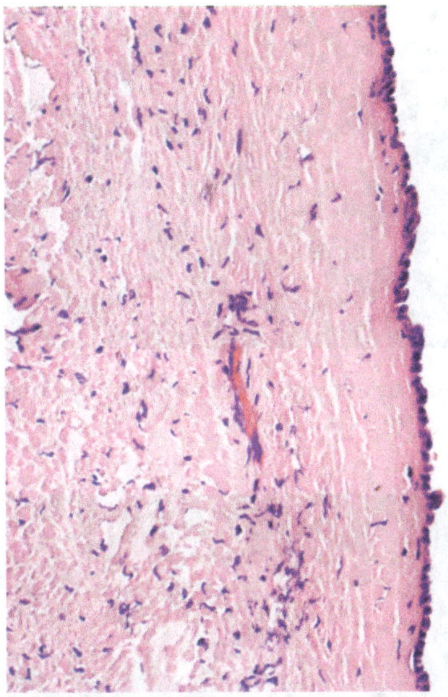

FIGURE 1: Cystic lesion with thin collagenous wall, lined by biliary type epithelium (flat to cuboidal). No pathohistological sign of inflammation or infection.

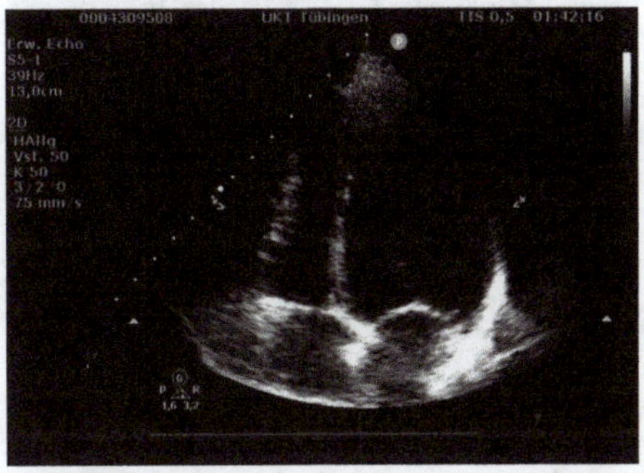

FIGURE 2: Echocardiogram, four-chamber view: extrinsic compression of the right ventricle.

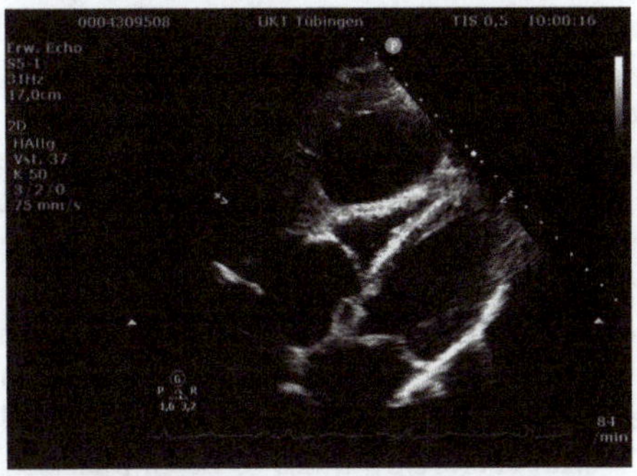

FIGURE 3: Echocardiogram, subxiphoidal view: cystic lesion of the liver compressing the right ventricle.

normal. The cysts can be detected by sonography, CT, or magnetic resonance imaging [8]. On ultrasound imaging, they appear as spherical or oval fluid-filled, nonseptated cavities with sharp and smooth borders (Figure 4). These distinct sonographic features combined with the lack of

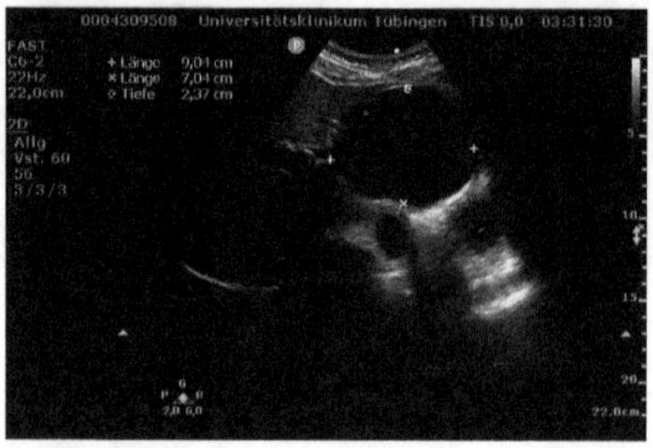

FIGURE 4: Sonography of the abdomen showing a cystic lesion in the liver (dimensions: 9×7 cm).

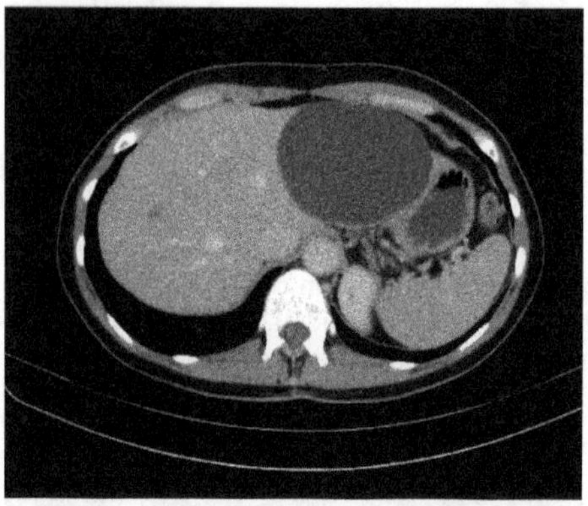

FIGURE 5: CT scan: large hepatic cyst in the left hepatic lobe.

dorsal shadowing distinguish them from potential harmful cystic lesions, such as the aforementioned echinococcosis, cystadenoma, and cystadenocarcinoma [8].

Exclusion of other differential diagnoses with cystic appearance on radiographic imaging such as hepatic abscess, hemangioma, hamartoma, and even necrotic malignant neoplasms can usually be made based upon a combination of sonographic findings, clinical presentation, and lab results [2, 8].

Treatment modalities of hepatic cysts in general range from mere observation and drainage to surgical measures such as laparoscopic or open unroofing and hepatic resection. The choice of procedure mainly depends on the type of cyst, size, and symptoms [1, 8]. The general therapeutic recommendation for simple but symptomatic hepatic cysts is wide unroofing, either by open or laparoscopic surgery [9], as was also performed in this case, due to the minimal recurrence rates of simple cysts after surgical treatment.

In this unique case, although neighboring abdominal structures, including the left-lobular cyst, are clearly visible on the CT scan (Figure 5), it has to be emphasized that the cyst's impact on the circulatory and cardiopulmonary system could not be determined by CT scan. This is due to the fact that a CT scan with focus on pulmonary embolism does not show the dynamics and alterations of the heart and potential impact on hemodynamics during an entire heart cycle.

With this case report, we presented an unusual cause of dyspnea and thoracic pressure. Although there were no evident alterations in preload or pulmonary pressure, the almost complete extrinsic compression of the right ventricle is the only explanation for the cardiorespiratory symptoms described by the patient. Right ventricular compression only became visible when performing an echocardiography, which also underlines its value as a radiation-free, economic, and convenient diagnostic tool in daily clinical practice.

Acknowledgments

We acknowledge the support by Deutsche Forschungsgemeinschaft and Open Access Publishing Fund of University of Tübingen. This project was also supported by the Deutsche Forschungsgemeinschaft (Klinische Forschungsgruppe-KFO-274: "Platelets-Molecular Mechanisms and Translational Implications") and by the Deutsche Forschungsgemeinschaft (DFG; German Research Foundation)—project number 374031971-TRR 240. We would like to thank Dr. Leonie Frauenfeld, Institute of Pathology, University Hospital Tuebingen, for the contribution and interpretation of the histological slides.

References

[1] A. Pitale, A. K. Bohra, and T. Diamond, "Management of symptomatic liver cysts," *The Ulster Medical Journal*, vol. 71, no. 2, pp. 106–110, 2002.

[2] A. Regev and K. R. Reddy, "Diagnosis and management in cystic lesions," January 2019, from https://www.uptodate.com/contents/diagnosis-and-management-of-cystic-lesions-of-the-liver#H17.

[3] M. Makar, G. Makar, and K. Yousef, "Large pericardial cyst presenting as acute cough: a rare case report," *Case Reports in Cardiology*, vol. 2018, Article ID 4796903, 3 pages, 2018.

[4] J. C. Mwita, P. Chipeta, R. Mutagaywa, B. Rugwizangoga, and E. Ussiri, "Pericardial cyst with right ventricular compression," *The Pan African Medical Journal*, vol. 12, 2012.

[5] D. E. Jaroszewski, T. A. Warsame, K. Chandrasekaran, and H. Chaliki, "Right ventricular compression observed in echocardiography from pectus excavatum deformity," *Journal of Cardiovascular Ultrasound*, vol. 19, no. 4, pp. 192–195, 2011.

[6] A. Tandon, D. Wallihan, A. M. Lubert, and M. D. Taylor, "The effect of right ventricular compression on cardiac function in pediatric pectus excavatum," *Journal of Cardiovascular Magnetic Resonance*, vol. 16, no. S1, 2014.

[7] C. Y. Li, M. Taylor, V. Garcia, R. Brown, and M. Rattan, "The effect of right ventricular compression on cardiac function in pediatric pectus excavatum patients," *Journal of the American College of Cardiology*, vol. 69, no. 11, p. 1571, 2017.

[8] M. A. Lantinga, T. J. G. Gevers, and J. P. H. Drenth, "Evaluation of hepatic cystic lesions," *World Journal of Gastroenterology*, vol. 19, no. 23, pp. 3543–3554, 2013.

[9] A. Tocchi, G. Mazzoni, G. Costa et al., "Symptomatic nonparasitic hepatic cysts: options for and results of surgical management," *Archives of Surgery*, vol. 137, no. 2, pp. 154–158, 2002.

Successful Treatment of Severe Paravalvular Leak by Repositioning a Self-Expandable Percutaneous Aortic Valve Bioprosthesis (Evolut PRO+) using the "Double Snare" Technique

Diego H. González-Bravo,[1] Pedro Colón-Hernández,[2] Melanie Quintana-Serrano,[1] Sergio Alegre-Boschetti,[1] Juan Vázquez-Fuster,[1] José J. Acevedo-Valles,[1,3] and Eric Avilés-Rivera[1,2]

[1]*Cardiovascular Division, Department of Medicine, VA Caribbean Healthcare System, San Juan, Puerto Rico, USA*
[2]*Cardiovascular Center, Menonita Medical Center, Cayey, Puerto Rico, USA*
[3]*Internal Medicine Division, Department of Medicine, VA Caribbean Healthcare System, San Juan, Puerto Rico, USA*

Correspondence should be addressed to Eric Avilés-Rivera; avileseric2@hotmail.com

Academic Editor: Yigit Canga

Significant (moderate or severe) paravalvular leak (PVL) after transcatheter aortic valve replacement (TAVR) remains a common phenomenon and has been associated with decrease survival and quality of life. Transcatheter valve embolization and migration (TVEM) is a rare post-TAVR complication that can occur in 1% of cases and has been associated with worse patient outcomes. Valve embolization or migration into the left ventricle can result in significant PVL causing hemodynamic instability, shock, heart failure, and hemolytic anemia. Although this complication most commonly occurs in the acute setting (90%) within 4 hours of TAVR, it can also present late (4 hr-43 days later) in 10% of cases. There are no clear guidelines as to how this condition should be managed; however, several percutaneous bailout techniques exist that can ultimately spare the patient from emergent cardiovascular surgery. We present a rare case of late ventricular transcatheter aortic valve migration 3 days after TAVR causing severe PVL and heart failure symptoms that was successfully treated using the percutaneous "double snare" technique.

1. Introduction

Transcatheter valve embolization and migration (TVEM) is a dismal complication that can occur in 1% of transcatheter aortic valve replacement (TAVR) cases [1]. It has been associated with increased morbidity and worse patient outcomes. Mortality rates have been reported as high as 40% at 30 days [1, 2]. This complication most commonly presents within the first 4 hours post-TAVR in 90% of TVEM cases; however, the remaining 10% can present late (4 hr-43 days later) for which a high clinical suspicion for diagnosis is imperative [2]. The ascending aorta (38%) is the most common site of valve embolization, followed by the left ventricle (31%) [2]. Among the risk factors for the development of this complication are the use of self-expandable valves, low implantation depths, valve undersizing, large aortic root dimensions, and the presence of a native bicuspid aortic valve [1].

Ventricular migration or embolization of a transcatheter aortic valve can result in significant paravalvular leak (PVL) causing hemodynamic instability, shock, heart failure, and hemolytic anemia [3, 4]. It is well known that post-TAVR significant (moderate or severe) PVL is associated with worse prognosis (17% mortality at 1 year) and poor quality of life [3]. Several percutaneous repair techniques exist that can be employed as "bail-out" procedures often sparing these patients from salvage and emergent cardiac surgery which carries a considerable higher risk of death at 30 days (32.7%) when compared to the percutaneous methods

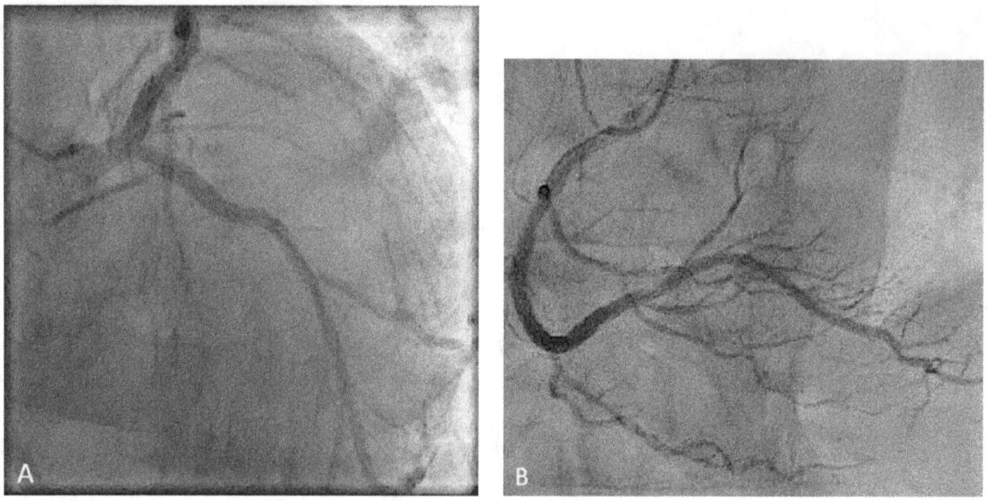

FIGURE 1: Coronary angiography. No evidence of obstructive coronary artery disease in the left coronary (a) and right coronary arteries (b).

(12.5%) [1]. However, comparative studies to establish superiority between these percutaneous "bail-out" techniques are lacking [4, 5]. Therefore, the selected approach for repair will mostly depend on the PVL mechanism (valve malapposition, undersizing, or malposition) and the capacity of the technique by itself to completely correct the problem as well as the operator's proficiency and familiarity with the selected technique.

We present a rare case of late ventricular TVEM 3 days after TAVR causing severe PVL and heart failure symptoms that was successfully treated using the percutaneous "double snare" technique. We aim to emphasize the importance of early recognition of this complication as we review its diagnosis and highlight its impact over patient morbidity and mortality, plus demonstrate how effective is the "double snare" technique for the treatment of these patients, as well as discuss our rationale behind the selection of this technique.

2. Case Presentation

2.1. History of Present Illness. A 74-year-old man who presented to our emergency department with symptoms of progressive exertional dyspnea and orthopnea for the last 24 hours. He was found afebrile (37.4°C), hemodynamically stable (heart rate = 81 beats/min and blood pressure = 121/58 mmHg) with a wide pulse pressure (63 mmHg), and tachypneic (22 breaths/min) without hypoxia (96%). Clinical examination revealed signs of central congestion, a grade 3 diastolic decrescendo murmur at the left upper sternal border, and warm extremities without edema. He underwent transcatheter aortic valve replacement (TAVR) 3 days prior at another institution and was discharged home the following day without complications.

2.2. Past Medical History. Medical history was significant for mesenteric low-grade follicular B-cell lymphoma, nonobstructive coronary artery disease (Figure 1), and severe aortic valve stenosis with 20-25% left ventricular (LV) systolic function. He underwent TAVR with a 34 mm Medtronic Evolut PRO+ bioprosthesis (supra-annular and self-expanding valve), with plans to proceed with chemotherapy subsequently.

2.3. Investigations. Electrocardiography revealed sinus rhythm without new ischemic changes (Figure 2). There was no angina or new wall motion abnormalities to favor a type 1 myocardial infarction despite elevated high-sensitive troponins (399 → 362 → 420 ng/L; >22 ng/L abnormal value). No anemia or leukocytosis was present, and pro-BNP was elevated (10,407 pg/mL). Chest X-ray and CT scan (Figure 3) showed a right moderate pleural effusion, pulmonary congestion, and no evidence of pulmonary embolism, aortic dissection, or pericardial effusion.

2.4. Differential Diagnosis. Clinical scenario was suggestive of congestive heart failure possibly due to prosthetic valve dysfunction. Nevertheless, given his recent TAVR and hospitalization, pulmonary embolism, aortic dissection, pericardial effusion, pneumonia, anemia, and myocardial infarction were all considered.

2.5. Management. Patient was admitted to the intensive care unit, and aggressive diuresis was provided. Transthoracic (TTE) (Figure 4) and transesophageal echocardiogram (TEE) (Figure 5, Videos 1–3) confirmed ventricular transcatheter aortic valve migration causing severe paravalvular leak (PVL) (circumferential extent~50%, aortic holodiastolic flow reversal, large vena contracta (diameter = 0.6 cm, area = 0.57 cm^2), low pressure half-time (PHT) of 126 msec, and a dilated LV in diastole (7.3 cm)) without evidence of bioprosthesis stenosis (peak systolic velocity (PSV) = 273 cm/sec, acceleration time (AT) = 80 msec, mean pressure gradient (MPG) = 15 mmHg, dimensionless index (DI) = 0.42). Renal, liver, and respiratory systems became compromised (cardiac index = 2.1 L/min/kg and pulmonary wedge pressure = 28 mmHg) requiring dobutamine and noninvasive ventilation for stabilization. Case was presented to patient's

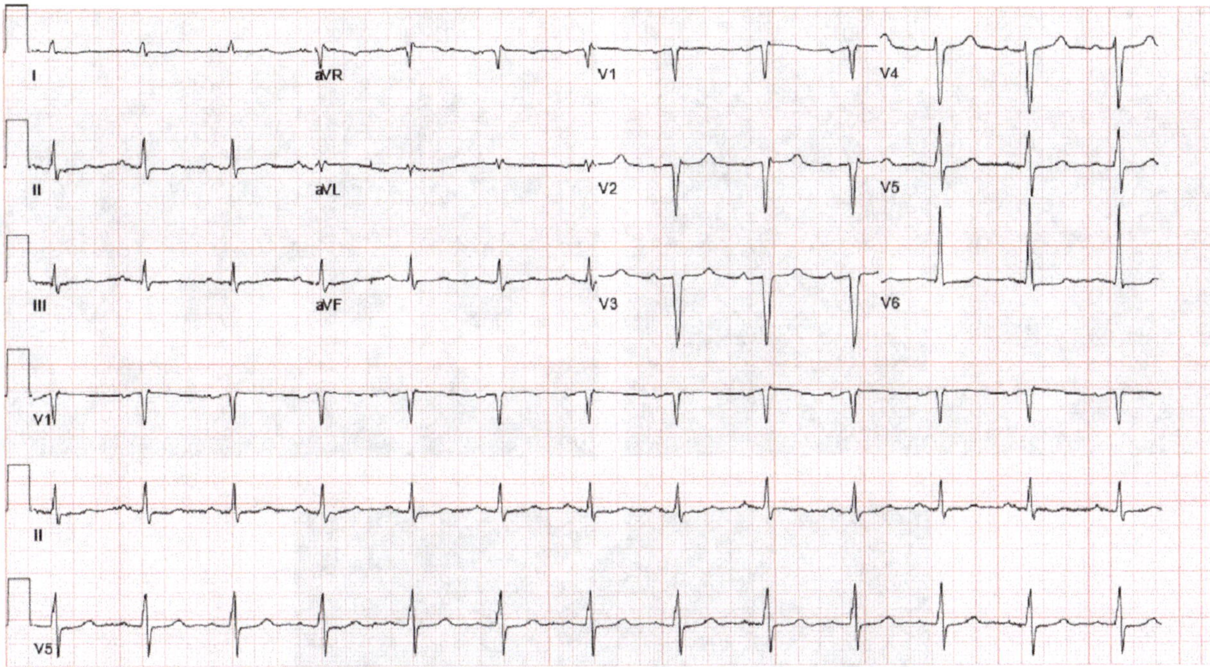

Figure 2: Electrocardiogram. Normal sinus rhythm with old nonspecific ST-segment changes in the lateral leads.

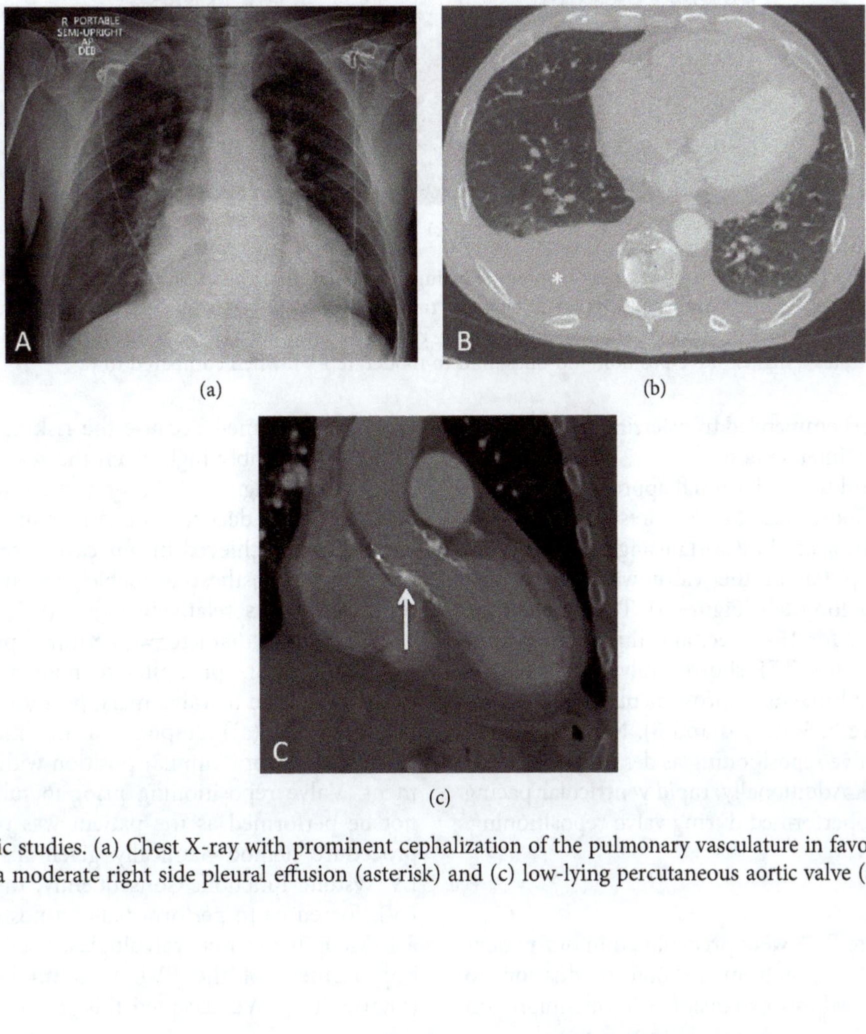

(a) (b)

(c)

Figure 3: Radiographic studies. (a) Chest X-ray with prominent cephalization of the pulmonary vasculature in favor of pulmonary edema. CT scan showing (b) a moderate right side pleural effusion (asterisk) and (c) low-lying percutaneous aortic valve (arrow).

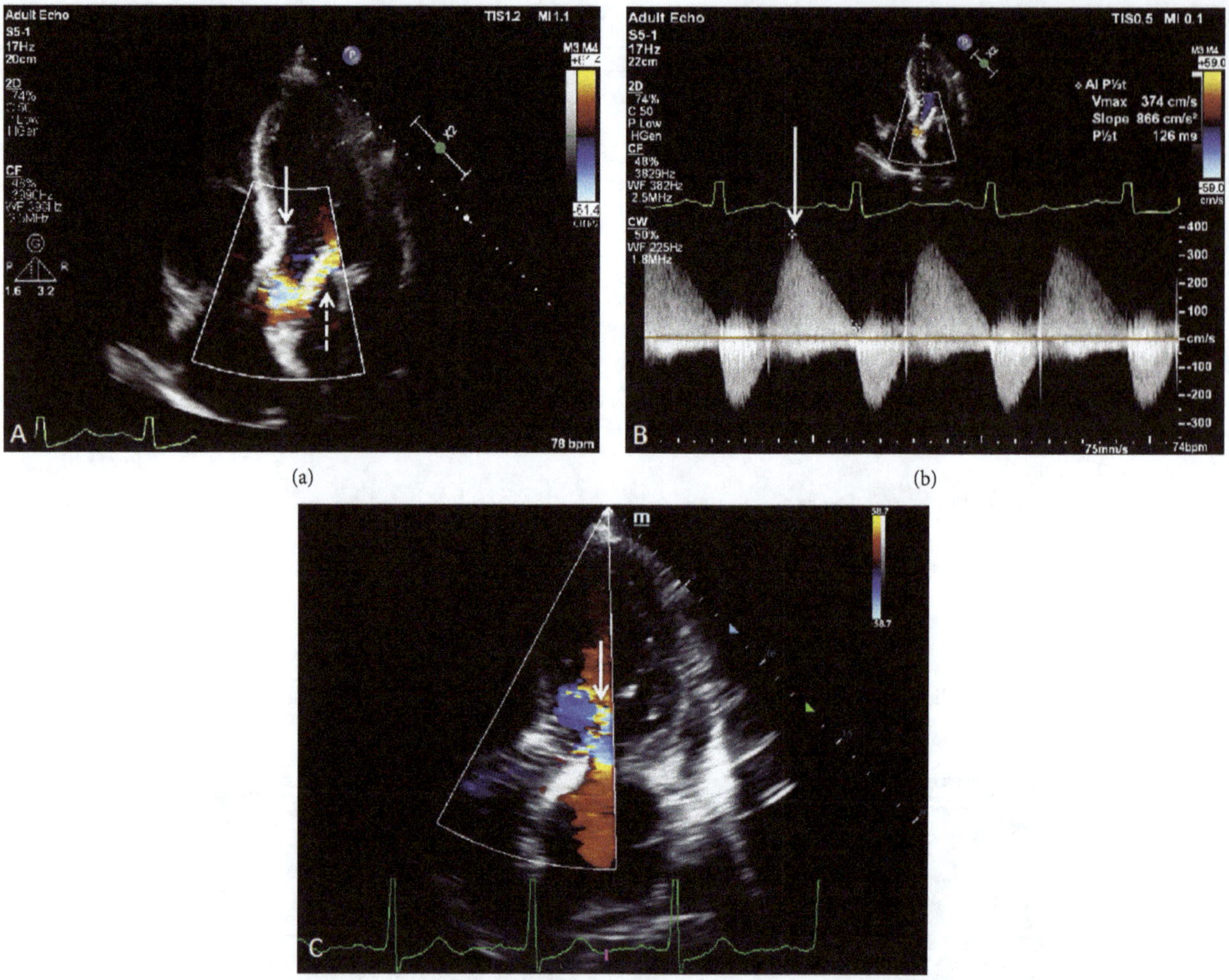

FIGURE 4: Transthoracic echocardiography. (a) Color Doppler showing left ventricular migration of an aortic bioprosthesis (solid arrow) resulting in PVL (dashed arrow). (b) Spectral Doppler showing a rapidly decelerating (triangle-shaped) aortic regurgitation jet (solid arrow) with a pressure half – time = 126 msec suggestive of severe PVL. (c) Transthoracic echocardiogram 24 hours post-TAVR for comparison. It demonstrates a higher valve position and only mild to moderate PVL when compared to (a).

TAVR operator who recommended transferring the patient to his institution for PVL intervention.

Via right radial and femoral arterial approach (6Fr), two Medtronic Amplatz Goose Neck Microsnares (15 × 120 mm) were advanced into the ascending aorta using two AL1 catheters. The inner loop tab of the valve was snared first followed by the outer loop tab (Figure 6). The snares were then pulled constantly for 15-20 sec, and this was repeated every 20 sec until real-time TEE showed valve repositioning to a higher level resulting in improvement of PVL from severe to mild (Figure 7, Videos 4 and 5). No postdilation was necessary after valve repositioning as described similarly in other reports [6–8]. Additionally, rapid ventricular pacing was not required nor performed during valve repositioning.

3. Discussion

Late TVEM and severe PVL were precipitated in our patient by several factors. First, upfront balloon predilation to ensure optimal bioprosthesis expansion without migration was not performed because the risk of stroke was believed to be unacceptably high given the severely complex calcific aortic valve (Figure 8). Second, valve oversizing > 10% has been shown to decrease the risk of future PVL; however, it could not be achieved in our case despite using the largest (34 mm) bioprosthesis available given that our patient's aortic annulus was relatively larger (CT measurements: area $= 771.4\,\text{mm}^2$, diameter = 31.8 mm, perimeter = 99.9 mm) [4]. Both factors precipitated moderate PVL immediately post-TAVR due to valve malapposition and a low malposition (Figure 6(a)) despite our intentions to implant the valve in the supra-annular position with commissural alignment. Valve repositioning prior to full deployment could not be performed as the patient was poorly tolerating the procedure hemodynamically given his severely decreased LV systolic function. Consequently, the residual moderate PVL forced us to perform balloon postdilation (BPD) with a Z-Med 30 × 40 mm valvuloplasty balloon resulting in the improvement of the PVL to a mild-to-moderate degree (Figure 4(c)). We accepted this result and opted to not be

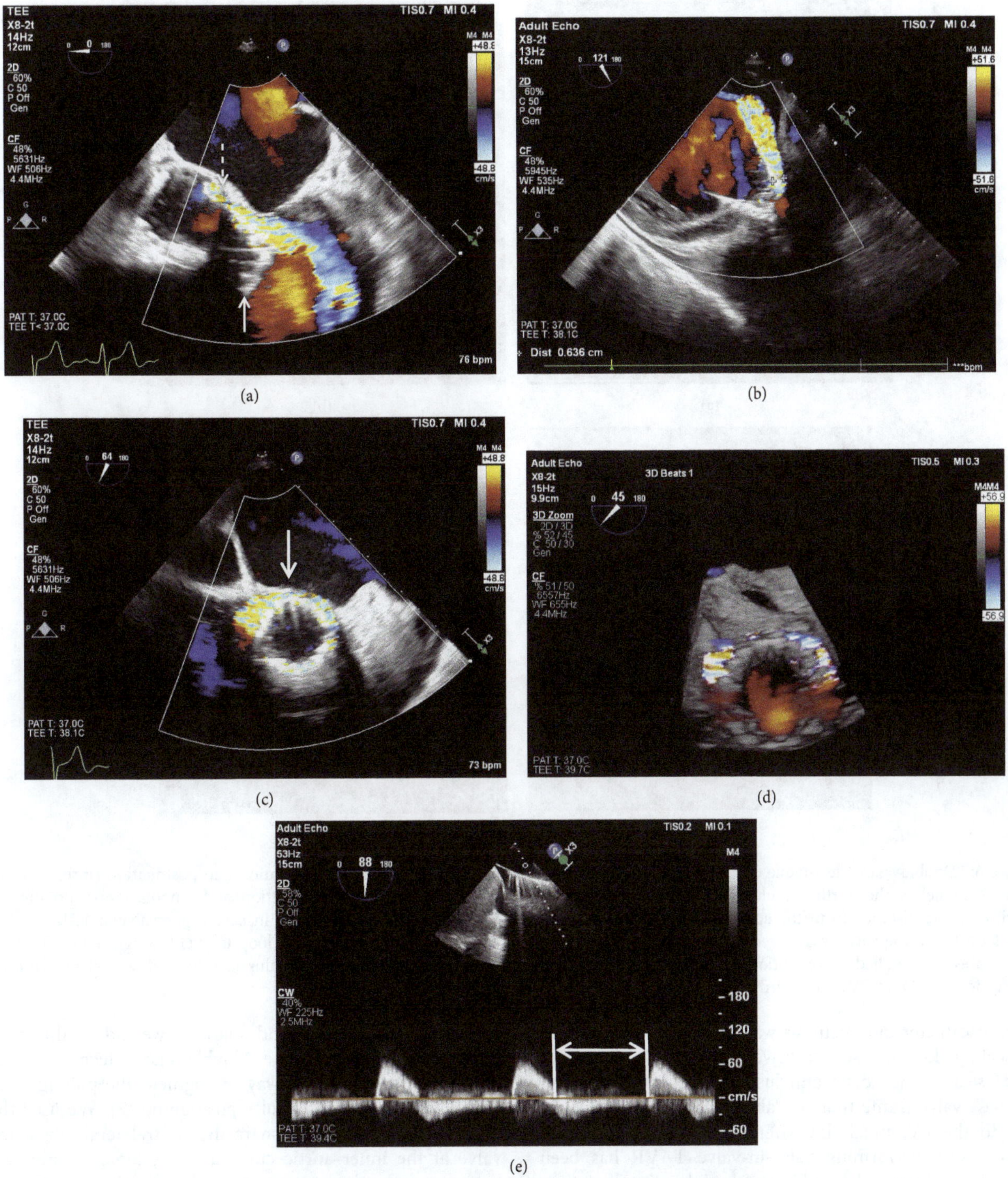

FIGURE 5: Transesophageal echocardiogram. (a) Aortic bioprosthesis ventricular migration (solid arrow) causing severe PVL (Videos 1–3) by color Doppler (dashed arrow). (b) Transgastric view showing a large vena contracta (0.636 cm). PVL circumferential extent (arrow) involving ~50% of the aortic annulus in the short-axis views in (c) 2D and (d) 3D color Doppler. (e) Thoracic aorta holodiastolic flow reversal consistent with severe PVL (arrow).

more aggressive with BPD as it has been shown to increase risk of stroke, leaflet injury, aortic rupture, and pacemaker implantation [4].

The relative size mismatch, lack of predilation, low malposition, and failure to perform a more aggressive BPD favored a "watermelon seeding" phenomenon that made the self-expanding valve slip into the LV resulting in late ventricular TVEM and severe PVL 3 days later after TAVR. At this stage, vascular plugs were not an option given the incorrect valve position, circumferential nature of the PVL, and its multiple jets [5]. Performing valve-in-valve TAVR was contemplated [4, 5]. Nevertheless,

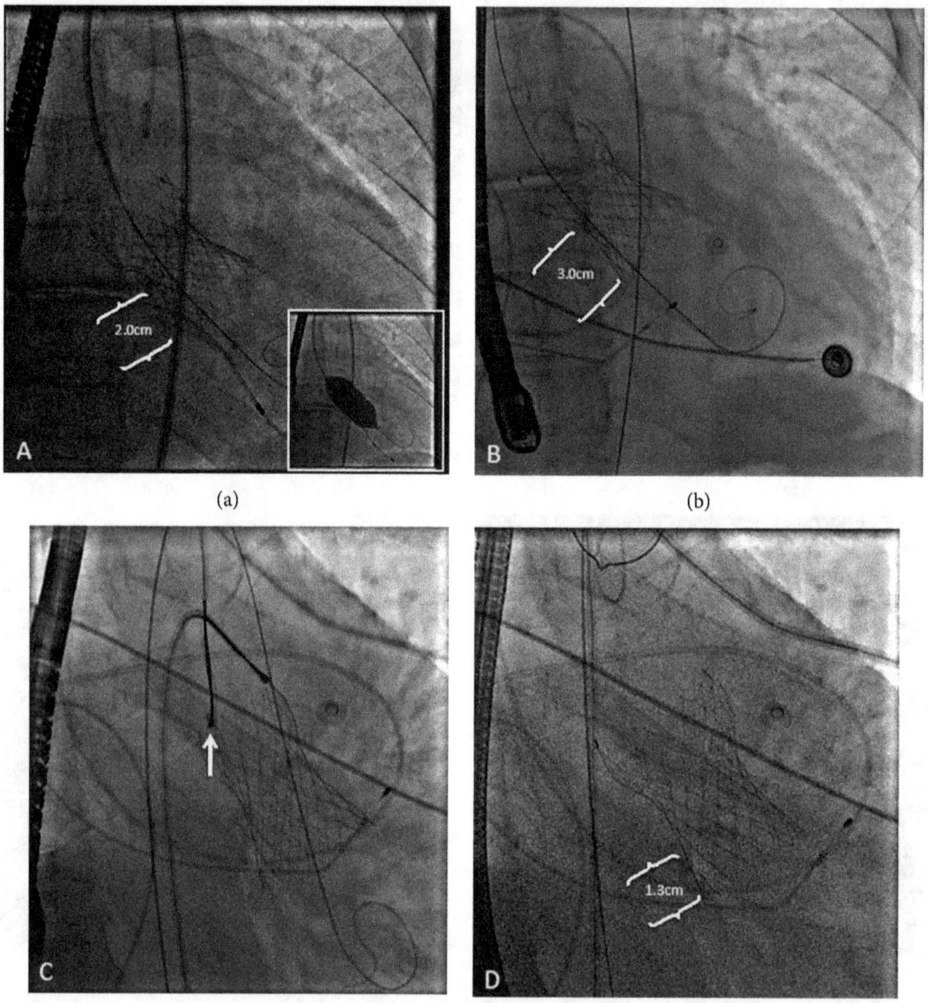

(a) (b) (c) (d)

Figure 6: "Double snare" technique (fluoroscopy). (a) Low-lying Evolut PRO+ after initial implantation and postdilation (inset) with its inflow 2 cm below the aortic annulus (braces) for comparison. (b) Late ventricular valve migration and embolization into the left ventricle as the distance from the aortic annulus to the valve inflow worsened (3.0 cm) resulting in severe paravalvular leak. (c) The inner loop tab of the valve was snared first (arrow) via the right radial artery followed by the outer loop tab via the right femoral artery. Both snares were pulled to reposition the valve cranially. (d) After repositioning, the aortic annulus-to-valve inflow distance (braces, 1.3 cm) decreased and PVL improved.

the transcatheter bioprosthesis was so deep in the LV that the sealing skirt of a second valve was going to be incapable of sealing the aortic annulus and the entire adjacent tissueless valve frame that was allowing blood to percolate back to the LV, much less overcome its radial strength. Furthermore, performing valve-in-valve TAVR has been shown to increase the risk of pacemaker implantation, acute coronary artery occlusion, may compromise future coronary access, and can indeed increase procedure cost [6]. Alternatively, the snare technique could bypass much of these challenges and correct the PVL effectively.

Vavouranakis et al. [6] were the first one to describe the snare technique by using a single Amplatz Goose Neck Microsnare (35 × 120 mm) to successfully reposition a low-implanted Medtronic CoreValve and resolve its PVL. This procedure is not to be confused with the snare technique used for facilitating advancement of the TAVR delivery system across challenging aortic anatomy and the aortic valve [9]. Adding a second snare as we did in this case, a maneuver known as the "double snare" technique, has also been described as a way to augment the pulling force and likelihood of successful repositioning [7]. We used the right radial approach to snare the contralateral tab of the valve at the inner aortic curve and the femoral approach to snare from the opposite side the remaining valve tab at the outer aortic curve. By using this configuration of contralateral forces crossing each other, the radial force of the valve was decreased as it was being forced to partially collapse on itself which in turn resulted in less friction and tissue damage as the valve was being pulled. Nonetheless, awareness should be made that aggressive pulling of the bioprosthesis could result in TVEM into the ascending aorta, embolic stroke, or aortic dissection [6–8]. Despite all these risks, a retrospective study by Won-Keun et al. [1] showed that the use of this percutaneous bailout strategy was found to have a lower 30-day

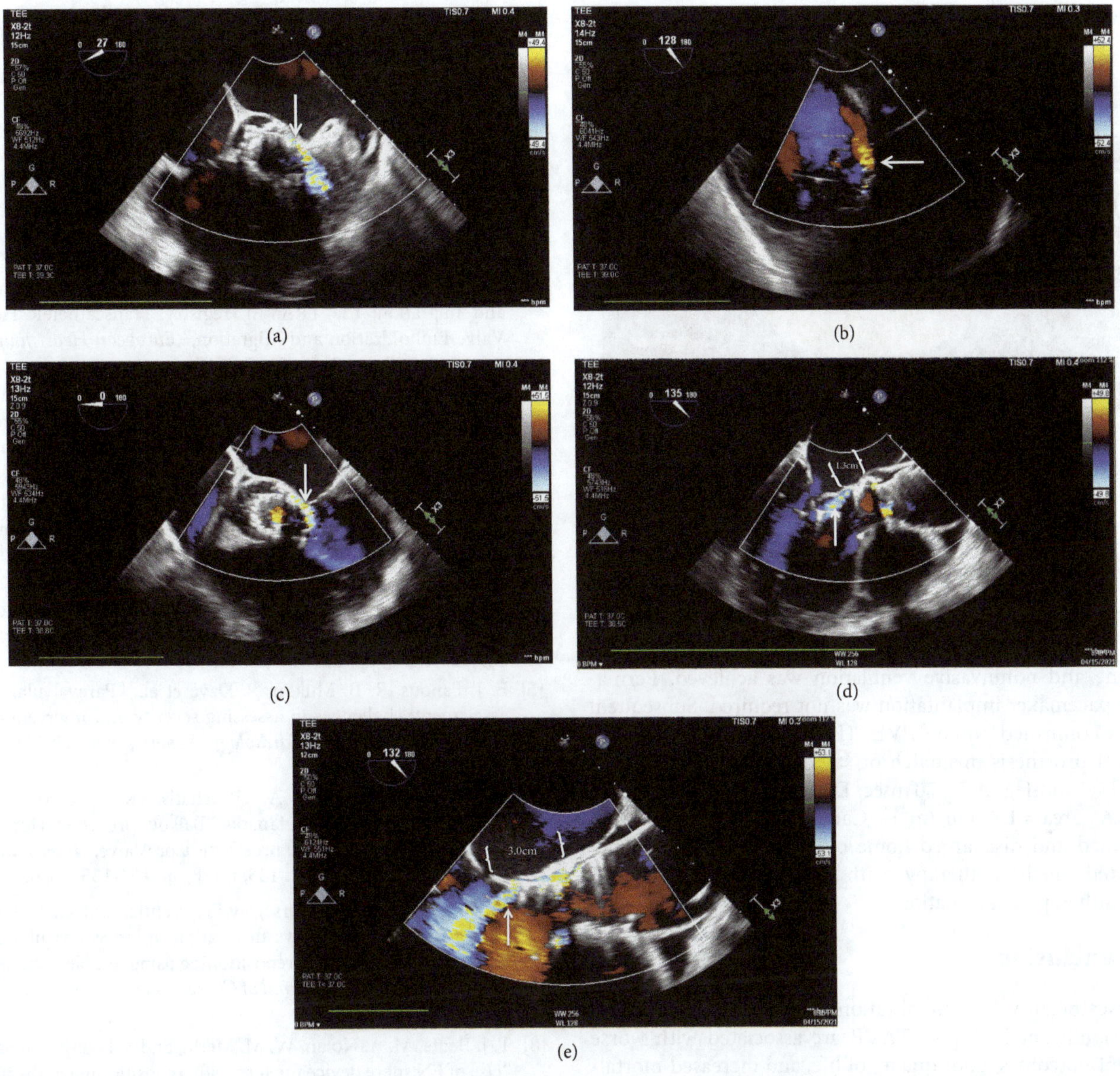

FIGURE 7: Transesophageal echocardiogram after valve repositioning. Mild PVL by color Doppler (arrow) in the (a) short-axis and (b) deep-transgastric views (Videos 4 and 5). (c) PVL circumferential extent (arrow) was reduced to 20%. (d) Long-axis view showing mild PVL (arrow). (e) Severe PVL (arrow) prior to valve repositioning for comparison. Postrepositioning, the aortic annulus-to-valve inflow distance (braces) was reduced from (e) 3.0 cm to (d) 1.3 cm.

mortality of 12.5% compared to performing a transcatheter valve-in-valve procedure (16.3%) and open-heart surgery (32.7%).

Postdilation after valve repositioning using the "double snare" technique was not performed for several reasons. First, we wanted to minimize further aggressive instrumentation of the ascending aorta knowing how severely calcific and friable the native aortic valve was, in order to decrease our risk of causing embolic complications, especially in our setting where we do not have available the cerebral embolic protection system (SENTINEL, Boston Scientific). Second, we believed that the risks (e.g., permanent pacemaker implantation, aortic rupture, and bioprothesis leaflet injury) were greater than the benefits, as we had used the largest diameter valvuloplasty balloon (30 × 40 mm, Z-MED) that we had available for postdilation after initial valve implantation, and it was unsuccessful in preventing late ventricular migration of the valve. And third, several similar reports using the "double snare" technique have demonstrated successful results without performing postdilation after valve repositioning [6–8].

The snare technique usefulness has been mostly described as a bailout procedure for the treatment of low valve implantation or acute (<1-4 hr) TVEM resulting in significant PVL. Our case is unique and exceptional since it shows that this technique can also be safe and effective for the treatment of late ventricular TVEM even when occurring days later after TAVR, as it was done successfully in our patient on day 7 post-TAVR sparing him from emergent open-heart surgery.

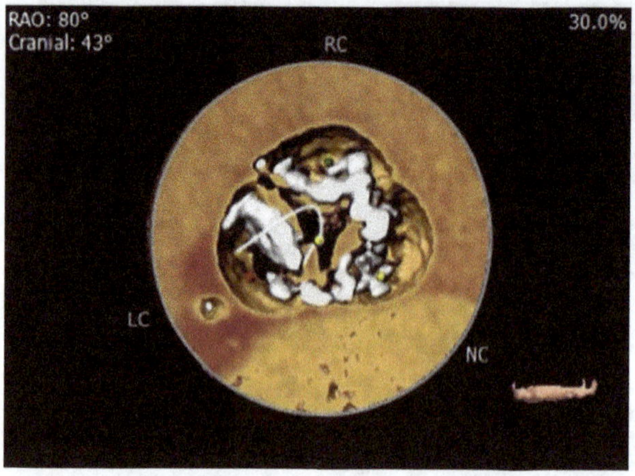

FIGURE 8: Extensive aortic valve calcifications (white). Right (RC), left (LC), and noncoronary (NC) cusps.

4. Follow-Up

After valve repositioning, patient's symptoms resolved, renal and liver function normalized, and discontinuation of dobutamine and noninvasive ventilation was achieved. Permanent pacemaker implantation was not required. Subsequent TTE confirmed mild PVL (PHT = 490 msec) without patient-prosthesis mismatch or stenosis (PSV = 151 cm/sec, MPG = 5 mmHg, AT = 70 msec, DI = 0.62, indexed effective orifice area = 1.47 cm^2/m^2). Cardiac rehabilitation was provided and discharged home on heart failure guideline-directed medical therapy with oncology follow-up for chemotherapy coordination.

5. Conclusion

Transcatheter valve embolization and migration (TVEM) and significant PVL post-TAVR are associated with worse patient outcomes, poor quality of life, and increased mortality. The "double snare" technique is a useful bailout procedure for the treatment of significant PVL post-TAVR due to low valve malposition and acute TVEM. However, this case is unique as it demonstrates that this technique may also be safe and effective for the treatment of late ventricular TVEM causing significant PVL.

Abbreviations

AT: Acceleration time
BPD: Balloon post-dilation
DI: Dimensionless index
MPG: Mean pressure gradient
LV: Left ventricle
PSV: Peak systolic velocity
PHT: Pressure half-time
PVL: Paravalvular leak
TAVR: Transcatheter aortic valve replacement
TEE: Transesophageal echocardiogram
TTE: Transthoracic echocardiogram
TVEM: Transcatheter valve embolization and migration.

Acknowledgments

This material is the result of work supported with resources and the use of facilities at the Veterans Affairs, Caribbean Healthcare System San Juan, P.R.

References

[1] W. K. Kim, U. Schäfer, D. Tchetche et al., "Incidence and outcome of peri-procedural transcatheter heart valve embolization and migration: the TRAVEL registry TranscatheteR HeArt Valve EmboLization and Migration," *European Heart Journal*, vol. 40, no. 38, pp. 3156–3165, 2019.

[2] U. N. Ibebuogu, S. Giri, O. Bolorunduro et al., "Review of reported causes of device embolization following transcatheter aortic valve implantation," *The American Journal of Cardiology*, vol. 115, no. 12, pp. 1767–1772, 2015.

[3] S. V. Arnold, Y. Zhang, S. J. Baron et al., "Impact of short-term complications on mortality and quality of life after transcatheter aortic valve replacement," *JACC Cardiovascular Interventions*, vol. 12, no. 4, pp. 362–369, 2019.

[4] S. Lerakis, S. S. Hayek, and P. S. Douglas, "Paravalvular aortic leak after transcatheter aortic valve replacement," *Circulation*, vol. 127, no. 3, pp. 397–407, 2013.

[5] E. J. Fanous, R. B. Mukku, P. Dave et al., "Paravalvular leak assessment: challenges in assessing severity and interventional approaches," *Current Cardiology Reports*, vol. 22, no. 12, p. 166, 2020.

[6] M. Vavouranakis, D. A. Vrachatis, K. P. Toutouzas, C. Chrysohoou, and C. Stefanadis, "Bail out procedures for malpositioning of aortic valve prosthesis CoreValve," *International Journal of Cardiology*, vol. 145, no. 1, pp. 154-155, 2010.

[7] M. Bunc, L. Vitez, S. Terseglav, T. Žlahtič, and G. P. Ussia, "Transcatheter aortic valve dislocation in left ventricular outflow tract with successful repositioning using double snare technique," *International Journal of Clinical Medicine*, vol. 12, no. 1, pp. 7–13, 2021.

[8] T. J. Beute, M. A. Nolan, W. M. Merhi, and S. Leung Wai Sang, "Use of EN snare device for successful repositioning of the newest self-expanding transcatheter heart valve," *SAGE Open Medical Case Reports*, vol. 6, article 2050313X1881993, 2018.

[9] K. J. Kunkel, P. Fiorilli, T. Kobayashi, N. D. Desai, S. Anwaruddin, and H. C. Herrmann, "Snare-assisted valve positioning of self-expanding valves for Transcatheter aortic valve replacement," *Case Reports*, vol. 3, no. 4, pp. 658–662, 2021.

43

Multiple Imaging and Surgical Characteristics in Cardiac Metastasis from Undifferentiated Uterine Sarcoma

Hiroka Sasahara,[1,2] Shoichiro Yatsu,[1] Hideki Wada,[1] Eiryu Sai,[3] Soshi Moriya,[1] Suguru Miyazaki,[4] Kan Kajimoto,[4] Manabu Ogita,[1] and Satoru Suwa[1]

[1]*Department of Cardiovascular Medicine, Juntendo University Shizuoka Hospital, Izunokuni-shi, Japan*
[2]*Department of Metabolism and Endocrinology, Juntendo University Graduate School of Medicine, Tokyo, Japan*
[3]*Department of Cardiovascular Biology and Medicine, Juntendo University Graduate School of Medicine, Tokyo, Japan*
[4]*Cardiovascular Surgery, Juntendo University Shizuoka Hospital, Izunokuni-shi, Japan*

Correspondence should be addressed to Shoichiro Yatsu; syatsu@juntendo.ac.jp

Academic Editor: Yuli Huang

Although cardiac metastasis of malignant tumors has often been reported, undifferentiated uterine sarcoma (UUS) is a rare and aggressive uterine tumor. Thus, little is known of the UUS as a primary site of cardiac metastasis. We report a case of a 66-year-old woman, with a history of uterine myoma for 30 years, who was hospitalized with a large uterine tumor and cardiac masses. Although we investigated cardiac masses using imaging modalities, such as ultrasound, cardiac computer tomography, and magnetic resonance imaging, it was challenging to determine the masses as metastasis or thrombi. Cardiac masses were removed by surgery to assess the tissue characteristics and were later identified as tumors due to their appearance. Then, pathological findings revealed that UUS spreads to the right ventricle. We attempted chemotherapy after surgery; however, the disease progressed very quickly and the patient died on the 49th day of admission. In this report, we described the case of a patient with a difficult diagnosis and rapid disease progression of cardiac metastasis from UUS.

1. Introduction

The incidence of cardiac metastases has increased over the last 30 years due to the increased life expectancy in oncologic patients owing to the advanced cancer diagnosis and management [1]. Uterine sarcomas are rare malignant tumors arising from the mesenchymal tissues of the uterus, i.e., the endometrial stroma, uterine muscle, and connective tissue [2]. Although it is estimated that 0.1–0.3% of the patients operated on for presumed uterine myoma have a uterine sarcoma, uterine sarcomas only represent 3–7% of all uterine malignances [3]. Thus, uterine sarcomas are relatively rare as the primary lesion of cardiac metastasis [1].

Undifferentiated uterine sarcoma (UUS) is one of the uterine sarcomas with a very poor prognosis, and most of the patients with UUS die within 2 years of diagnosis [2]. In addition, UUS is one of the rarest of the disease, with a prevalence of less than 10% among all uterine sarcomas [2]. Thus, due to its infrequent occurrence and adverse outcome, cardiac metastasis from UUS has never been reported. Although one report suggested the utility of ultrasound to differentiate the uterine sarcomas [4], approaches to UUS either in diagnosis or systemic therapy remain controversial despite the necessity for early diagnosis to treat this rapidly progressive disease. Herein, we presented a case of right ventricle metastases from UUS to report the imaging characteristics and state of rapid progress.

2. Case Report

A 66-year-old woman experienced abdominal pain and visited a private medical center. The patient had had a medical history of uterine myoma for 30 years, but no other history was reported. Computed tomography (CT) showed enlarged uterine myoma and a right ventricular mass and she was immediately transferred to our hospital. She had a blood pressure of 132/68 mmHg, a heart rate of 78 b.p.m.,

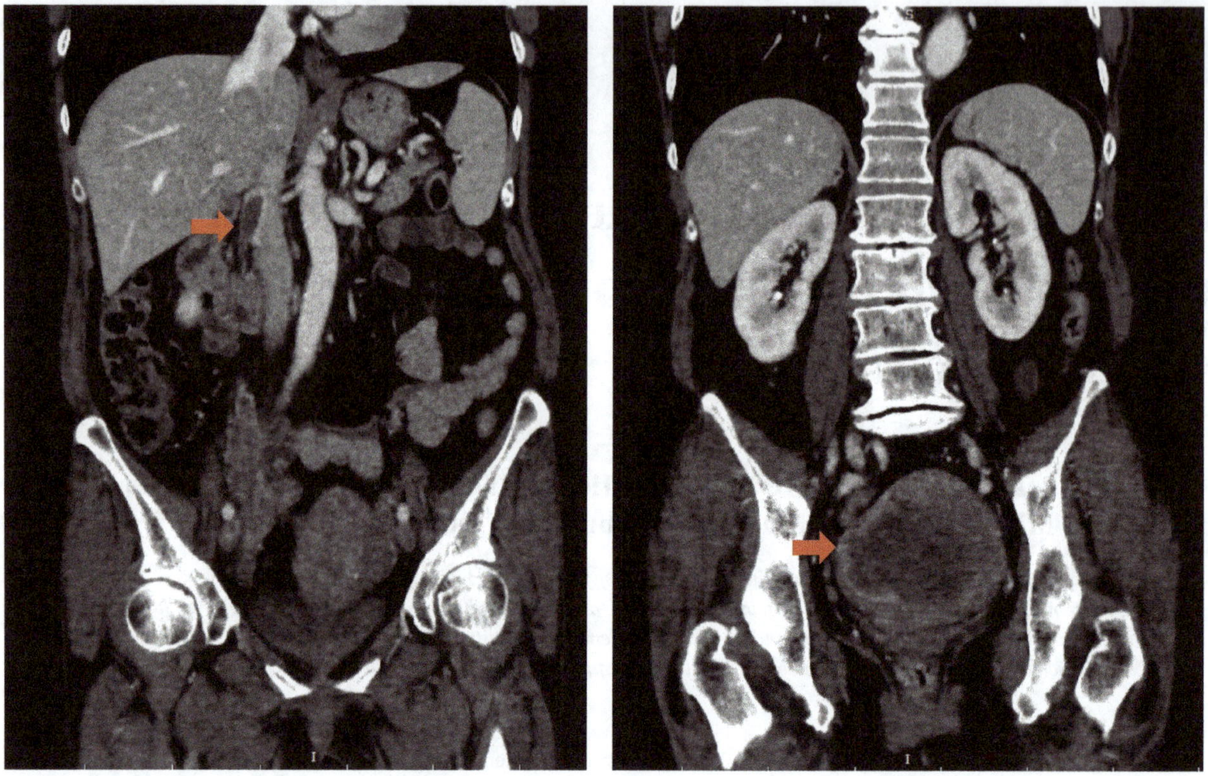

(a) (b)

Figure 1: Computed tomography on admission. Intraluminal filling defect from the right ovarian vein to the inferior vena cava (arrow) (a) and a large uterine mass (arrow) (b).

respiratory rate of 18 breaths/min, and oxygen saturation of 96% on room air at arrival. On initial physical examination, she had regular cardiac rhythm with no heart murmurs and no significant pretibial edema. Chest radiography showed neither congestion nor infiltrative shadows. Electrocardiography showed normal sinus rhythm without any ST segment change. Blood tests indicated a hemoglobin level of 10.7 g/L, C-reactive protein level of 1.10 mg/dL, and a D-dimer level of 8.3 μg/mL. Tumor markers were within normal limits, including CA125 of 8 U/mL. A transthoracic echocardiogram showed an elongated mass-like structure in the right ventricle without any other complications. Transabdominal and transvaginal ultrasound showed multiple uterine solid masses (60 mm) with well-defined margins and mild extracellular fluid space. Contrast-enhanced CT revealed a very large uterine mass (107.5 mm), intraluminal filling defect via the right ovarian vein to the inferior vena cava (Figure 1), and right ventricle masses.

Experienced gynecologists and radiologists discussed and evaluated the CT scan findings. Although the uterine mass seemed to be a malignant tumor based on its configuration, tissue diagnosis was necessary to choose the adequate treatment. Multiple transvaginal biopsies were performed, but a diagnosis of normal uterine tissue was reached by a dedicated pathologist. However, diagnosing uterine mass with transvaginal biopsy has a low accuracy. Surgical mass resection was required, but the presence of cardiac masses made a surgical approach for uterine mass difficult due to the risk of embolization.

Thus, cardiologists were consulted and conducted further assessments for the cardiac mass. Transesophageal echocardiography revealed a well-defined, mobile mass below the pulmonary artery valve (Figures 2(a) and 2(b)). The cardiac CT scan and cardiac magnetic resonance imaging (MRI) were performed by experienced cardiologists and radiologists to assess further the anatomical and qualitative details. The cardiac CT revealed a well-defined mass with a lack of contrast enhancement in the right ventricle below the pulmonary artery valve (Figure 2(c)). The cardiac MRI showed some masses in the right ventricle, which had hypersignal intensity on fat-saturated T2-weighted image (Figure 2(d)), isointensity on T1-weighted image (Figure 2(e)), and no suppressed signal by fat suppression on T1-weighted image (Figure 2(f)). Based on these images, it was difficult to identify them as either tumors or thrombi. In addition, the mass did not respond well to anticoagulants, with its size remaining unchanged after one week of rivaroxaban (15 mg twice daily: Japanese standard dose for venous thromboembolism).

Our cardiologists and gynecologists repeatedly discussed the approach on this case and decided to perform an open-heart mass removal for tissue diagnosis and to remove the embolic source. On the 20th day of hospitalization, cardiac surgery was performed with median sternotomy by making

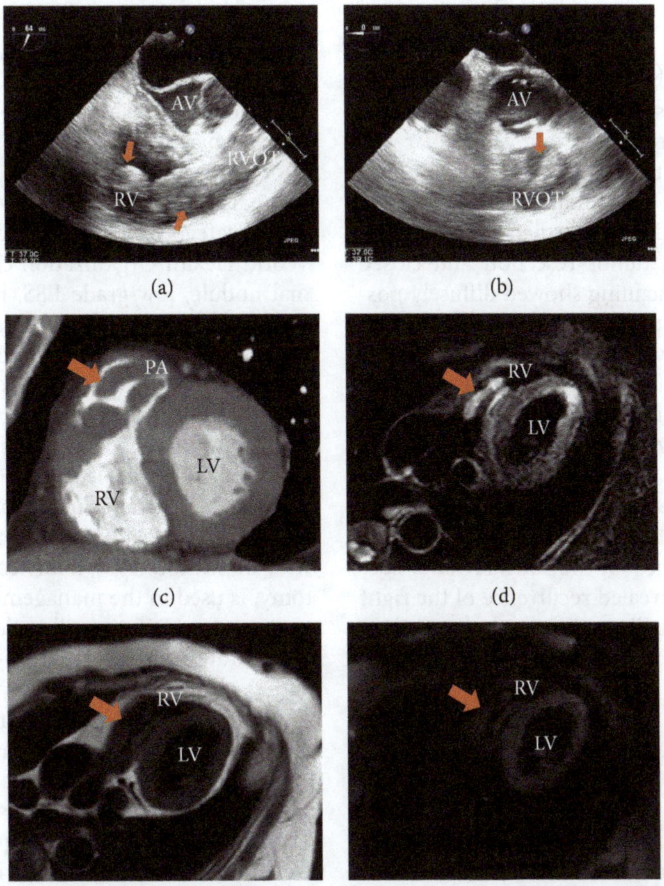

(a) (b) (c) (d) (e) (f)

FIGURE 2: Transesophageal echocardiography, cardiac CT, and MRI appearance. Transesophageal echocardiography showed elongated mass-like structure (arrow) in the right ventricle (a, b). Short axis view of cardiac computed tomography scan revealed a well-defined mass lacking contrast enhancement in the right ventricle below the pulmonary artery valve (c), and cardiac magnetic resonance imaging showed some masses which had hypersignal intensity on fat-saturated T2-weighted image (d), isointensity on T1-weighted image (e), and no suppressed signal on fat-saturated T1-weighted image (f). (AV: atrioventricular; RV: right ventricle; RVOT: right ventricular outflow tract; LV: left ventricle; RV: right ventricle).

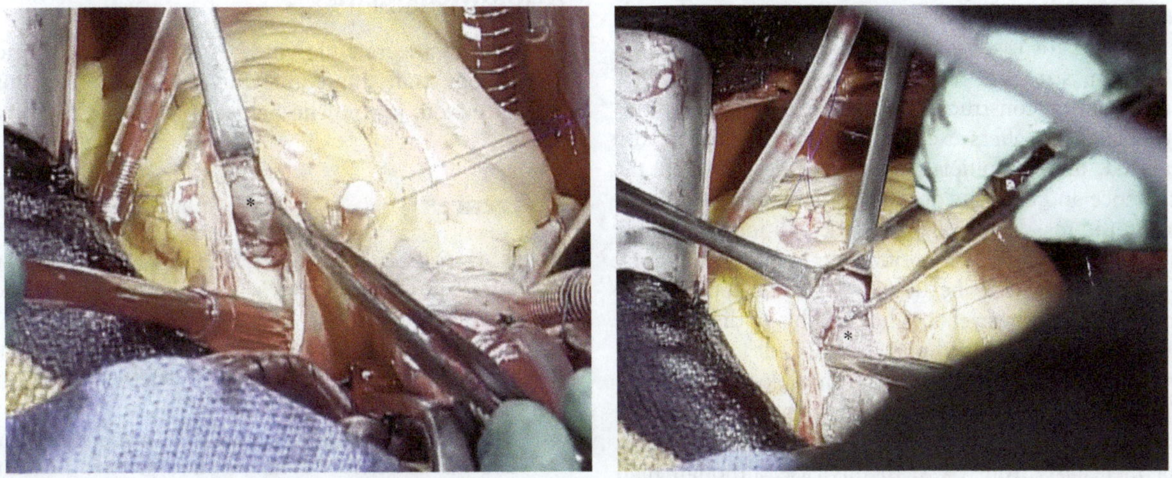

(a) (b)

FIGURE 3: Surgical images via pulmonary artery incision. A large mass (asterisk) in the main pulmonary artery and in the right ventricle via the pulmonary artery incision (a) was removed from the right ventricle (b).

an incision along the right atrium and main pulmonary artery. A large mass was observed in the main pulmonary artery and right ventricle. The mass was identified as a tumor due to a solid and elastic appearance. It perforated the pulmonary valve and infiltrated the right ventricular wall (Figure 3). Intraoperative rapid pathological findings showed hemorrhagic necrosis, interstitial edema, and dense growth of anaplastic cells, indicating cardiac metastasis. At this stage, we had done only tumor resection and closed her chest. Moreover, immunostaining showed diffusely positive staining for vimentin, partially positive for CD10, CD68, and Ki-67, and negative results for desmin, CD34, factor VIII, and estrogen receptor, which led to the diagnosis of undifferentiated sarcoma. These results suggest that UUS spreads to the right ventricle via the right ovarian vein and inferior vena cava.

The patient's postoperative recovery was uneventful and she decided to undergo chemotherapy. However, she experienced severe nausea and dyspnea on the 15th day after surgery. Contrast-enhanced CT revealed recurrence of the right ventricle mass, pulmonary embolism, intestinal obstruction, and multiple pulmonary metastases. The patient died 29 days postsurgery.

3. Discussion

This case presents a rapidly deteriorating condition with difficulty in diagnosing cardiac metastasis from UUS, which was pathologically diagnosed after open cardiac surgery. Cardiac metastases of malignant tumors are relatively common, ranging from 0.7% to 3.5% in autopsy cases, despite low diagnosis rates in individuals during their lives [1]. Although cardiac metastasis is highly reported in lung cancer, breast cancer, leukemia, malignant lymphoma, and malignant melanoma, only few cases have been reported on metastasis in uterine sarcoma [5, 6]. While imaging studies are important, the usage of these modalities in diagnosing cardiac mass has not been determined. Echocardiography is the first choice for assessing cardiac masses and it verifies their location, size, and mobility [7, 8]. Also, cardiac CT reveals anatomical construction with excellent spatial resolution whereas MRI offers excellent contrast resolution and unparalleled, direct multiplanar assessment. However, the low incidence and diversity of cardiac mass make it difficult to identify the mass and diagnose the condition using only imaging modalities [9, 10]. Positron emission tomography (PET) CT is known as the useful diagnostic tool for the malignant disease; however, it is not suitable to discriminate uterine myoma and sarcoma and it is difficult to judge cardiac malignant tumors because of the physiological accumulation in the heart. To our knowledge, this is the first case report that describes the characteristics of cardiac CT and MRI of metastasis from UUS. In this case, although high T2- and isointensity T1-weighted signals were indicative of metastatic tumors, thrombus could not be ruled out due to the characteristics of clots in MRI findings which gradually changed according to the duration from the onset of thrombus [9]. Therefore, improving the accuracy of the imaging modalities of cardiac metastasis from UUS is required to manage patients with cardiac masses.

Uterine sarcomas are rare tumors that constitute 3%–7% of uterine neoplasms [3]. They are heterogeneous pathological neoplasms characterized by a more aggressive and poorer prognosis than endometrial cancer. Endometrial stromal sarcoma (ESS) is a uterine mesenchymal tumor that can be categorized into four categories according to the 2014 World Health Organization classification: endometrial stromal nodule, low-grade ESS, high-grade ESS, and UUS [2]. UUS is classified as a high-grade sarcoma and is one of the most aggressive uterine tumors that typically arises in the endometrium and is cytologically atypical and highly mitotic. UUS usually develops in postmenopausal women with common manifestations including a pelvic mass and abnormal vaginal bleeding. Patients with UUS are usually present with extrauterine involvement at the time of diagnosis and are quite advanced [2]. Although total hysterectomy, with or without lymphadenectomy and bilateral oophorectomy, is used in the management of UUS, nonsurgical interventions for UUS are still under investigation because of lack of accurate evidence regarding UUS sensitivity to radiation and chemotherapy [3].

In the present case, the preoperative diagnosis of endocardial and uterine masses was difficult and open-heart surgery led to the diagnosis of a metastatic cardiac tumor and UUS. Due to the highly invasive nature of cardiac surgery, a nonsurgical approach is required for the diagnosis of cardiac mass. UUS is a very rare disease with rapid progression and therefore, early diagnosis and therapeutic intervention are necessary. To the best of our knowledge, this is the first to report the case of cardiac metastasis from UUS. In the future, accumulating further similar cases is important to discuss the diagnostic and therapeutic processes of cardiac metastasis from UUS.

Acknowledgments

The authors are grateful to the Department of Obstetrics and Gynecology staff, Juntendo University Shizuoka Hospital, Izunokuni-shi, Japan, who helped us treat the patients.

References

[1] A. D. Goldberg, R. Blankstein, and R. F. Padera, "Tumors metastatic to the heart," *Circulation*, vol. 128, no. 16, pp. 1790–1794, 2013.

[2] C. M. Conklin and T. A. Longacre, "Endometrial stromal tumors," *Advances in Anatomic Pathology*, vol. 21, no. 6, pp. 383–393, 2014.

[3] I. Ríos, Á. Rovirosa, J. Morales et al., "Undifferentiated uterine sarcoma: a rare, not well known and aggressive disease: report of 13 cases," *Archives of Gynecology and Obstetrics*, vol. 290, no. 5, pp. 993–997, 2014.

[4] M. Ludovisi, F. Moro, T. Pasciuto et al., "Imaging in gynecological disease (15): clinical and ultrasound characteristics of uterine sarcoma," *Ultrasound in Obstetrics & Gynecology*, vol. 54, no. 5, pp. 676–687, 2019.

[5] M. G. Silva, N. Banazol, P. Coelho, and J. I. G. Fragata, "Metastatic endometrial stromal sarcoma: a rare cause of right-sided intracardiac mass," *Journal of Cardiac Surgery*, vol. 36, no. 6, pp. 2143–2145, 2021.

[6] A. Maebayashi, M. Nagaishi, T. Nakajima, M. Hata, T. Xiaoyan, and K. Kawana, "Successful surgical treatment of cardiac metastasis from uterine leiomyosarcoma: a case report and literature review," *The Journal of Obstetrics and Gynaecology Research*, vol. 46, no. 5, pp. 795–800, 2020.

[7] K. Reynen, U. Köckeritz, and R. H. Strasser, "Metastases to the heart," *Annals of Oncology*, vol. 15, no. 3, pp. 375–381, 2004.

[8] D. Auger, J. Pressacco, F. Marcotte, A. Tremblay, A. Dore, and A. Ducharme, "Cardiac masses: an integrative approach using echocardiography and other imaging modalities," *Heart*, vol. 97, no. 13, pp. 1101–1109, 2011.

[9] C. Aggeli, Y. Dimitroglou, L. Raftopoulos et al., "Cardiac masses: the role of cardiovascular imaging in the differential diagnosis," *Diagnostics*, vol. 10, no. 12, p. 1088, 2020.

[10] C. S. Restrepo, A. Largoza, D. F. Lemos et al., "CT and MR imaging findings of malignant cardiac tumors," *Current Problems in Diagnostic Radiology*, vol. 34, no. 1, pp. 1–11, 2005.

44

Giant Thrombosis at Left Anterior Descending Artery Aneurysm in a 10-Year Old Boy with Granulomatosis with Polyangiitis

Ehsan Aghaei Moghadam,[1,2] Nahid Aslani,[3] Helia Mojtabavi,[2] Farnoosh Larti,[2] Azin Ghamari,[4] and Vahid Ziaee[1,2,5]

[1] *Department of Pediatrics, Tehran University of Medical Science, Tehran, Iran*
[2] *Children's Medical Center, Pediatrics Center of Excellence, Tehran, Iran*
[3] *Department of Pediatrics, Isfahan University of Medical Science, Isfahan, Iran*
[4] *Growth and Development Research Center, Tehran University of Medical Science, Tehran, Iran*
[5] *Pediatric Rheumatology Research Group, Rheumatology Research Center, Tehran University of Medical Sciences, Tehran, Iran*

Correspondence should be addressed to Vahid Ziaee; ziaee@tums.ac.ir

Academic Editor: Ertugrul Ercan

Granulomatosis with polyangiitis (GPA), necrotizing vasculitis of small and medium-sized vessels, is traditionally believed to mainly affect respiratory tract with additional focal kidney involvements as its primary manifestations with a relatively rare annual incidence rate of 20-50 cases per million. Six percent of the affected cases have cardiac involvements; among which, aneurysms comprise the lowest penetrance. By this paper, we aim to cast light on clinical diagnostic and treatment methods of a rare case presentation, a 10-year-old male GPA patient, diagnosed with massive thrombosis at his coronary artery aneurysm. GPA should be considered as differential diagnosis of prolong fever and coronary aneurysms in adolescents.

1. Introduction

Granulomatosis with polyangiitis (GPA) or Wegener's granulomatosis as a necrotizing vasculitis of small and medium-sized vessels is traditionally believed to mainly affect respiratory tract with additional focal kidney involvements as its primary manifestations with a relatively rare annual incidence rate of 20-50 cases per million. Multiorgan involvements including renal 18%, gastrointestinal tract 10-12%, cardiac 6%, and neurologic 5% have been described recently by the literature. Despite the low incidence, uncommon organ involvements are severe and could be fatal in case remain untreated [1–3].

Definitive granulomatosis with polyangiitis (GPA) diagnosis lies on fulfilling three out of six following criteria: compatible histopathology with granulomatosis inflammation within the wall of an artery or in the perivascular region, oral or nasal chronic involvement, laryngo-tracheobronchial stenosis, radiographic findings suggestive for pulmonary lesions, positive enzyme-linked immunosorbent assay (ELISA) test for antineutrophil cytoplasmic antibodies (ANCAs), and renal involvement [4]. The most common clinical and laboratory features present at the time of diagnosis were constitutional symptoms, upper and lower respiratory tract, mucosa, and skin and musculoskeletal involvement. In the pediatric population, the disease occurs in the second decade of life, with a female preponderance [5].

Cardiac complications of GPA include pericarditis, coronary arteritis, aortic regurgitation, aortic valvular lesions simulating endocarditis, heart block, and aneurysms [6].

By this paper, we aim to cast light on clinical diagnostic and treatment methods of a rare case presentation, a 10-

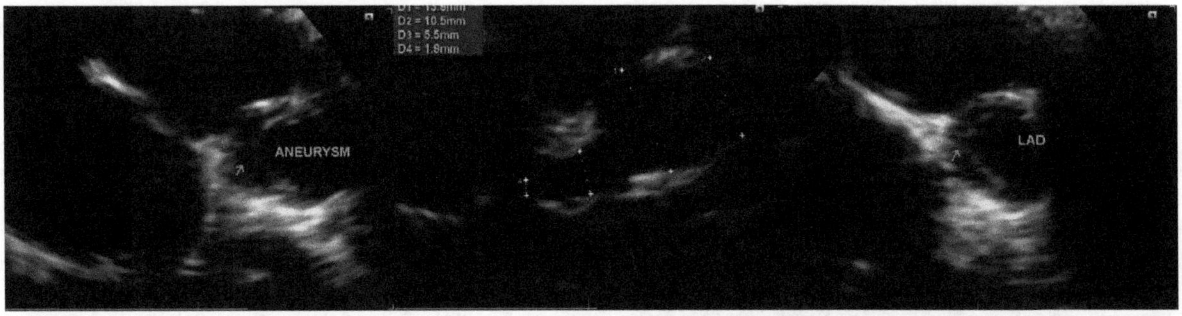

FIGURE 1: Short axis view (SAX) of transthoracic echocardiography (TTE) in our patient shows ectasia at left anterior descending (LAD) artery and huge aneurysm with large circular nonorganized thrombosis occupying the majority of the aneurysm, narrowing the internal lumen of the artery.

year-old patient, diagnosed with massive thrombosis at his coronary artery aneurysm.

2. Case Presentation

The patient was a ten-year-old boy who had been referred to children's medical center as a pediatric center of excellence for diagnostic and therapeutic evaluation due to persistent fever associated with upper respiratory infection symptoms and lower limb pain. In the previous medical center, he was treated with antibiotic as bacterial pneumonia that resulted in poor clinical response. After which, antituberculosis regimen was initiated mainly based on endemic region ethnicity for the mycobacterium and cavitary pulmonary lesion on radiographic studies. He also had an episode of perforated otitis media with effusion (OME) with additional mastoiditis receiving ventilation tube as the treatment. Alongside the disease course, he experienced antibiotic-resistant sinusitis for 2 months requiring surgical treatment. By this point, the diagnosing team focused on immunologic work up; hence, his recurrent infections which revealed our child had a competent immune system. It is noteworthy that the patient and his family reside in a different city than our clinic so not all the therapy happened under our supervision.

After 6 months, he was referred to Children's Medical Center, Pediatric Center of Excellence in Tehran as a tertiary referral center for more diagnostic evaluation and treatment. There was no arthritis in the lower extremity examination, but due to the difference in lower limb size, an evaluation for thrombosis was performed that was suggestive of deep vein thrombosis (DVT). Due to prolonged fever and increased inflammatory markers such as elevated erythrocyte sedimentation rate (ESR = 105), C-reactive protein (CRP = 95), leukocytosis (WBC = 17,600), and thrombocytosis (Plt = 635,000), pediatrics rheumatologists were consulted for the possibility of rheumatologic diseases and collagen vascular disorder. Transthoracic echocardiography was performed showing diffuse ectasia and dilation with huge aneurysm in the left anterior descending artery (LAD) with the size of 14 mm (Figure 1). Although, there was no other clinical signs in favor of Kawasaki disease other than prolonged fever, due to the high inflammatory markers and age of patient and the possibility of atypical neglected atypical Kawasaki disease or other rare vasculitis.

Other positive findings include antinuclear antibody (ANA) with titer of 1/640 and coarse speckled pattern in indirect immune fluorescent assay (IIF) and antineutrophil cytoplasmic antibodies (ANCAs) with perinuclear pattern. Regarding thrombosis, an assessment for antiphospholipid antibodies and antiphospholipid syndrome was performed, which was negative. Serum immunoglobulins, complements, and nitroblue tetrazolium were normal.

Finally, based on the history of severe upper airway infection, pulmonary cavitary lesion, saddle nose (Figure 2), elevated ESR and CRP, positive ANA and ANCA with perinuclear pattern (P-ANCA), granulomatosis with polyangiitis (Wegener granulomatosis) was diagnosed for this patient. Initial treatment as induction therapy was methylprednisolone pulse (30 mg/kg/day for 3 days/monthly) and cyclophosphamide pulse 750 mg/m2/monthly for 6-month duration. Oral medication was administered with prednisolone (1/mg/kg/day) and mycophenolate mofetil (1,200 mg/m2/day). An additional aspirin (5 mg/kg) plus warfarin (0.1 mg/kg) was administered to prevent further thrombotic events by maintaining the INR level at the range of 2-3.

On a follow-up, transthoracic and transesophageal echocardiographic evaluation, large circular nonorganized thrombosis occupying the majority of the aneurysm was noted that was confirmed by CT angiography despite the anticoagulation prophylaxis (Figure 3). To target the thrombosis, high dose of methylprednisolone and 10 mg/kg of heparin were applied initially, then warfarin was added subsequently to maintain INR level at 3-4. In interventional cardiology consult suggested medical therapy without any intervention due to high risk thrombotic complications.

In a longtime follow-up, he is under maintenance therapy for GPA (with low-dose prednisolone, mycophenolate mofetil, and antithrombotic therapy for 1.5 years without any flare up of underlying disease, but serial transthoracic echocardiography showed minimal improvement in the size of aneurism and thrombosis).

3. Discussion

GPA is one of the most common necrotizing vasculitides. The prevalence of the disease is 3 in 100,000 populations with male to female ratio of 3 : 2, and peak incidence is at the age of

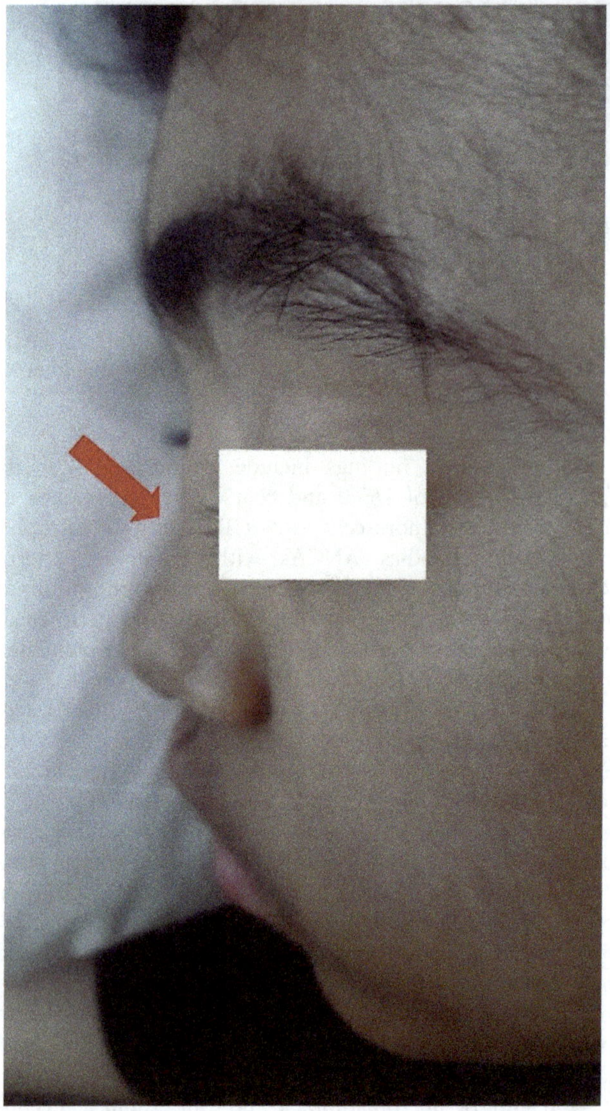

FIGURE 2: Saddle nose in our patient with granulomatosis with polyangiitis.

50-60 [7]. GPA is a rare rheumatologic disorder in Iranian children with prevalence less than 1 per million children [8].

Etiology still remains unknown, but it is usually associated with antineutrophil cytoplasmic antibody (ANCA) that was detected in predominantly cytoplasmic form (cANCA). Granulomatous lesions of the upper and lower airways and the kidneys are predominant features of the disease [9].

GPA is a very rare condition in pediatric population, despite the fact that it appears to be the same disease observed in adults, clinical presentations vary in both population. In children, high frequency of constitutional symptoms, upper and lower respiratory tract, mucosa, and skin and musculoskeletal involvement could be considered as characteristics of the disease based on an analysis of 56 affected children [5].

It has long been known that kidney and lung involvement are major predictors of mortality, and cardiac involvement is relatively infrequent in GPA [10, 11]. In one study of all patients with GPA diagnosis who were referred to all Iranian Pediatric Rheumatology Division from 2002 to 2011, in total of 11 patients, the most common organ system involvement was upper respiratory tract (81.8%), and lower respiratory tract involvement was seen in 63.9%. Six children (54.4%) had abnormal imaging in chest X-ray or chest CT-scan. Renal involvement in 4 children (36.3%) and venous thrombosis in 1 patient (9%) were observed [8].

In one cohort of 158 patients with GPA, cardiac manifestations (predominantly pericarditis) were present in 10 patients (6%), and, of these, 3 patients had coronary artery involvement [12].

Although the leading cause of coronary aneurysms is atherosclerosis, it also could be seen as an uncommon feature among some connective tissue disorders. Kawasaki disease (KD) and polyarthritis nodosa (PAN) constitute most cases of coronary aneurysms in the presence of connective tissue diseases; however, other small vessel vasculitis can also develop relatively large aneurysms [13]. Hence, GPA, classified as small to medium vessel vasculitis which is associated with positive ANCA titer, is capable of evolving aneurysms in branches of renal, hepatic, gastric, splanchnic, subclavian, and cerebral most commonly with some rare incidence of affecting walls of coronary arteries [14, 15]. Moreover, thrombosis is not frequently associated with GPA yet was reported to occur commonly at large and small intracranial vessels, deep veins of extremities, sinuses, lungs, and kidneys. The presence of any systemic predisposition for hypercoagulability state is still a debating subject [16]. In the most cases of GPA, atherosclerotic vascular disease, particularly that seen in systemic lupus erythematous (SLE) and rheumatoid arthritis (RA), has not been documented, reflecting the fact that vascular inflammation and thrombosis, including coronaritis and coronary thromboembolism, as more characteristics for GPA [17–19].

In our case, the onset of the disease with recurrent upper and lower respiratory infections was frequent and had deep vein thrombosis (DVT) in the course of the disease.

The association between respiratory infection and risk of heart attacks and strokes is well established. However, less evidence exists for an association between respiratory infection and venous thromboembolism (VTE) and probably is an increased risk following infection for pericardial effusion (PE) as well as for DVT and that this may be related to the severity of the infection [20].

Another diagnosis initially given to the patient due to fever and evidence of coronary involvement (diffuse ectasia and dilation with huge aneurysm in the left anterior descending artery with the size of 14 mm) was KD.

Kawasaki disease (KD) is a vasculitis of medium-sized vessels the majority of cases occurs in children under 5 years of age. The dreaded cardiac complication is coronary artery involvement, present in 20% of cases, resulting in myocardial infarction and aneurysm formation. Hence, KD should be considered as the possible cause of acute coronary syndromes in young adults, particularly when aneurysms are found. In the absence of generalized atherosclerotic disease, a history of KD-like illness in childhood should always be sought in these cases [6].

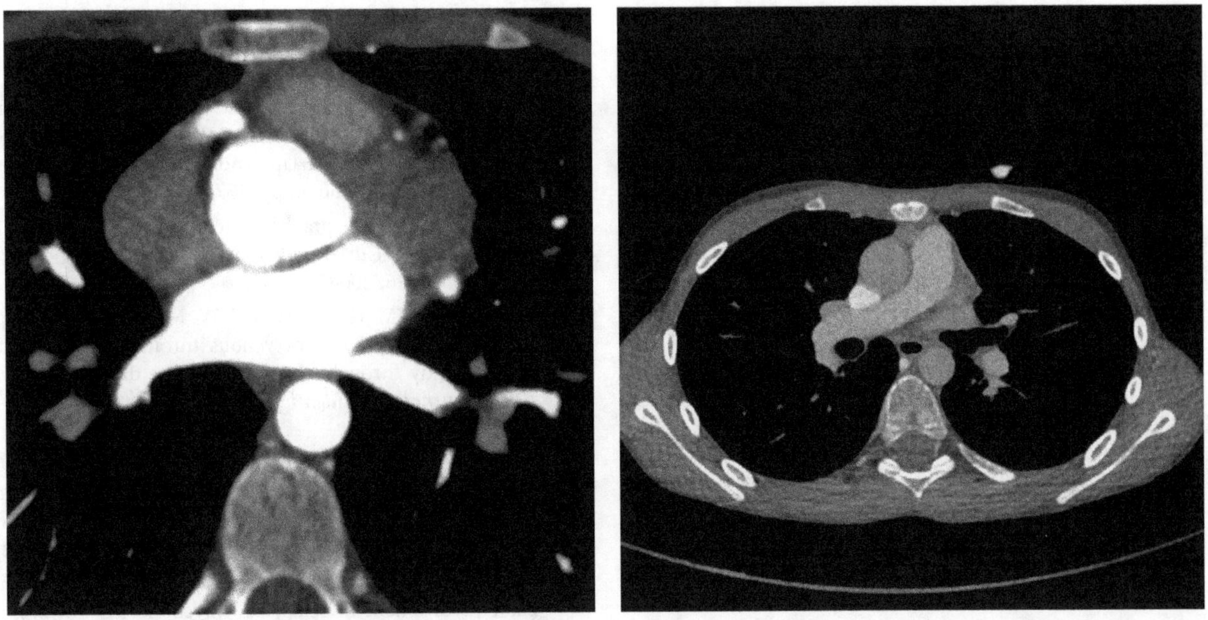

(a) (b)

FIGURE 3: (a) High-resolution, ECG-synchronized computed tomography of the heart with attention to the coronary arteries showed left main coronary ectasia (4.2 mm), fusiform aneurysmal dilation measured 19 mm length, and14 mm transverse diameter with partial thrombosis in the lumen measured 17 × 10 mm in proximal segment of left anterior descending artery (LAD) and aneurysmal dilatation in proximalpart of left circumflex (LCX) in 5 mm diameter. (b) A cavity formation in the left lung apex measure 36 × 27 × 21 mm and some fibrotic and atelectatic bands in bases of both lung.

KD and PAN are the systemic vasculitis that more often present coronary artery aneurysms [6]. Mavrogeni et al. using magnetic resonance angiography showed discrete fusiform coronary aneurysms in patients with PAN and microscopic polyangiitis, but they did not find them in patients with GPA or eosinophilic GPA (Churg-Strauss syndrome) [21].

Relapsing polychondritis (RP) is another cause of coronary artery aneurysm that frequently has saddle-nose deformity as an otolaryngological manifestation [22]; 24% of these patients could present low titles of ANCA, especially P-ANCA, that showed myeloperoxidase antigen specificity [23].

In our case, patient's age, the absence of aneurysms in the kidneys and abdomen, and positive ANCA C with high levels of proteinase-3 suggested that the coronary artery aneurysms observed were caused by diseases other than RP, KD, or PAN, such as ANCA-associated vasculitis, in particular, GPA.

Finally, GPA was diagnosed for him based on history of severe upper airway infection, saddle nose, ANCA and P-ANCA positivity, and cavitary pulmonary lesion. Thrombosis occurred within the enlarged space, 8 months after salicylate administration which required high-dose methylprednisolone application for three subsequent days, 10 mg/kg of heparin, and warfarin maintenance therapy to reach INR level of 3. The mass resembling thrombosis at the echocardiographic study was reduced by 10 days following mixed anticoagulation therapy and resolved 3 months later.

The risk of thromboembolic events increases in patients with WD [24], but pulmonary hypertension is exceptionally described up till now [25]. Atherosclerosis is the main cause of coronary artery aneurysm; however, they can be observed in connective tissue diseases such as systemic lupus erythematosus and vasculitis. KD and polyarteritis nodosa (PAN) are the systemic vasculitis that more often present coronary artery aneurysms.

There are descriptions in the literature that small vessel vasculitis such as microscopic polyangiitis and PAN could develop coronary artery aneurysm, which are infrequent in other ANCA-associated vasculitis. Musuruana et al. report a 25-year-old with WG and extensive anterior myocardial infarction. Coronary artery aneurysms were shown in cardiac angiography and were resolved after treatment with high doses of corticosteroids and cyclophosphamide [13].

In conclusion, coronary aneurysms and vascular thrombosis are rare presentations of GPA. So, GPA should be considered as differential diagnosis in patients with prolong fever and coronary aneurysms as atypical Kawasaki disease in children and adolescents. We suggest that the desirable therapeutic management of aneurysm of GPA lies in administering the combination of ASA and warfarin, as initial treatment even though no giant coronary aneurysms are detectable with the presence of merely small-sized aneurysms so to prevent consecutive thrombotic complication.

References

[1] M. Mortazavi and H. Nasri, "Granulomatosis with polyangiitis (Wegener's) presenting as the right ventricular masses: a case report and review of the literature," *Journal of Nephropathology*, vol. 1, no. 1, pp. 49–56, 2012.

[2] R. A. Watts, "Wegener's granulomatosis: unusual presentations," *Hospital Medicine*, vol. 61, no. 4, pp. 250–253, 2000.

[3] P. Korantzopoulos, D. Papaioannides, and K. Siogas, "The heart in Wegener's granulomatosis," *Cardiology*, vol. 102, no. 1, pp. 7–10, 2004.

[4] S. Ozen, A. Pistorio, S. M. Iusan et al., "EULAR/PRINTO/PRES criteria for Henoch-Schönlein purpura, childhood polyarteritis nodosa, childhood Wegener granulomatosis and childhood Takayasu arteritis: Ankara 2008. Part II: final classification criteria," *Annals of the Rheumatic Diseases*, vol. 69, no. 5, pp. 798–806, 2010.

[5] M. Bohm, M. Gonzalez Fernandez, S. Ozen et al., "Clinical features of childhood granulomatosis with polyangiitis (Wegener's granulomatosis)," *Pediatric Rheumatology Online Journal*, vol. 12, no. 1, p. 18, 2014.

[6] D. C. Knockaert, "Cardiac involvement in systemic inflammatory diseases," *European Heart Journal*, vol. 28, no. 15, pp. 1797–1804, 2007.

[7] A. S. Fauci and S. M. Wolff, "Wegener's granulomatosis: studies in eighteen, patients and a review of the literature. 1973," *Medicine*, vol. 73, no. 6, pp. 315–324, 1994.

[8] F. Tahghighi, M. H. Moradinejad, Y. Aghighi et al., "Evaluation of 10-year experience of Wegener's granulomatosis in Iranian children," *ISRN Rheumatology*, vol. 2013, Article ID 694928, 4 pages, 2013.

[9] J. C. Jennette, R. J. Falk, K. Andrassy et al., "Nomenclature of systemic Vasculitides," *Arthritis and Rheumatism*, vol. 37, no. 2, pp. 187–192, 1994.

[10] G. Cocco and A. Y. Gasparyan, "Myocardial ischemia in Wegener's granulomatosis: coronary atherosclerosis versus vasculitis," *The Open Cardiovascular Medicine Journal*, vol. 4, pp. 57–62, 2010.

[11] E. Reinhold-Keller, N. Beuge, U. Latza et al., "An interdisciplinary approach to the care of patients with Wegener's granulomatosis: long-term outcome in 155 patients," *Arthritis and Rheumatism*, vol. 43, no. 5, pp. 1021–1032, 2000.

[12] G. S. Hoffman, G. S. Kerr, R. Y. Leavitt et al., "Wegener granulomatosis: an analysis of 158 patients," *Annals of Internal Medicine*, vol. 116, no. 6, pp. 488–498, 1992.

[13] J. L. Musuruana, J. A. Cavallasca, J. Berduc, and J. Vicario, "Coronary artery aneurysms in Wegener's granulomatosis," *Joint, Bone, Spine*, vol. 78, no. 3, pp. 309–311, 2011.

[14] J. B. Arlet, D. le Thi Huong, A. Marinho, P. Cluzel, B. Wechsler, and J. C. Piette, "Arterial Aneurysms in Wegener's Granulomatosis: Case Report and Literature Review," *Seminars in arthritis and Rheumatism*, vol. 37, no. 4, pp. 265–268, 2008.

[15] D. Shitrit, A. B. G. Shitrit, D. Starobin et al., "Large vessel aneurysms in Wegener's granulomatosis," *Journal of Vascular Surgery*, vol. 36, no. 4, pp. 856–858, 2002.

[16] E. Von Scheven, T. T. Lu, H. M. Emery, M. E. Elder, and D. W. Wara, "Thrombosis and pediatric Wegener's granulomatosis: acquired and genetic risk factors for hypercoagulability," *Arthritis and Rheumatism*, vol. 49, no. 6, pp. 862–865, 2003.

[17] G. Emmi, E. Silvestri, D. Squatrito et al., "Thrombosis in vasculitis: from pathogenesis to treatment," *Thrombosis Journal*, vol. 13, no. 1, 2015.

[18] P. Morbini, B. Dal Bello, and E. Arbustini, "Coronary artery inflammation and thrombosis in Wegener's granulomatosis-polyarteritis nodosa overlap syndrome," *Giornale Italiano di Cardiologia*, vol. 28, no. 4, pp. 377–382, 1998.

[19] P. Seo, "Wegener's granulomatosis: managing more than inflammation," *Current Opinion in Rheumatology*, vol. 20, no. 1, pp. 10–16, 2008.

[20] T. C. Clayton, M. Gaskin, and T. W. Meade, "Recent respiratory infection and risk of venous thromboembolism: case-control study through a general practice database," *International Journal of Epidemiology*, vol. 40, no. 3, pp. 819–827, 2011.

[21] S. Mavrogeni, M. N. Manoussakis, T. C. Karagiorga et al., "Detection of coronary artery lesions and myocardial necrosis by magnetic resonance in systemic necrotizing vasculitides," *Arthritis and Rheumatism*, vol. 61, no. 8, pp. 1121–1129, 2009.

[22] A. Del Rosso, N. R. Petix, M. Pratesi, and A. Bini, "Cardiovascular involvement in relapsing polychondritis," *Seminars in Arthritis and Rheumatism*, vol. 26, no. 6, pp. 840–844, 1997.

[23] T. Papo, J. C. Piette, D. le Thi Huong et al., "Antineutrophil cytoplasmic antibodies in polychondritis," *Annals of the Rheumatic Diseases*, vol. 52, no. 5, pp. 384-385, 1993.

[24] P. A. Merkel, G. H. Lo, J. T. Holbrook et al., "Brief communication: high incidence of venous thrombotic events among patients with Wegener granulomatosis: the Wegener's Clinical Occurrence of Thrombosis (WeCLOT) Study," *Annals of Internal Medicine*, vol. 142, no. 8, pp. 620–626, 2005.

[25] G. C. Colin, A. C. Pouleur, C. Lefebvre, and B. Ghaye, "Unexpected 'pulmonary hypertension' in a patient with granulomatosis with polyangiitis," *European Heart Journal*, vol. 35, no. 44, p. 3141, 2014.

Acute Lower Limb Ischemia in COVID-19 Patient with Delayed Presentation

Sangam Shah,[1] Rukesh Yadav,[1] Rajan Chamlagain,[2] Yagya Raj Adhikari,[2] Sanjit Kumar Sah,[2] Bipin Kandel,[2] Subash Basnet,[2] and Sutap Yadav[3,4]

[1]Maharajgunj Medical Campus, Institute of Medicine, Tribhuvan University, Maharajgunj 44600, Nepal
[2]Tribhuvan University Teaching Hospital, Maharajgunj 44600, Nepal
[3]Department of Cardiology, Institute of Medicine, Tribhuvan University, Maharajgunj 44600, Nepal
[4]Department of Cardiology, Manmohan Cardiothoracic Vascular and Transplant Center, Maharajgunj 44600, Nepal

Correspondence should be addressed to Sangam Shah; sangam.shah.1997@gmail.com

Academic Editor: Yigit Canga

Thromboembolism is a common complication of SARS-CoV-2, which generally involves venous thromboembolism, although there have been reported cases of arterial thrombosis affecting cerebral, coronary, and visceral arteries, as well as arteries in the extremities. We discuss a case of a 45-year-old diabetic man with COVID-19 who developed late-onset acute lower limb ischemia.

1. Introduction

Coronavirus disease 19 (COVID-19) is a contagious disease caused by severe acute respiratory syndrome coronavirus-2 (SARS-CoV-2) that was first reported on December 2019 in Wuhan, China. As of July 2021, about 19 million cases have been reported across the world with approximately 4 million deaths. The presentation of COVID-19 ranges from asymptomatic to a rapidly progressive fatal disease, which may result from multiorgan failure, mainly involving the respiratory system. Severe acute respiratory syndrome coronavirus-2 causes coagulation problems that lead to thromboembolic consequences (SARS-CoV-2) [1]. High D-dimer, von Willebrand factor antigen and activity, and factor VIII activity are noted in patients with COVID-19 having coagulation disorders. Endothelial dysfunction, inflammation, cytokine release, hypercoagulability, and hypoxia all have been linked to thrombosis [2]. We discuss the case of a 45-year-old diabetic man who developed left lower leg ischemia eighteen days after the diagnosis of COVID pneumonia.

2. Case Presentation

A 45-year-old diabetic male presented to our center with chief complaints of bluish discoloration and cold left lower limb for five days. He also complained of left lower limb pain and subsequent difficulty in walking. He had COVID-19 that was confirmed from nasopharyngeal swab by reverse transcriptase polymerase chain reaction (RT-PCR) 18 days prior to admission to our center. He was managed conservatively with ceftriaxone, azithromycin, and dexamethasone. He consumed 4-6 cigarettes per day for 20 years but did not consume alcohol.

He was ill looking and not well oriented to time, place, and person with Glasgow Coma Scale (GCS) of 12/15. His axillary temperature was 97.9°F, blood pressure was 100/70 mm Hg, respiratory rate was 24 breaths/minute, pulse rate was 120 beats per minute, and oxygen saturation was 90% in the room air. On general physical examination, he had no pallor, icterus, clubbing, edema, and cyanosis. Dorsalis pedis artery and posterior tibial artery of the left lower limb were feeble on palpation.

Laboratory examination revealed hemoglobin 11.6 gm%, total leukocyte count 15800 cells/mm^3, platelets 506000 cells/mm^3, urea 7 mg/dl, creatinine 0.6 mg/dl, Na^{+132} mEq/l, and K$^{+4.1}$ mEq/l at the time of presentation. His random blood sugar was 283 mg/dl, and activated partial thromboplastin time (APTT) was 110 seconds. Arterial blood gas (ABG) analysis revealed respiratory alkalosis and hypoxemia. High-resolution computed tomography (HRCT) of chest showed multifocal consolidation with ground glass opacities, interlobular septal thickening, and fibrotic bands in the lungs (Figure 1). CT angiogram of abdominal aorta and bilateral lower limbs showed partially occluded thrombus in bilateral profunda femoris artery, completely occluding thrombus in left popliteal artery and tibioperoneal trunk and partially extending to left anterior tibial artery with collateral reformation of left posterior tibial artery and peroneal artery (Figure 2).

Clinically, he had Rutherford class I acute limb ischemia, and hence, he was planned for anticoagulation with unfractionated heparin (UFH). Furthermore, the patient was managed with intravenous antibiotic (ceftriaxone), analgesic (paracetamol and tramadol), rosuvastatin, metformin, aspirin (75 mg OD), cilostazol (100 mg BD), and insulin. He was kept on UFH for 10 days during hospital stay. The patient showed improvement as pain subsided and patient could walk without difficulty again, and following this, he was discharged on warfarin for a month.

On a follow-up visit after one month, he had difficulty in walking along with pain and swelling in the left lower limb. Power was 4/5 in the left knee flexion and extension, ankle extension, and dorsiflexion. Sensation for touch and temperature was decreased in the left leg. Angiogram and Doppler study showed organized clot at the level of the popliteal artery with distal flow. He was diagnosed with occlusive disease of left popliteal artery. Following this, he was managed by distal embolectomy of left superficial femoral artery. He was discharged after five days on oral medications (rivaroxaban (20 mg OD), rosuvastatin (20 mg OD), and metformin (500 mg BD)). On a follow-up after 12 days of embolectomy, he had no complications and was able to walk without pain.

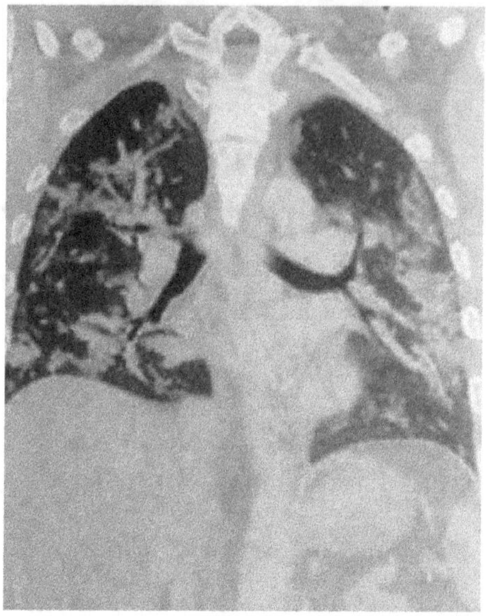

Figure 1: HRCT of chest showing multifocal consolidation with ground glass opacities, interlobular septal thickening, and fibrotic bands in the lungs.

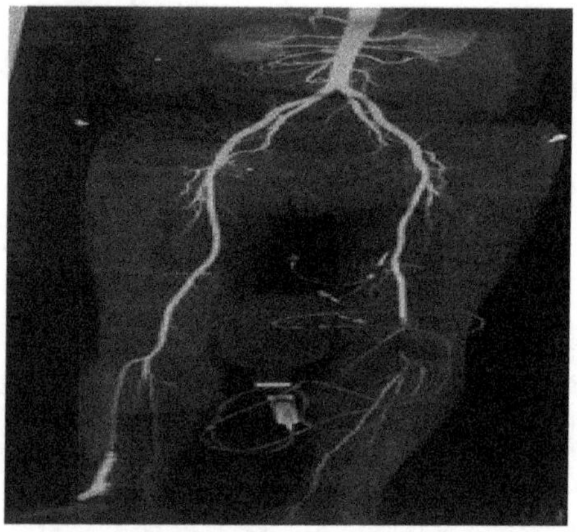

Figure 2: CT angiogram of abdominal aorta and bilateral lower limbs showing partially occluded thrombus in bilateral profunda femoris artery, completely occluding thrombus in left popliteal artery and tibioperoneal trunk.

3. Discussion

Even with mild symptoms, COVID-19 patients might develop acute limb ischemia as seen in our case. Although acute respiratory distress syndrome (ARDS) is the most common consequence in patients with severe COVID-19, cardiovascular, thromboembolic, inflammatory, and neurologic complications are being reported more recently. Comorbidities such as cardiovascular disease, diabetes mellitus, obesity, smoking, cancer, chronic renal disease, chronic obstructive pulmonary disease, solid organ or hematopoietic stem cell transplantation, and advanced age are the risk factors for developing severe COVID-19 infection [3, 4]. Coagulation disorders that lead to thromboembolic events are linked to a poor prognosis. According to the study by Fournier et al. conducted in France, COVID patients with arterial thrombosis had a threefold greater mortality [5].

Embolization of a cardiac or aneurysmal thrombus or thrombophilic conditions such as antiphospholipid antibody syndrome, malignancy, or heparin-induced thrombocytopenia are the most common differential diagnoses in a patient with thrombotic abnormality. Given the huge clot size and the absence of clinical signs of endocarditis, arrhythmia, or congestive heart failure, a cardioembolic cause was ruled out in our patient. Similarly, his clinical presentation, laboratory testing, and chest imaging did not indicate the existence of a malignancy, and once COVID-19 was diagnosed, no further workup was done [6, 7]. Patients with comorbidities including hypertension, diabetes, chronic respiratory disease, renal disease, and obesity have a higher risk of adverse outcomes [8].

While the majority of patients with arterial thrombosis in the literatures had the aforementioned preexisting comorbidities, it is important to note that a minority of patients had no prior health problems or arterial disease [9]. Furthermore, the majority of documented cases of acute limb ischemia occurred in hospitalized patients to patients admitted in high dependency or intensive care units. The most common thrombotic event is venous thromboembolism, but there have been instances of arterial events such as stroke, myocardial infarction, and acute limb ischemia. Acute limb ischemia can occur with asymptomatic to moderately symptomatic patients who are hospitalized in the intensive care unit (ICU) due to severe COVID-19 infection.

Virchow triad explains the pathophysiology of arterial and venous thrombosis (hypercoagulability, stasis, and endothelial injury). Endothelial damage caused direct invasion of endothelial cells, and complement activation has been identified as another mechanism [10]. Endothelial damage can also be caused by acute-phase reactants and acute inflammatory response mediators. Blood stasis plays a role in critically ill patients with longer period of immobilization. COVID-19 patients have hyperviscosity, increased levels of factor VIII, fibrinogen, circulating thrombotic microparticles, and neutrophil extracellular traps. The suppression of complement activation prevents the thromboembolic events that also include limb ischemia and end-organ damage [11]. Bellosta et al. recently published a study that found a low revascularization success rate in a group of 20 patients [12]. Due to the low success rate of revascularization, conservative treatment with anticoagulation is indicated. Our treatment was consistent with the European Society of Vascular Surgery (ESVS) guidelines, which encourage conservative management in patients with class I acute limb ischemia [13]. However, our patient's symptoms did not improve; therefore, embolectomy was performed later.

4. Conclusion

Even with mild symptoms, COVID-19 patients might develop acute limb ischemia, thrombotic events like venous thromboembolism, thrombotic stroke, and acute myocardial infection. If the limb is not urgently threatened, it can be treated conservatively with UFH and with surgical embolectomy as a last resort if the symptoms do not improve. Anticoagulation alone may not be enough to relieve the symptoms of acute limb ischemia, and the ischemia may progress to the point where the limb cannot be saved. As observed in our patient, thrombotic events can occur even late in the course after COVID-19 detection.

Consent

The report was published with the written informed consent of the patient.

Authors' Contributions

SS conceptualized the study, reviewed, edited the manuscript, and was in charge of the case. SS and RY wrote the original, reviewed, and edited the manuscript. SS, RY, RC, YRA, SKS, BK, SB, and SY were in charge of the case and reviewed the manuscript.

References

[1] M. Panigada, N. Bottino, P. Tagliabue et al., "Hypercoagulability of COVID-19 patients in intensive care unit: a report of thromboelastography findings and other parameters of hemostasis," *Journal of Thrombosis and Haemostasis*, vol. 18, no. 7, pp. 1738–1742, 2020.

[2] D. Giannis, I. A. Ziogas, and P. Gianni, "Coagulation disorders in coronavirus infected patients: COVID-19, SARS-CoV-1, MERS-CoV and lessons from the past," *Journal of Clinical Virology*, vol. 127, p. 104362, 2020.

[3] S. L. Harrison, E. Fazio-Eynullayeva, D. A. Lane, P. Underhill, and G. Y. H. Lip, "Comorbidities associated with mortality in 31,461 adults with COVID-19 in the United States: a federated electronic medical record analysis," *PLoS Medicine*, vol. 17, p. 10.1371/JOURNAL.PMED.1003321, 2020.

[4] C. M. Petrilli, S. A. Jones, J. Yang et al., "Factors associated with hospital admission and critical illness among 5279 people with coronavirus disease 2019 in New York City: prospective cohort study," *BMJ*, vol. 369, p. 10.1136/bmj.m1966, 2020.

[5] M. Fournier, D. Faille, A. Dossier et al., "Arterial thrombotic events in adult inpatients with COVID-19," *Mayo Clinic Proceedings*, vol. 96, no. 2, pp. 295–303, 2021.

[6] Y. Zhang, M. Xiao, S. Zhang et al., "Coagulopathy and antiphospholipid antibodies in patients with Covid-19," *New England Journal of Medicine*, vol. 382, no. 17, p. e38, 2020.

[7] I. Harzallah, A. Debliquis, and B. Drénou, "Lupus anticoagulant is frequent in patients with Covid-19," *Journal of Thrombosis and Haemostasis*, vol. 18, no. 8, pp. 2064-2065, 2020.

[8] "What's new | COVID-19 Treatment Guidelines," 2021, https://www.covid19treatmentguidelines.nih.gov/about-the-guidelines/whats-new/.

[9] O. Thompson, D. Pierce, D. Whang, M. O'Malley, B. Geise, and U. Malhotra, "Acute limb ischemia as sole initial manifestation of SARS-CoV-2 infection," *Journal of Vascular Surgery Cases and Innovative Techniques*, vol. 6, no. 4, pp. 511–513, 2020.

[10] J. Yu, X. Yuan, H. Chen, S. Chaturvedi, E. M. Braunstein, and R. A. Brodsky, "Direct activation of the alternative complement pathway by SARS-CoV-2 spike proteins is blocked by factor D inhibition," *Blood*, vol. 136, no. 18, pp. 2080–2089, 2020.

[11] S. Voicu, C. Ketfi, A. Stépanian et al., "Pathophysiological processes underlying the high prevalence of deep vein thrombosis in critically ill COVID-19 patients," *Frontiers in Physiology*, vol. 11, p. 10.3389/FPHYS.2020.608788, 2021.

[12] R. Bellosta, L. Luzzani, G. Natalini et al., "Acute limb ischemia in patients with COVID-19 pneumonia," *Journal of Vascular Surgery*, vol. 72, no. 6, pp. 1864–1872, 2020.

[13] M. Björck, J. J. Earnshaw, S. Acosta et al., "Editor's Choice - European Society for Vascular Surgery (ESVS) 2020 Clinical Practice Guidelines on the Management of Acute Limb Ischaemia," *European Journal of Vascular and Endovascular Surgery*, vol. 59, no. 2, pp. 173–218, 2020.

Novel Product for the Management of Coronary Ruptures Happening during Percutaneous Coronary Interventions

Arash Hashemi,[1] Ashkan Hashemi,[2] Arsis Ahmadieh,[1] Azin Alizadehasl,[3] and Mohammad Mostafa Ansari Ramandi[4,5]

[1]*Erfan General Hospital, Tehran, Iran*
[2]*Weill Cornell Medicine, New York, New York, USA*
[3]*Rajaie Cardiovascular, Medical and Research Center, Iran University of Medical Sciences, Tehran, Iran*
[4]*Cardiovascular Diseases Research Center, Birjand University of Medical Sciences, Birjand, Iran*
[5]*Network of Immunity in Infection, Malignancy and Autoimmunity (NIIMA), Universal Scientific Education and Research Network (USERN), Tehran, Iran*

Correspondence should be addressed to Mohammad Mostafa Ansari Ramandi; dr.mm.ansari@gmail.com

Academic Editor: Expedito E. Ribeiro

Coronary artery perforation during percutaneous coronary interventions is a rare but dreaded complication. One of the treatment methods for this complication is the injection of an obliterating material into the ruptured vessel. We will introduce a novel material named "Spongostan" for embolization with significant advantages over available treatment options.

1. Introduction

Coronary perforation is a potentially fatal complication of PCI [1]. It is a rare complication with more prevalence in females and patients with hypertension, previous coronary artery bypass grafting, and those admitted with NSTEMI [2]. It also has a higher incidence during complex procedures like bifurcation stenting, very tortuous or heavily calcified vessels, use of atheroablation devices, or CTO procedures [1, 2]. The most common cause of these perforations is wire tip induced [3]. This complication can be fatal and needs to be addressed properly. With more and more aggressive and advanced techniques or wires like heavy CTO-dedicated wires used, the rate of this complication rises [1–3]. Ellis classification (Table 1) shows the different types of coronary perforations [4].

Its incidence is between 0.35 and 0.52 percent [5]. A very high index of suspicion, timely diagnosis, and often definitive treatment are required to minimize adverse outcomes from this complication [5, 6].

2. Case Presentation

A 50-year-old female presented to our hospital with increased intensity of exertional retrosternal chest pain. She had exertional chest pain from a few days before and experienced a more severe form of pain from 3 hours before admission with slight exertion. The pain had a compressive nature without radiation and was accompanied by diaphoresis. On physical examination, she had a blood pressure of 135/85 mmHg, a heart rate of 86 beats/minute, and a respiratory rate of 20/minute. She had no fever. There was no remarkable finding in the physical examination.

2.1. Past Medical History. She had a history of controlled hypertension from 10 years before. She was a smoker for

Table 1: Ellis classification.

Ellis classification	Description
Type I	Extraluminal crater without extravasation
Type II	Epicardial fat or myocardial blush without extravasation
Type III	Extravasation through a frank (>1 mm) perforation
Type IIICS	Extravasation through a frank (>1 mm) perforation into a circulatory chamber (e.g., left ventricle or coronary sinus)

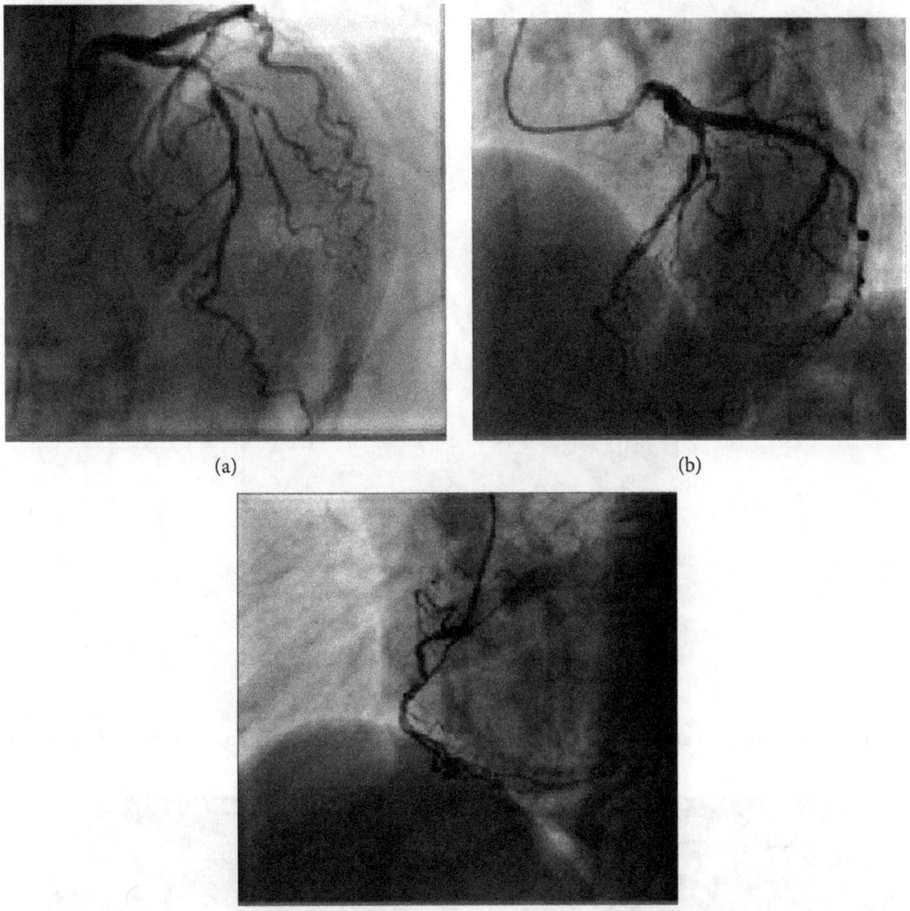

(a) (b) (c)

Figure 1: (a) Anterior-posterior (AP) cranial projection showing the stenosis in LAD-diagonal bifurcation. (b) Left anterior oblique (LAO) cranial projection showing the stenosis in LAD-diagonal bifurcation. (c) Right anterior oblique projection showing stenosis in RCA.

15 years (7.5 pack-year). No history of cardiac disease or diabetes mellitus was present.

2.2. Differential Diagnosis. Considering her past medical history and sign and symptoms, acute coronary syndrome was the main diagnosis.

2.3. Investigations. Electrocardiography was done for the patient that revealed ST-segment depression in anterior and lateral precordial leads.

On laboratory testing, she had troponin I elevated to five-folds of the normal upper limit.

Considering the diagnosis of non-ST-segment elevation-myocardial infarction (NSTEMI) and due to the refractory angina after the event, she underwent diagnostic coronary angiography which revealed two-vessel diseases with significant stenosis in left anterior descending- (LAD-) diagonal bifurcation (Video 1) and proximal right coronary artery (RCA) and a low SYNTAX score (Figure 1).

Therefore, she was planned to undergo stage percutaneous coronary intervention (PCI) on LAD-diagonal bifurcation and then proximal RCA.

2.4. Management. Our plan for LAD-diagonal bifurcation was to perform provisional stenting and after wiring both branches' predilation in both vessels and finally, provisional stenting in LAD (Video 2) with postdilation, and final proximal optimization technique (POT) was done (Figure 2(a)). After final POT, the patient developed severe refractory chest pain and ST-segment changes due to closure of the jailed

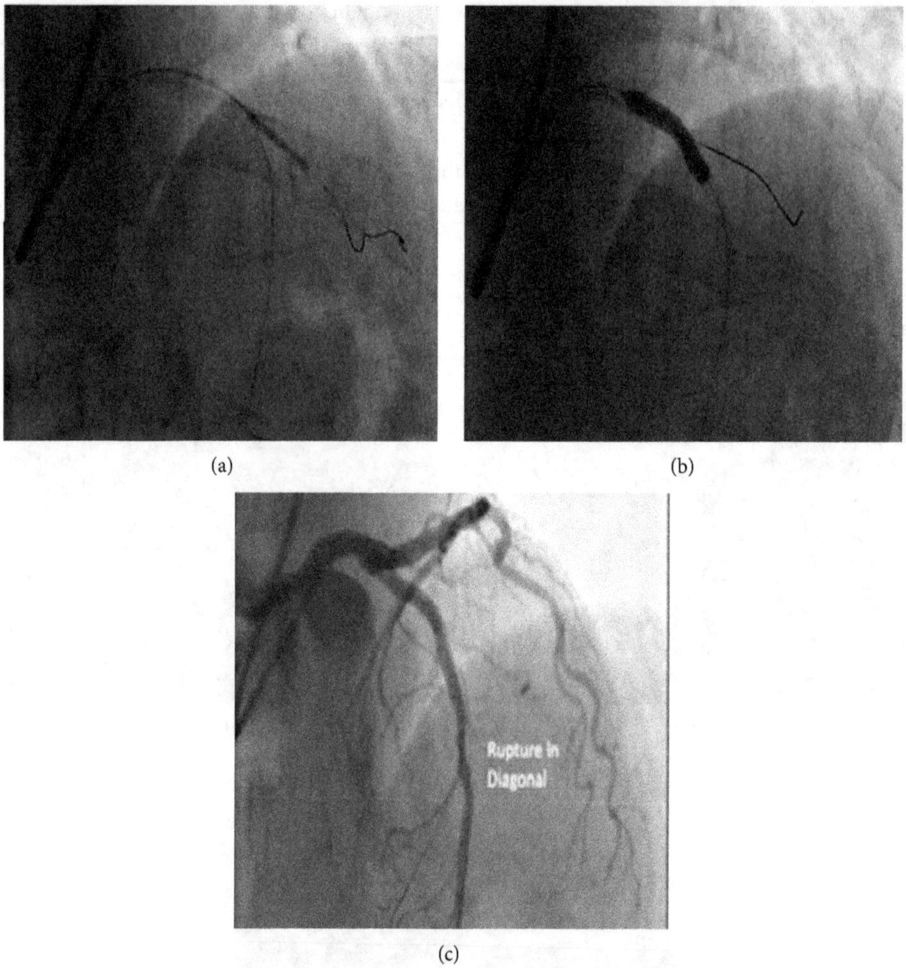

FIGURE 2: (a) Stenting in LAD and POT. (b) Rewiring in diagonal after its total occlusion. (c) Diagonal rupture.

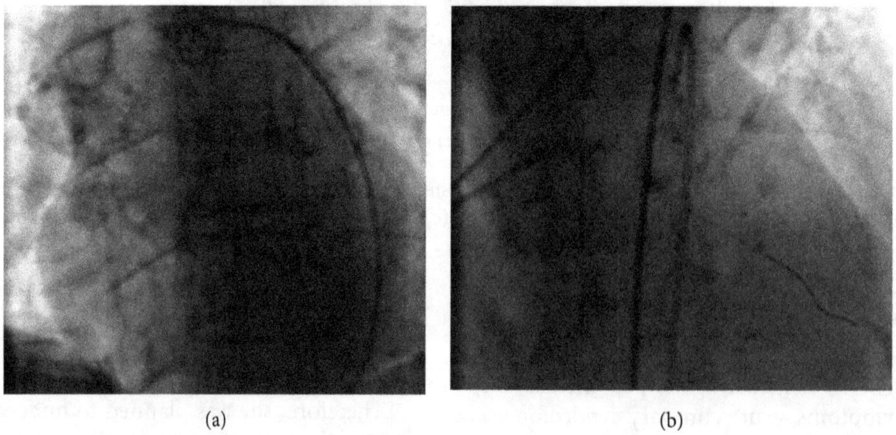

FIGURE 3: (a) Pigtail insertion. (b) Repeated wiring of the diagonal and prolonged balloon inflation.

diagonal artery so we decided to perform rewiring (Video 3) and balloon opening of the occluded diagonal (Figure 2(b)). After rewiring and ballooning the diagonal, we noticed an iatrogenic rupture in the diagonal artery caused by the wire tip (Video 4, 5) (Figure 2(c)).

We started step-wise actions for treatment and management of this rupture including prolonged balloon inflation (Video 6) and serial echocardiographic evaluations. After three episodes of prolonged balloon inflations using a 2×20 mm balloon, it seemed that we managed to seal the perforation and there was no more leakage (Video 7). The echocardiographic evaluation showed mild to moderate pericardial effusion, and we terminated the procedure and sent the patient to the coronary care unit (CCU) and kept her under observation.

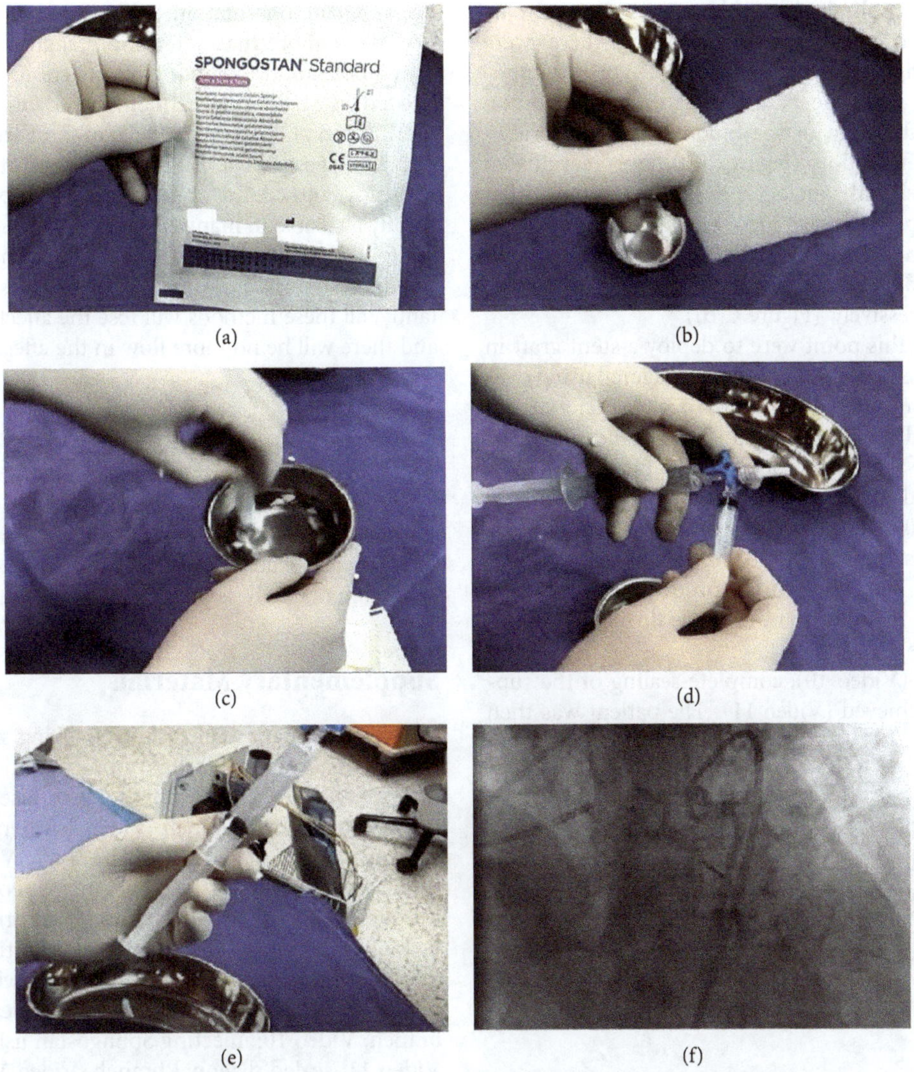

FIGURE 4: (a) Spongostan package. (b) Spongostan sponge. (c) Stirring and soaking one-fifth of the sponge in contrast media. (d) Dissolving the sponge using two syringes. (e) Dissolved Spongostan in the contrast. (f) Injection through microcatheter tip.

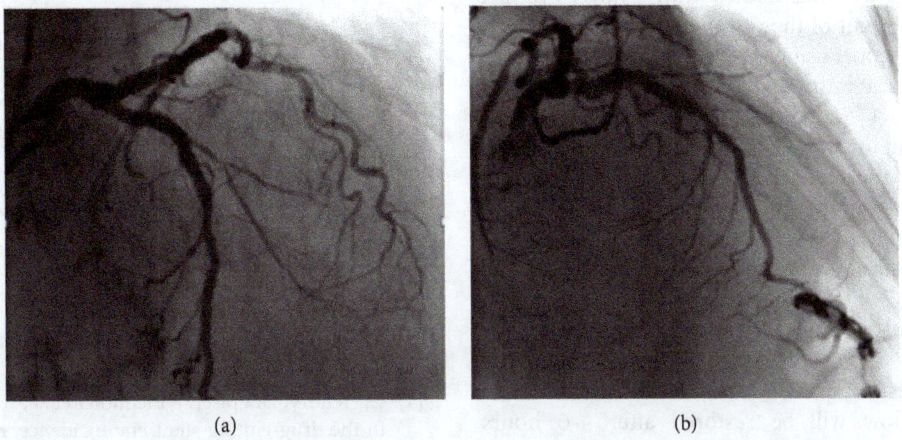

FIGURE 5: (a) AP cranial projection showing complete restoration of flow in the ruptured diagonal artery and no residual leakage after 48 hours. (b) LAO caudal projection showing complete restoration of flow in the ruptured diagonal artery and no residual leakage after 48 hours.

Four hours later, she had low blood pressure and paradoxical pulse. On serial echocardiography, there were right atrium and right ventricle collapse in favor of tamponade. We quickly sent the patient to the catheterization laboratory. After drainage of the blood from the pericardium and pigtail insertion (Figure 3(a)), we reevaluated the ruptured vessel with angiography and found out that the leakage was persistent (Video 8). Repeated diagonal wiring and prolonged balloon inflation were done again with no luck (Video 9), and we decided to manage the rupture more aggressively (Figure 3(b)).

Our options at this point were to deploy a stent graft in the main LAD vessel or try to occlude the diagonal using coils or polyvinyl alcohol (PVA) or standard glue material. All these materials and methods have their costs and pitfalls so we decided to use a novel product for sealing the rupture. This product is called "Spongostan" and is a form of Gel foam commonly used by ear, nose, and throat (ENT) surgeons. It is very easy to use, and its preparation takes under two minutes. First, we dissolved the product with standard contrast, and then, the injection was made through a microcatheter tip (Figure 4).

After injection (Video 10), complete sealing of the ruptured vessel was achieved (Video 11). The patient was then sent to the CCU.

2.5. Follow-Up. After 24 hours the pigtail was removed, the repeated echocardiography showed no pericardial effusion. Repeated angiography was done the next day which showed complete restoration of flow in the diagonal artery and no leakage (Video 12) (Figure 5). During the following three years after her procedure, she had no angina symptoms and is doing well.

3. Discussion

In this case, wire-induced coronary rupture happened during bifurcation stenting in a female patient with history of hypertension admitted for NSTEMI. Due to failed conservative management, the patient was treated with a novel product for sealing and treatment of the rupture. To our knowledge, this is the first case report using this material via intracoronary root for hemostatic purposes.

Our novel product "Spongostan" is an absorbable, sterile, water-insoluble, and malleable hemostatic gelatin sponge, intended for hemostatic use by applying to a bleeding surface.

This product is routinely used by ENT surgeons for hemostatic purposes [7]. It has also been used recently for endovascular hemostasis and controlling bleeding in thyroid surgeries [8, 9].

It has a couple of advantages over standard treatment. It is very inexpensive, very easy to use, needs a very short time to prepare, achieves complete sealing very fast, and most importantly, the flow will be restored after 4-6 hours completely after the ruptured vessel was sealed and will achieve complete sealing simply with increasing the injected material in a stepwise manner.

Although conservative management like wait and watch, prolonged balloon inflations using appropriate sized low-pressure balloon inflation, and reversal of heparin are among first steps, more than often more aggressive treatments like fat embolization, coiling, glue injection, or stent grafts are needed as standard treatment based on the situation and localization of the rupture. Each of these treatments has some disadvantages [6, 10]. Fat embolization is time-consuming to get ready, and coiling or glues are very expensive and are not readily available in many centers and are technically demanding to deploy. Stent grafts are expensive and have a very high rate of restenosis and poor long term results. Most importantly, all these methods will lose the affected artery for good and there will be no more flow in the affected vessel [6, 10].

4. Conclusions

Although coronary rupture can be a fatal complication, stepwise actions can help to overcome it. Having a high index of suspicion, timely diagnosis and management are important for managing such patients. The use of novel products can help us manage these patients with a better outcome.

Supplementary Materials

Video 1: coronary angiography showing significant stenosis in LAD artery and diagonal branch. Video 2: stent placed in LAD and side branch flow compromised. Video 3: rewiring of the diagonal branch. Video 4: when tip of the wire is causing rupture of the diagonal branch. Video 5: leakage in the diagonal branch. Video 6: using balloon inflation to seal the rupture. Video 7: rupture under control after prolonged balloon inflation. Video 8: pigtail insertion after 4 hours due to tamponade and angiography showing diagonal leakage. Video 9: using balloon inflation for sealing the diagonal branch. Video 10: injecting Spongostan using microcatheter. Video 11: sealed diagonal branch. Video 12: coronary angiography after 48 hours showing restored diagonal flow without leakage. *(Supplementary Materials)*

References

[1] G. Fogarassy, D. Apró, and G. Veress, "Successful sealing of a coronary artery perforation with a mesh-covered stent," *The Journal of Invasive Cardiology*, vol. 24, no. 4, article E80, 2012.

[2] R. al-Lamee, A. Ielasi, A. Latib et al., "Incidence, predictors, management, immediate and long-term outcomes following grade III coronary perforation," *JACC: Cardiovascular Interventions*, vol. 4, no. 1, pp. 87–95, 2011.

[3] I. Stathopoulos, G. Panagopoulos, K. Kossidas, M. Jimenez, and K. Garratt, "Guidewire-induced coronary artery perforation and tamponade during PCI: in-hospital outcomes and impact on long-term survival," *The Journal of Invasive Cardiology*, vol. 26, no. 8, pp. 371–376, 2014.

[4] C. Hendry, D. Fraser, J. Eichhofer et al., "Coronary perforation in the drug-eluting stent era: incidence, risk factors, management and outcome: the UK experience," *EuroIntervention*, vol. 8, no. 1, pp. 79–86, 2012.

[5] A. Shimony, L. Joseph, S. Mottillo, and M. J. Eisenberg, "Coronary artery perforation during percutaneous coronary intervention: a systematic review and meta-analysis," *Canadian Journal of Cardiology*, vol. 27, no. 6, pp. 843–850, 2011.

[6] A. H. Jamali, M. S. Lee, and R. R. Makkar, "Coronary perforation after percutaneous coronary intervention successfully treated with local thrombin injection," *The Journal of Invasive Cardiology*, vol. 18, no. 4, pp. E143–E145, 2006.

[7] C. J. Massey and A. Singh, "Advances in absorbable biomaterials and nasal packing," *Otolaryngologic Clinics of North America*, vol. 50, no. 3, pp. 545–563, 2017.

[8] F. Libra, D. Falsaperla, C. M. Desiderio, S. S. Signorelli, S. Palmucci, and A. Basile, "Spontaneous bleeding in systemic lupus erythematosus: endovascular treatment of two rare cases," *Radiology Case Reports*, vol. 15, no. 7, pp. 992–998, 2020.

[9] M. Scaroni, U. von Holzen, and C. A. Nebiker, "Effectiveness of hemostatic agents in thyroid surgery for the prevention of postoperative bleeding," *Scientific Reports*, vol. 10, no. 1, article 1753, 2020.

[10] A. Shimony, D. Zahger, M. van Straten et al., "Incidence, risk factors, management and outcomes of coronary artery perforation during percutaneous coronary intervention," *The American Journal of Cardiology*, vol. 104, no. 12, pp. 1674–1677, 2009.

47

Chest Pain from Pneumopericardium with Gastropericardial Fistula

Abdullah Rathur, Hussein Al-Mohamad, Jeffrey Steinhoff, and Ronald Walsh

Department of Cardiology, HCA Healthcare/USF Morsani College of Medicine GME Programs/Largo Medical Center, Largo, FL, USA

Correspondence should be addressed to Abdullah Rathur; abdullah.rathur@hcahealthcare.com

Academic Editor: Luigi Sciarra

Introduction. Gastropericardial fistula, a connection between the upper gastrointestinal tract and pericardium, is a rare clinical finding most commonly associated with postsurgical complications, as well as direct tissue invasion from gastric cancer. *Case Report.* We report a case of a 58-year-old Caucasian woman with metastatic colon cancer treated with FOLFOX, a combination chemotherapy regimen, and bevacizumab who presented with chest pain. She was ruled out for acute coronary syndrome, aortic dissection, or pulmonary embolism. A computed tomography (CT) scan of her chest showed pneumopericardium. A barium swallow ruled out esophageal ulceration, and esophagogastroduodenoscopy (EGD) showed a large penetrating gastric ulcer with no evidence of gastric dysplasia or malignancy or evidence of Helicobacter pylori (H. pylori). The patient underwent median sternotomy with gastric ulcer resection and repair, as well as pericardial washout and pericardial chest tube placement. After an uncomplicated course, she was safely discharged home. *Conclusion.* Given that gastrointestinal ulceration and perforation are known phenomena in patients taking vascular endothelial growth factor (VEGF) inhibitors, surveillance endoscopy may be beneficial to discover them before they result in potentially fatal complications such as gastropericardial fistulas.

1. Introduction

Pneumopericardium is the presentation of air within the pericardial cavity and can be caused by trauma, thoracic surgery, thoracentesis, infectious pericarditis, foreign body aspiration, cocaine inhalation, and fistula formation between the pericardium and other structures [1]. Gastropericardial fistula, a rare condition caused by pathological communication between the upper gastrointestinal tract and the pericardium, is one of the causes of pneumopericardium. The gastropericardial fistula is associated with significant morbidity and mortality, reaching as high as 69% in one study [2]. The presentation of gastropericardial fistulas varies, with acute dyspnea, chest pain, hemodynamic instability from cardiac tamponade, or even cardiac arrest from tension pneumopericardium [3]. Conditions most commonly associated with gastropericardial fistulas include prior gastroesophageal surgery such as Nissen fundoplication or hernia repair, gastroesophageal cancer [2], and even ulcers associated with gastroesophageal reflux disease, NSAID use, and Zollinger-Ellison syndrome [4–6]. This case highlights a very rare diagnosis of gastropericardial fistula in a patient on VEGF-inhibitor chemotherapy for metastatic colon cancer, in the absence of gastric cancer, prior gastroesophageal surgery, or significant risk factors for peptic ulcer disease.

2. Case Presentation

A 58-year-old Caucasian woman with a past medical history of stage IV colon cancer being treated actively with FOLFOX and bevacizumab presented to the emergency department (ED) with complaint of left-sided chest pain and left shoulder pain which started over a year ago but acutely increased in intensity and frequency over the past three weeks. The pain was inconsistently worse with position, associated with dyspnea, left-sided neck pain, and belching, without fever, chills, cough, abdominal pain, nausea, vomiting, diarrhea, dysphagia, melena, or hematochezia. Her last chemotherapy treatment was five days prior. She was initially diagnosed with the cancer 2.5 years ago with metastasis to the liver and was treated initially with diverting colostomy and chemotherapy with bevacizumab, later modified to include FOLFOX. The patient denied nonsteroidal anti-inflammatory drug (NSAID) use or alcohol or illicit drug abuse.

In the ED, initial vital signs showed blood pressure 174/83 mmHg, heart rate 101/minute, respiratory rate 24/minute, SpO_2 97% on room air, temperature 96.9°F. Physical examination was unremarkable except for decreased breath sounds and regular tachycardia. Labs showed hemoglobin (16 g/dL), alkaline phosphatase (299 U/L), and negative urine drug screen. Serial troponins six hours apart were negative, and initial ECG showed sinus rhythm without ischemic changes. Thoracic CT angiogram ruled out pulmonary embolism and showed pneumopericardium, gastropericardial fistula, and three liver lesions suspicious for metastatic disease, as shown in Figure 1.

A transthoracic echocardiogram showed a left ventricular (LV) ejection fraction of 55-60%, no valvular disease, and a normal pulmonary pressure and suggested the presence of pericardial air due to significant acoustic attenuation in otherwise previously normal windows. A barium swallow was performed with no visible esophageal stricture or ulceration, but the field of view did not include the stomach.

An EGD was done and showed a normal esophagus and 3 cm penetrating gastric cardia ulcer with surrounding edema and nonbleeding vessel in the center; biopsy was negative for dysplasia, metaplasia, malignancy, or H. pylori.

Surgical intervention was performed by cardiothoracic and general surgery teams, including median sternotomy, laparotomy, intraoperative transesophageal echocardiogram (TEE) to delineate the area of ulceration, posterior pericardial debridement of tissue adhesions, gastric ulcer resection and primary repair with omental patch, gastrojejunostomy feeding tube insertion, diaphragmatic patch with mesh, pericardial washout, and pericardial/pleural chest tube placement. She was transferred to the intensive care unit (ICU) and placed on total parenteral nutrition. After a few days, she was discharged home without any postoperative complications.

3. Discussion

Gastropericardial fistula is a rare condition typically associated with prior gastroesophageal surgery or gastroesophageal cancer [2]. Presentation is highly variable, ranging from benign left shoulder pain to cardiac arrest from tension pneumopericardium [3].

Our patient presented with chest pain and long-standing left shoulder pain, initially attributed to rotator cuff pathology. However, long-standing shoulder pain is an important symptom associated with nontraumatic gastric perforation into the pericardium [7], and chest or left shoulder pain is the presenting symptom in 66% of cases of gastropericardial fistula [2]. Overall, the prognosis is typically poor with this condition due to late recognition in an acute chest pain setting. Gastropericardial fistula is frequently associated with infection and sepsis, requiring surgical intervention for repair [8, 9]. Pneumopericardium is often first diagnosed by chest X-ray, but the finding is nonspecific in identifying the etiology. Contrast CT imaging is useful for identifying a fistulous tract between the GI tract and the pericardium [3]. Endoscopy allows diagnosis and localization of a fistula by direct visualization and is beneficial in those unidentified by contrast imaging, and it also allows for biopsy of the ulcer to look for malignancy. Per literature review by Davidson et al., fluoroscopic contrast studies to detect gastropericardial fistula should be reserved for cases with negative initial CT or in equivocal cases. Transthoracic echocardiography is not usually effective for diagnosing pneumopericardium due to air attenuation artifact [10].

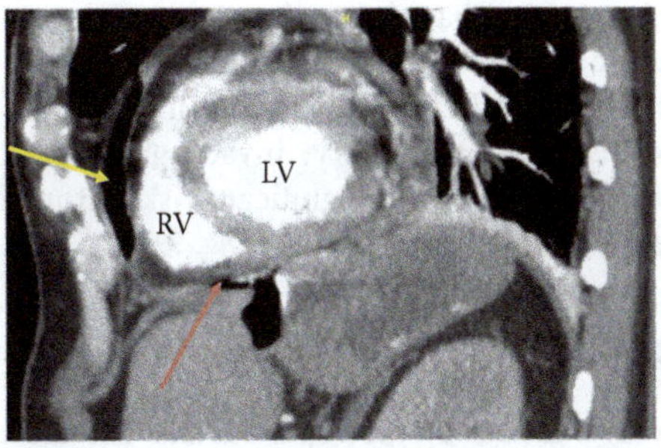

FIGURE 1: Sagittal view of chest CT showing pneumopericardium (yellow arrow) and gastropericardial fistula (red arrow).

Gastrointestinal perforation is a known side effect of bevacizumab, a humanized monoclonal antibody against the vascular endothelial growth factor (VEGF). Vasoactive agents such as prostaglandins and nitrous oxide are activated by VEGF, and inhibition of growth factors can lead to weakened mucosal defense [11]. Animal models showed the regression of capillaries of intestinal villi which could contribute to perforation if exacerbated by other pathologic processes [12]. In a study by Hendrick et al., 1.7% of patients being concomitantly treated with bevacizumab and first-line chemotherapy had gastrointestinal perforation, with 68% occurring in the first 60 days. Our literature review did not show any prior reported cases of gastropericardial fistula in the setting of VEGF-inhibitor usage without any other risk factors.

Gastropericardial fistula in the absence of gastric malignancy, prior gastrointestinal surgery, or combination chemotherapy and radiation therapy is a very rare clinical syndrome. In one previously reported case, the patient had no prior gastric malignancy or surgery, and the only risk factor for gastric ulceration was alcohol abuse [13], which has been shown to be a risk factor for ulcer perforation [13]. Despite having metastatic colon cancer, our patient's gastric biopsy was negative for malignancy or H. pylori, and she denied a history of significant NSAID or alcohol use, making peptic ulcer disease a less likely cause. Gastropleural, gastropericardial, and gastropleuropericardial fistula formations have been reported with combination radiation therapy and chemotherapeutic agents such as fluorouracil, oxaliplatin, and sunitinib [14]. Radiation treatment results in vessel destruction and tumor necrosis, causing endothelial cytotoxicity and potential adhesion between the gastric fundus and diaphragm, leading to possible gastropericardial fistula formation [15–17]. As per standard of care, our patient did not need to receive radiation therapy. Pericardial metastasis can cause pericardial effusion, clinical pericarditis, and sometimes tamponade, but this was not the case in our patient as per biopsy. Again, based on literature review, our case appears to be the first reported case of gastropericardial fistula as a result of VEGF-inhibitor use in a patient without prior gastroesophageal surgery, invading gastroesophageal or pericardial cancer, or any significant risk factors for peptic ulcer disease.

4. Conclusion

Clinical presentation of gastropericardial fistulas can vary from mild chest pain and shortness of breath to cardiac arrest from tension pneumopericardium, and there is usually little to no clinical suspicion for such an uncommon diagnosis. Given that this clinical diagnosis can be difficult, a more useful approach may be prevention before a gastropericardial fistula can form. Although there are currently no such guidelines, it may be prudent to consider surveillance endoscopy in patients taking combination VEGF inhibitors and other chemotherapeutic agents to assess for gastrointestinal ulceration in order to intervene before complications like gastropericardial fistula can occur.

References

[1] V. Chopra, N. Garg, and P. Mrigpuri, "Spontaneous pneumopericardium an unusual complication in a patient of HIV and pulmonary tuberculosis," *Lung India*, vol. 30, no. 2, pp. 148–150, 2013.

[2] V. Azzu, "Gastropericardial fistula: getting to the heart of the matter," *BMC Gastroenterology*, vol. 16, no. 1, p. 96, 2016.

[3] K. Hervik, I. Vognild, L. M. Bjerke, and S. M. Almdahl, "Gastropericardial fistula presenting with cardiac arrest: a case report," *European Heart Journal-Case Reports*, vol. 2, no. 2, 2018.

[4] Z. C. Farkas, S. Pal, G. P. Jolly, M. M. D. Lim, A. Malik, and R. Malekan, "Esophagopericardial fistula and pneumopericardium from caustic ingestion and esophageal stent," *The Annals of Thoracic Surgery*, vol. 107, no. 3, pp. e207–e208, 2019.

[5] S. Park, J.-H. Kim, Y. C. Lee, and J. B. Chung, "Gastropericardial fistula as a complication in a refractory gastric ulcer after esophagogastrostomy with gastric pull-up," *Yonsei Medical Journal*, vol. 51, no. 2, pp. 270–272, 2010.

[6] T. M. Grandhi, D. Rawlings, and C. G. Morran, "Gastropericardial fistula: a case report and review of literature," *Emergency Medicine Journal*, vol. 21, no. 5, pp. 644-645, 2004.

[7] N. Sailing, A. M. Falensteen, and L. G. Larsen, "Non-traumatic perforation of gastric ulcer in a hiatal hernia to the pericardium," *Acta Medica Scandinavica*, vol. 213, no. 3, pp. 225-226, 1983.

[8] M. Weng, J. Wu, and K. Chiu, "Gastropericardial fistula-caused pneumopericardium," *Clinical Gastroenterology and Hepatology*, vol. 11, no. 9, pp. e64–e65, 2013.

[9] S. A. Azam, A. G. Wilcox, K. G. King, and G. Whang, "Gastropericardial fistula," *Surgery*, vol. 167, no. 4, pp. e3–e4, 2020.

[10] J. P. Davidson, T. M. Connelly, E. Libove, and R. Tappouni, "Gastropericardial fistula: radiologic findings and literature review," *Journal of Surgical Research*, vol. 203, no. 1, pp. 174–182, 2016.

[11] M. Schmidinger, "Understanding and managing toxicities of vascular endothelial growth factor (VEGF) inhibitors," *EJC Supplements*, vol. 11, no. 2, pp. 172–191, 2013.

[12] T. Kamba and D. M. McDonald, "Mechanisms of adverse effects of anti-VEGF therapy for cancer," *British Journal of Cancer*, vol. 96, no. 12, pp. 1788–1795, 2007.

[13] I. B. Andersen, T. Jørgensen, O. Bonnevie, M. Grønbæk, and T. I. A. Sørensen, "Smoking and alcohol intake as risk factors for bleeding and perforated peptic ulcers: a population-based cohort study," *Epidemiology*, vol. 11, no. 4, pp. 434–439, 2000.

[14] A. Neri, Y. Lambert, D. Marrelli et al., "Gastro-pleuro-pericardial fistula following combined radiation and chemotherapy for lung metastases from renal cell carcinoma: report of a case," *Surgery Today*, vol. 43, no. 12, pp. 1457–1460, 2013, Epub 2013 Jan 12.

[15] C. Emmanouilides, G. Sfakiotaki, N. Androulakis et al., "Front-line bevacizumab in combination with oxaliplatin, leucovorin and 5-fluorouracil (FOLFOX) in patients with metastatic colorectal cancer: a multicenter phase II study," *BMC Cancer*, vol. 7, no. 1, article 91, 2007.

[16] "Colon cancer treatment, by stage| how to treat colon cancer," 2020, November 2020, https://www.cancer.org/cancer/colon-rectal-cancer/treating/by-stage-colon.html.

[17] S. J. Jang, Y. K. Cha, J. S. Kim, D. Y. Kim, and D. B. Kim, "A gastro-pleuro-pericardial fistula that occurred following palliative chemoradiotherapy for tongue cancer: a case report," *Journal of the Korean Society of Radiology*, vol. 80, no. 4, p. 815, 2019.

Percutaneous Closure of Patent Foramen Ovale after Anterior Spinal Cord Infarction

João Ferreira Reis,[1] Petra Loureiro,[2] Rita Lopes Silva,[3] and José Diogo Martins[2]

[1]*Department of Cardiology, Hospital de Santa Marta, Centro Hospitalar Universitário de Lisboa Central, Lisbon, Portugal*
[2]*Department of Pediatric Cardiology, Hospital de Santa Marta, Centro Hospitalar Universitário de Lisboa Central, Lisbon, Portugal*
[3]*Pediatric Neurology Unit, Pediatric Department, Hospital de Dona Estefânia, Centro Hospitalar Universitário de Lisboa Central, Lisbon, Portugal*

Correspondence should be addressed to João Ferreira Reis; 72761@chlc.min-saude.pt

Academic Editor: Christopher S. Snyder

In patients with a patent foramen *ovale* (PFO) who have had a cryptogenic ischemic stroke, percutaneous closure reduces its recurrence risk. However, its role in spinal cord infarction (SCI) is less well-established. A few case reports describe the putative causative role of PFO in SCI. We present a case of a teenager with cryptogenic anterior SCI in the setting of a deep vein thrombosis and a high risk-PFO who underwent successful percutaneous closure.

1. Introduction

Spinal cord infarction is an uncommon, but important cause of acute myelopathy; however, a definite cause is not found in a significant proportion of cases (60–75% of the cases) [1, 2]. The presence of a patent foramen *ovale* is a well-established risk factor for cryptogenic brain infarction due to paradoxical embolism; however, the physiopathological link of right-to-left shunting in spinal cord ischemia is less clearly defined.

2. Case Report

2.1. History of Presentation. We describe the case of a 16-year-old male patient who presents to the emergency department with cervical pain radiating to both arms, followed by bilateral upper limb weakness and numbness, which began after performing a Valsalva maneuver (intense physical exercise—abdominal crunches). The paresthesias rapidly progressed to the abdomen and lower extremities, despite intact lower limb strength, and sphincter dysfunction developed. He denied having suffered a relevant trauma in the previous days.

A comprehensive neurological exam revealed flaccid paralysis of both upper extremities, with muscle power of 2/5 on the Medical Research Council (MRC) scale in 3 upper right arm adduction and right forearm flexion and muscle power 3/5 in upper left arm adduction and left forearm flexion, downward drift of both outstretched arms (Barré test), bilateral bicipital hyperreflexia, and pain and temperature sensation impairment in both upper and lower extremities. Proprioception, lower extremity strength, and cranial nerve examination were normal.

2.2. Past Medical History. The patient is overweight (body mass index -32 kg/m^2) and had a right tibial fracture in the previous year, treated with osteosynthesis. There is familial history of venous thromboembolism and premature atherosclerotic disease.

2.3. Differential Diagnosis. The clinical presentation is that of a "man-in-the-barrel syndrome," which translates an anterior spinal cord syndrome and can have several possible etiologies, including ischemic, inflammatory, traumatic, or neoplastic.

2.4. Investigations. Laboratory tests were remarkable for a borderline positive antinuclear antibodies' titer of 1 : 160 (speckled pattern) with positive anti-DFS70 autoantibodies, but the remainder of the autoimmune workup was negative,

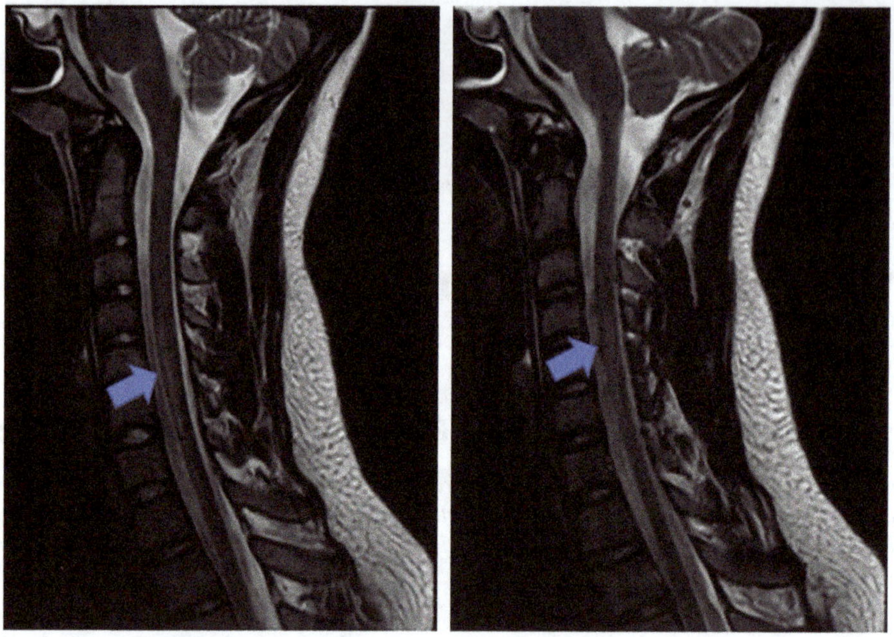

Figure 1: Spine MRI showing an extensive multisegmental T2-weighted hyperintense signal between the median plane of C4 and the transition from C7 to D1 (arrows) with symmetrical anterior medullary involvement and restricted diffusion on DWI, but without spinal cord expansion or signs of spinal cord compression. There was a normal T2 vertebral artery flow void, with no apparent signs of acute vertebral artery dissection or intramural hematoma.

including antiphospholipid antibodies and high factor VIII levels (182%). The workup was otherwise normal, including hypercoagulability, vasculitis, infectious, and transverse myelitis workups were negative. Cerebrospinal fluid examination was unremarkable.

T2-weighted sagittal MRI of the cervical spine disclosed a hyperintense lesion extending from C4 to D1 involving the anterior horns of the spinal cord, without signs of spinal cord compression and no apparent signs of acute vertebral artery dissection or intramural hematoma (Figure 1). Brain MRI was unremarkable.

Chest and CT angiography of supra-aortic arteries failed to identify an etiology and excluded acute aortic syndrome or supra-aortic vessel dissection. Digital subtraction spinal and supra-aortic artery angiography excluded abnormalities of the spinal cord vascular system, namely, arteriovenous malformations and vessel dissection, despite a slow filling of the anterior spinal artery. Lower Extremity Venous Doppler Study revealed thrombotic occlusion of the left posterior tibial artery.

Transcranial Doppler showed patency of major cerebral arteries, and saline bolus detected a right-to-left at-rest grade I shunt according to the Spencer grading scale during rest that increased with Valsalva maneuver. In order to evaluate for the presence of an intracardiac shunt, the patient underwent a transesophageal echocardiogram (TEE) that revealed the presence of a PFO with a tunnel length of 18 mm and an additional 2 mm ostium secundum atrial septal defect and an exuberant persisting Eustachian valve.

2.5. Management. Upon diagnosis of deep venous thrombosis, anti-Xa assay-guided low molecular weight heparin was started, requiring multiple dose adjustments due to subtherapeutic levels. The patient underwent successful physical rehabilitation.

The patient was referred to our cardiac center for percutaneous closure (PC). Under general anesthesia and TEE guidance, a Cardia Ultrasept PFO 20 mm device was successfully implanted, with no residual leak (Figures 2 and 3). The procedure was undertaken 8 months after spinal cord infarction, and a lower extremity venous Doppler was repeated prior to PFO closure in order to document resolution of deep venous thrombosis and ensure the safety of the procedure.

Due to a probable underlying thrombophilia, it was decided to maintain anticoagulation.

3. Discussion

We report one of the first percutaneous closure of a PFO in a patient with a cryptogenic medullar infarction, involving the youngest patient described in literature.

PFO affects about 25% of the adult population. It has a role in cryptogenic stroke in young adults, by providing a conduit to paradoxical embolism or by serving as a nidus for *in situ* thrombus formation, particularly in long-tunneled PFO with exuberant Eustachian valves. Recent randomized controlled trials (RCTs) [3–6] have demonstrated superiority of PC in comparison with medical therapy alone for prevention of recurrent stroke.

The vast majority of strokes associated with PFO are of cortical pattern, and the major RCTs evaluating the efficacy and safety of its percutaneous closure excluded patients with strokes due to small-vessel occlusive disease. Spinal cord infarction (SCI) due to paradoxical embolism is rare, and a

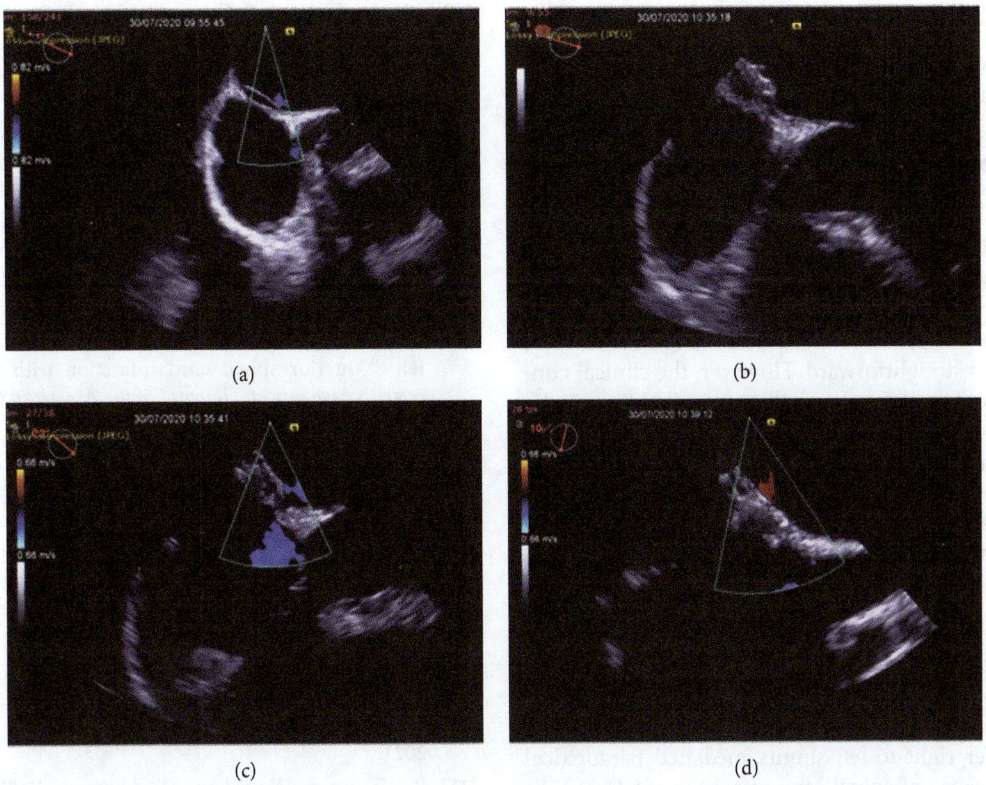

FIGURE 2: (a) TEE revealing a long-tunneled PFO. (b–d) TEE showing the final position of Cardia Ultrasept PFO 20 mm device, with no residual leak.

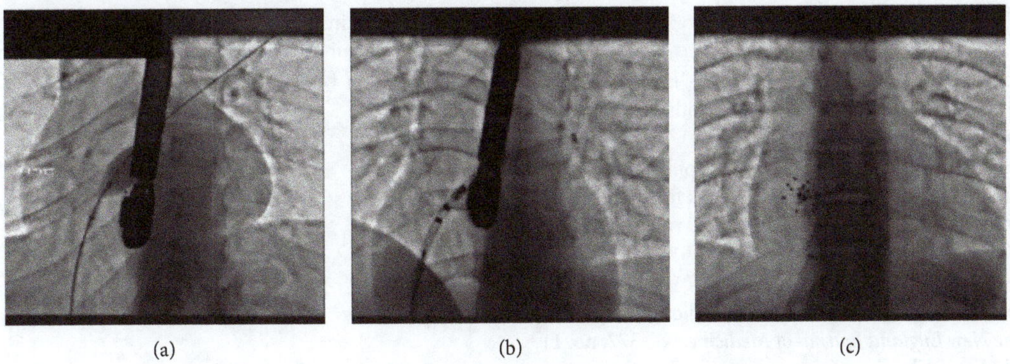

FIGURE 3: (a–c) Cardia Ultrasept PFO 20 mm device implantation.

few recent case reports [7–12] have postulated a possible physiopathological link between PFO-mediated paradoxical embolism and SCI.

We debated carefully the decision to close our patient's PFO. Contrary to closure, patients under 18 years old are largely underrepresented or have been excluded from the major RCTs [3–6]; there is tenuous clinical data that support this intervention after cryptogenic SCI; the long-term arrhythmic burden associated with PC including permanent postprocedural atrial fibrillation (AF) is largely unknown. Data on AF after transcatheter PFO closure are sparse; however, according to a recent meta-analysis, PFO closure increased the risk of new-onset AF at 4.6 times compared to medical therapy (4.2% vs. 0.7%; risk ratio 4.55, CI 95% 2.16-9.6, and $p = 0.0001$) [13]. In the REDUCE clinical study, postprocedural AF was mostly early onset, transient, and with no later recurrence and occurred more frequently among patients with higher age and larger devices [14].

Favoring closure, our patient presented with several features highly suggestive of a PFO-related paradoxical embolic event: the presence of lower limb deep venous thrombus; the temporal association between a Valsalva maneuver and symptom onset; the presence of high-risk characteristics associated with the PFO (exuberant Eustachian valve, long tunnel) [15], and, finally, the elevated levels of factor VIII, which are an established independent risk factor for thrombotic events, especially if the levels are above 150% [16].

4. Follow-Up

In the short-term follow-up, the patient is doing well, with no additional neurological events.

5. Conclusions

Our case describes the first percutaneous PFO closure in SCI in a young patient after a deep vein thrombosis and with a positive family history for venous thromboembolism. Due to the lack of randomized controlled trials on the management of SCI in the presence of PFO, the decision to close the PFO was not straightforward. However, the clinical context suggestive of paradoxical embolism, a probable underlying prothrombotic predisposition, the high-risk features of the PFO, and operator's experience played a role in the decision to close the PFO, despite patient's young age. Our work seeks to raise awareness to the role of right-to-left shunts and paradoxical embolism in cryptogenic ischemic spinal disorders.

Additional Points

Learning Objectives. (i) To recognize patent foramen *ovale* (PFO) and other right-to-left shunts mediated paradoxical embolism as a cause of spinal cord infarction (SCI). (ii) To be able to identify the ideal candidates for percutaneous PFO closure.

References

[1] K. Nedeltchev, T. J. Loher, F. Stepper et al., "Long-term outcome of acute spinal cord ischemia syndrome," *Stroke*, vol. 35, no. 2, pp. 560–565, 2004.

[2] M. Y. Cheng, R. K. Lyu, Y. J. Chang et al., "Spinal cord infarction in Chinese patients. Clinical features, risk factors, imaging and prognosis," *Cerebrovascular Diseases*, vol. 26, no. 5, pp. 502–508, 2008.

[3] J. L. Saver, J. D. Carroll, D. E. Thaler et al., "Long-term outcomes of patent foramen ovale closure or medical therapy after stroke," *The New England Journal of Medicine*, vol. 377, no. 11, pp. 1022–1032, 2017.

[4] J. L. Mas, G. Derumeaux, B. Guillon et al., "Patent foramen ovale closure or anticoagulation vs. antiplatelets after stroke," *The New England Journal of Medicine*, vol. 377, no. 11, pp. 1011–1021, 2017.

[5] L. Søndergaard, S. E. Kasner, J. F. Rhodes et al., "Gore REDUCE Clinical Study Investigators. Patent foramen ovale closure or antiplatelet therapy for cryptogenic stroke," *The New England Journal of Medicine*, vol. 377, no. 11, pp. 1033–1042, 2017.

[6] P. H. Lee, J. K. Song, J. S. Kim et al., "Cryptogenic stroke and high-risk patent foramen ovale: the DEFENSE-PFO trial," *Journal of the American College of Cardiology*, vol. 71, no. 20, pp. 2335–2342, 2018.

[7] R. He, Q. Huang, X. Yan, Y. Liu, J. Yang, and X. Chen, "A case of paradoxical embolism causing anterior spinal cord syndrome and acute myocardial infarction following the intradiscal oxygen-ozone therapy," *Frontiers in Neurology*, vol. 10, no. 10, p. 137, 2019.

[8] M. Mendonça, A. S. Correia, A. Luís, P. Soares, S. Calado, and M. Viana-Baptista, "Spinal cord infarction and patent foramen ovale: is there a link?," *Case Reports in Neurology*, vol. 6, no. 2, pp. 188–192, 2014.

[9] S. Mori, S. Sadoshima, K. Tagawa, K. Iino, and M. Fujishima, "Massive spinal cord infarction with multiple paradoxical embolism: a case report," *Angiology*, vol. 44, no. 3, pp. 251–256, 1993.

[10] R. B. Domingues and M. F. Vilas-Novas, "Cervical spinal cord infarct associated with patent foramen ovale," *Arquivos de Neuro-Psiquiatria*, vol. 70, no. 5, pp. 381-382, 2012.

[11] B. X. Nguyen, T. Gullatt, N. Subah, S. Gilani, and T. A. Sharifeh, "Anterior spinal cord infarction with patent foramen ovale: a case report," *Journal of the American College of Cardiology*, vol. 75, no. 11, p. 2855, 2020.

[12] M. Petruzzellis, A. Fraddosio, M. Giorelli et al., "Posterior spinal artery infarct due to patent foramen ovale," *Spine*, vol. 35, no. 5, pp. E155–E158, 2010.

[13] T. K. M. Wang, M. T. M. Wang, and P. Ruygrok, "Patent foramen ovale closure versus medical therapy for cryptogenic stroke: meta-analysis of randomised trials," *Heart, Lung & Circulation*, vol. 28, no. 4, pp. 623–631, 2019.

[14] A. Andersen, K. L. Matzen, G. Andersen et al., "Atrial fibrillation after closure of patent foramen ovale in the REDUCE clinical study," *Catheterization and Cardiovascular Interventions*, 2021.

[15] R. Nakayama, Y. Takaya, T. Akagi et al., "Identification of high-risk patent foramen ovale associated with cryptogenic stroke: development of a scoring system," *Journal of the American Society of Echocardiography*, vol. 32, no. 7, pp. 811–816, 2019.

[16] P. V. Jenkins, O. Rawley, O. P. Smith, and J. S. O'Donnell, "Elevated factor VIII levels and risk of venous thrombosis," *British Journal of Haematology*, vol. 157, no. 6, pp. 653–663, 2012.

49

Acute Nonatherosclerotic Coronary Thromboembolism Presenting with an Inferior STEMI in a Patient on Oral Contraception

Nabil Braiteh,[1] **Raheel Chaudhry**,[2] **Ibraheem Rehman**,[3] **Jowana Breiteh**,[4] **and Alon Yarkoni**[1]

[1]*Department of Cardiology, United Health Services Hospitals, Wilson Regional Medical Center, NY, USA*
[2]*Department of Internal Medicine, United Health Services Hospitals, Wilson Regional Medical Center, NY, USA*
[3]*Emory University School of Medicine, Atlanta, Georgia, USA*
[4]*Department of Nutrition and Food Sciences, American University of Beirut, Beirut, Lebanon*

Correspondence should be addressed to Nabil Braiteh; nab.braiteh@gmail.com

Academic Editor: Yigit Canga

Background. Direct coronary embolism in the setting of oral contraceptive pill (OCP) use is a rare adverse effect. It is known for OCP to increase the risk of thrombosis; however, leading to an inferior ST elevated myocardial infarction (STEMI) due to an acute occlusive embolism is a rare entity. Coronary embolism occurs in about 3% of patients with acute coronary syndrome. *Case Report.* We present a case of a young 41-year-old female with a past medical history significant for dysfunctional uterine bleeding on oral contraceptive pills, who presented to the hospital with chest pain. Her workup was significant for troponin elevation and an electrocardiogram showing inferior ST elevations. The patient was taken emergently to the cardiac catheterization lab. A coronary angiogram revealed a coronary thrombus involving the distal left main and proximal left anterior descending (LAD) with no evidence of atherosclerotic disease. The patient subsequently received anticoagulation therapy leading to complete resolution of symptoms and ST elevations. *Conclusion.* Coronary embolism is rare and often not considered in the differential of acute coronary syndrome. It is of utmost importance for clinicians to keep a wide differential of nonatherosclerotic causes of STEMI especially when the patient is young, without significant cardiac risk factors.

1. Introduction

Nonatherosclerotic causes of STEMI may be life-threatening and can occur even in the absence of significant cardiovascular risk factors. A nonatherosclerotic direct coronary thromboembolism is a rare occurrence. It requires further investigation and the initiation of appropriate therapy immediately.

Coronary embolism occurs in about 3% of patients with acute coronary syndrome [1]. It may be paradoxical, direct, or iatrogenic. An embolism breaks off an initial source such as a thrombus and then causes a decrease or blockage of blood flow upstream.

Oral contraceptive pills (OCPs) are used widely to prevent unwanted pregnancies and dysfunctional uterine bleeding. There has been much research on the increased risk of thromboembolic events from these drugs. Norgestimate/ethinyl estradiol is a progesterone and estrogen combination used to prevent ovulation and pregnancy. OCPs including norgestimate/ethinyl estradiol are known to significantly increase the risk of clot formation in female smokers who are above the age of 35 [2]. Estrogen is also known to cause downregulation of protein S creating a hypercoagulable state [3].

Herein we report a 41-year-old female who presented with an inferior STEMI and was found to have a saddle clot (thrombus) involving the distal left main artery, left circumflex, and proximal LAD. Her only cardiac risk factors were smoking and the use of oral contraceptives.

2. Case Report

A 41-year-old gravida 6 para 3 female (uncompleted pregnancies due to miscarriages) presented to the emergency department with a chief complaint of chest pain. Pain started two hours prior to presentation, was dull, left sided, substernal, radiated to her left arm, and with a severity of 7/10. One month prior to presentation the patient was complaining of an abnormal uterine bleeding and was started on oral norgestimate/ethinyl estradiol pills.

The patient has no significant past medical history. Her social history is significant for smoking 1/2 a pack per day for the past 10 years. Her family history is not significant for premature coronary artery disease or thrombosis. Her past surgical history is significant for dilatation and curettage two weeks prior to presentation. Home medications include daily oral norgestimate/ethinyl estradiol pills. Her only cardiac risk factors were smoking and the use of oral contraceptives.

Upon arrival to the emergency department, the patient was vitally stable. Her physical exam was noncontributory. Cardiac and lung exams were unremarkable. A twelve-lead ECG showed 1 mm ST elevations in inferior leads with no reciprocal changes and a sinus rhythm at a rate of 60 beats/minute (Figure 1). A STEMI code was called, and the patient was taken emergently to the Cath Lab. She was started on acute coronary syndrome (ACS) treatment including oral aspirin 324 milligrams, oral clopidogrel 600 milligrams, and intravenous heparin 5000 U. Significant laboratory data showed a troponin of 0.615 ng/mL (0-0.04 ng/mL), hemoglobin of 8.7 g/dL (12.0-15.5 g/dL), and white blood cell count of 13.7×10^9/L ($4.5 - 11.0 \times 10^9$/L).

Coronary angiogram revealed a saddle clot (thrombus) involving the distal left main artery, left circumflex, and proximal LAD (Figure 2). TIMI flow grade was 3 throughout, and no intervention took place during the coronary angiogram. There was also an occlusion in the apical portion of the LAD. The right coronary artery did not have any abnormalities. An echocardiogram revealed an estimated ejection fraction of 55-60% with apical septal hypokinesis and a normal diastolic function. There was no evidence of an intra-atrial shunt or left atrial appendage. Patient was admitted to the cardiac care unit (CCU) and was started on intravenous tirofiban for 10 hours, oral aspirin 81 milligrams daily, oral clopidogrel 75 milligrams daily, and intravenous heparin drip as per ACS protocol. Troponin peaked at 11 ng/mL. The patient was given 2 units of PRBC due to persistent vaginal bleeding. Doppler of the lower extremities did not reveal any evidence of a DVT. Telemetry over 48 hours of the hospital stay did not show any evidence of cardiac arrhythmia.

Thrombophilia testing lab results showed antithrombin activity of 88% (80-120%), antithrombin III AG 79%, cardiolipin AB IGA < 9.4 APL (<20.0 APL), beta – 2 glycoprotein IGG < 9.4 U/mL (<20.0 U/mL), beta – 2 glycoprotein IGM < 9.4 U/mL (<20.0 U/mL), cardiolipin AB IGM MCLIP < 9.4 MPL (<15 MPL), cardiolipin AB IGG GCLIP < 9.4 GPL (<15 GPL), prothrombin G20210A gene negative, beta – 2 glycoprotein AB IGA < 9.4 U/mL (<15.0 U/mL), PS/PT IGG < 9.4 U (<30.0 U), PS/PT IGM 20.0 U (<30.0 U), and platelet count of 376 K/μL (149-400 K/μL).

OBGYN were consulted, and placement of IUD was recommended to help prevent bleeding. After 48 hours, heparin was discontinued. EKG prior to discharge showed resolution of ST elevations (Figure 3). A repeat angiography was not done as symptoms had resolved and EKG showed resolution of STEMI. OCPs were held, and patient was discharged on oral anticoagulation.

3. Discussion

Coronary embolism occurs in about 3% of patients with acute coronary syndrome. However, it is a rare occurrence in a patient without a cardiac history of endocarditis, arrhythmia, or family history. Coronary embolism is of three main types: direct, paradoxical, and iatrogenic.

Direct embolism usually results from a thrombus originating in the left ventricle or left atrium or due to endocarditis involving the mitral or aortic valve. Paradoxical embolism occurs from the venous circulation through a patent foramen ovale. Iatrogenic embolism occurs after a cardiac procedure [1].

Risk factors include evidence of blood stasis (i.e., left ventricular aneurysm, atrial fibrillation, and deep vein thrombosis with ASD or PFO), hypercoagulable state (i.e., cancer, thrombophilia, oral contraceptive use, and heparin-induced thrombocytopenia), endothelial injury (i.e., angioplasty, valvuloplasty, and aortic/coronary surgery), and anatomic predisposition (i.e., ASD/PFO, endocarditis, and mitral stenosis). Smoking itself is considered to increase the risk of ischemic vascular events such as myocardial infarction and ischemic strokes [4–6].

Diagnosis of coronary embolism can be made using a scoring system proposed by Shibata et al. [7]. Major criteria include (1) angiographic evidence of coronary embolus, (2) concomitant systemic embolization without evidence of left ventricular thrombus, (3) concomitant coronary emboli in multiple coronary territories, (4) evidence of an embolic source based on imaging, and (5) histological evidence of venous origin of coronary embolic material.

Minor criteria include (1) <25% stenosis on angiography in the nonculprit vessels, (2) presence of atrial fibrillation, and (3) presence of embolic risk factors.

Patients with 2 or more major criteria, 1 major and 2 minor, or 3 minor criteria were considered to have a definite coronary embolus. Patients with 1 major and 1 minor or 2 minor criteria were considered to have a probable coronary embolus [1, 7].

Our patient is a young female with tobacco abuse, on norgestimate/ethinyl estradiol pills for dysfunctional uterine bleeding who presented with an inferior STEMI secondary to a clot (thrombus) involving the distal left main artery, left circumflex, and proximal and distal LAD.

ECG changes were mainly seen in the inferior rather than the anterior or anterolateral leads. That can be explained by two theories. (1) There might have been a right coronary artery clot that was dislodged prior to the

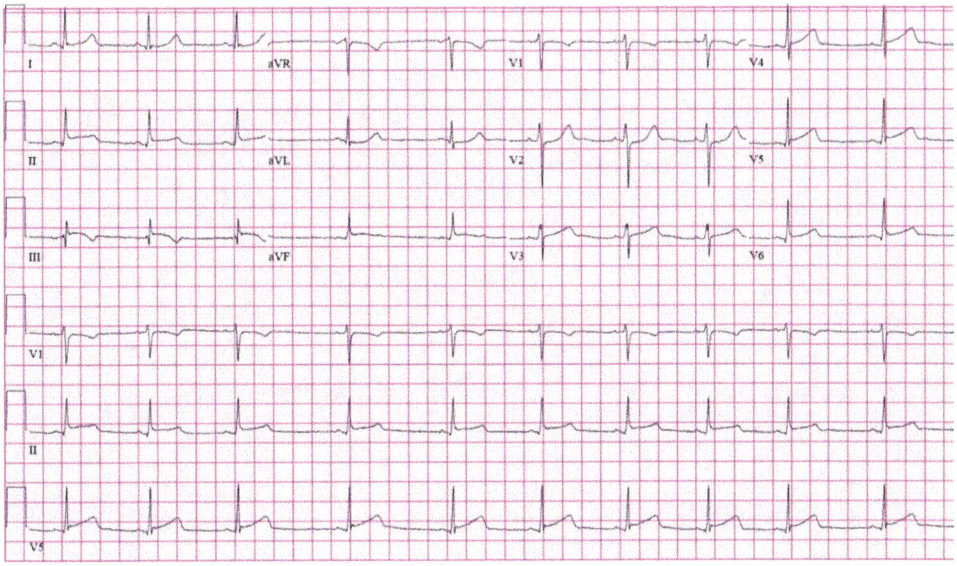

FIGURE 1: Electrocardiogram showing 1 mm ST elevations in inferior leads with no reciprocal changes and a sinus rhythm at a rate of 60 beats/minute.

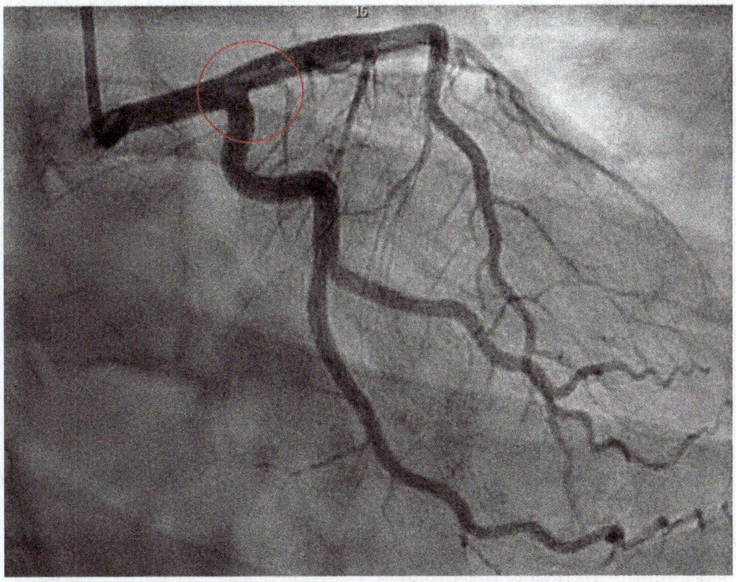

FIGURE 2: Coronary angiogram revealed a saddle clot (thrombus) involving the distal left main artery, left circumflex artery, and proximal left anterior descending artery (red circle).

angiogram especially that the repeat ECG showed resolution of inferior ST elevations. (2) There was a complete occlusion of the distal LAD artery (which is a wrap-around artery), with evidence of continued flow in the left main and proximal LAD artery.

She did not have a history of atrial fibrillation; no evidence of clot, valvular heart disease, wall motion abnormality, or an intra-atrial shunt with rest and provocation on TTE; and no evidence of DVT. The primary hypothesis for our case is that she had a direct arterial thromboembolism that developed secondary to the combination of oral contraception and smoking which is a rare entity, since most thromboembolisms due to acquired thrombophilia are rather venous. Although the patient was monitored on telemetry over 48 hours without cardiac arrhythmias, she was recommended to have a long-term cardiac monitoring (by an event monitor) to rule out paroxysmal atrial fibrillation as a possible cause of this thromboembolism. A transesophageal echocardiogram was recommended to be done in the outpatient setting to further assess the presence of a clot in the left atrial appendage.

Although thrombophilia workup is seldom indicated as part of the coronary embolism workup [1], it was performed during her admission and was negative. The patient did have

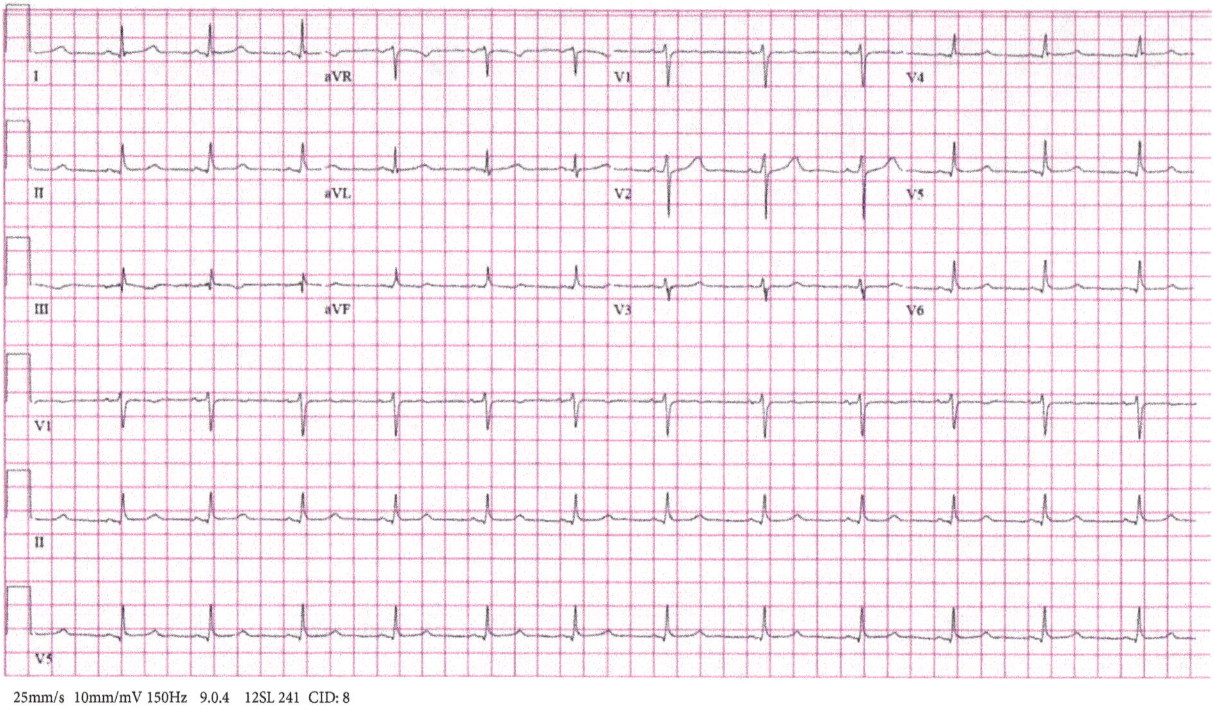

FIGURE 3: Electrocardiogram showing evidence of ST elevation resolution in the inferior leads.

miscarriages in the past, but it is less likely due to a hypercoagulable state since that workup was negative in the past. Long-term cohort studies revealed increased risk of venous rather than arterial thromboembolism in patients with inherited thrombophilias [8].

Antiplatelet therapy was continued in our case due to the presence of a distal LAD (apical) occlusion which is most likely due to the presence of a clot (thrombus), but we were unable to completely rule out the presence of atherosclerotic disease in that area.

Although estrogen and progesterone therapy may be an effective method of dysfunctional uterine bleeding, it is an oral contraceptive which is known to create a hypercoagulable state in combination with smoking, thereby increasing the risk for a thromboembolic event [9–11].

Vendittelli et al. performed a literature review on a total of 214 cases of coronary thromboembolism with the etiology being atrial fibrillation (26%), endocarditis (24%), iatrogenic emboli (21%), prosthetic valve thrombi (12%), hypercoagulable state with PFO (6%), aortic atheroma (5%), myxoma (2%), fat emboli (2%), and coronary stent emboli (2%) [12].

Treatment of coronary embolism depends on the root cause. Patients with atrial fibrillation or recurrent coronary embolism should be offered long-term anticoagulation regardless of their CHADS2-VASc score. Patients with a reversible risk factor such as smoking or OCP use should receive oral anticoagulation for 3 months [1].

After review of the literature, there have been only a couple of case reports to describe a case of a STEMI due to coronary embolism in a patient who is taking OCPs without evidence of a DVT or a patent foramen ovale [13, 14].

4. Conclusion

Atherosclerotic coronary artery disease is the main cause of STEMI. While coronary embolism is rare and often not considered in the differential of acute coronary syndrome, it is of utmost importance for clinicians to keep a wide differential of nonatherosclerotic causes of STEMI especially when the patient is young, without significant cardiac risk factors.

References

[1] C. E. Raphael, J. A. Heit, G. S. Reeder et al., "Coronary Embolus: An Underappreciated Cause of Acute Coronary Syndromes," *JACC: Cardiovascular Interventions*, vol. 11, no. 2, pp. 172–180, 2018.

[2] W.-S. Chan, "Risk of stroke in women exposed to low-dose oral contraceptives," in *Archives of Internal Medicine*, American Medical Association, 2004, Available from: https://jamanetwork.com/journals/jamainternalmedicine/fullarticle/216898.

[3] A. Suzuki, N. Sanda, Y. Miyawaki et al., "Down-regulation of *PROS1* Gene Expression by 17 β-Estradiol via Estrogen Receptor α (ERα)-Sp1 Interaction Recruiting Receptor-interacting Protein 140 and the Corepressor-HDAC3 Complex," *Journal of Biological Chemistry*, vol. 285, no. 18, pp. 13444–13453, 2010.

[4] Z. Vasiljevic, M. Scarpone, M. Bergami et al., "Smoking and sex differences in first manifestation of cardiovascular disease," *Atherosclerosis*, vol. 330, pp. 43–51, 2021.

[5] A. Hackshaw, J. K. Morris, S. Boniface, J. L. Tang, and D. Milenković, "Low cigarette consumption and risk of coronary heart disease and stroke: meta-analysis of 141 cohort studies in 55 study reports," *BMJ*, vol. 360, p. j5855, 2018.

[6] E. Prescott, M. Hippe, P. Schnohr, H. O. Hein, and J. Vestbo, "Smoking and risk of myocardial infarction in women and men: longitudinal population study," *BMJ*, vol. 316, no. 7137, pp. 1043–1047, 1998.

[7] T. Shibata, S. Kawakami, T. Noguchi et al., "Prevalence, clinical features, and prognosis of acute myocardial infarction attributable to coronary artery embolism," *Circulation*, vol. 132, no. 4, pp. 241–250, 2015.

[8] I. Martinelli, P. M. Mannucci, V. De Stefano et al., "Different risks of thrombosis in four coagulation defects associated with inherited thrombophilia: a study of 150 families," *Blood*, vol. 92, no. 7, pp. 2353–2358, 1998.

[9] J. L. Kujovich, "Hormones and pregnancy: thromboembolic risks for women," in *Wiley Online Library*, John Wiley & Sons, Ltd, 2004, April 20 Available from: https://onlinelibrary.wiley.com/doi/full/10.1111/j.1365-2141.2004.05041.x.

[10] R. Peragallo Urrutia, R. R. Coeytaux, A. J. McBroom et al., "Risk of acute thromboembolic events with oral contraceptive Use," *Obstetrics & Gynecology*, vol. 122, no. 2, pp. 380–389, 2013.

[11] D. Keeling, "Combined oral contraceptives and the risk of myocardial infarction," *Annals of Medicine*, vol. 35, no. 6, pp. 413–418, 2003.

[12] P. S. Vendittelli, B. Botros, H. S. Rosman, V. Govindaraju, A. Zaitoun, and T. S. Marroush, "Coronary artery embolism: two case reports and a review of the literature," *The American Journal of the Medical Sciences*, vol. 357, no. 4, pp. 333–337, 2019.

[13] A. Rahhal, F. Khir, M. Adam, A. Aljundi, M. K. Mohsen, and J. Al-Suwaidi, "Low dose combined oral contraceptives induced thrombotic anterior wall myocardial infarction: a case report," *BMC Cardiovascular Disorders*, vol. 20, no. 1, p. 182, 2020.

[14] A. N. Aslan, H. Süygün, S. Sivri, and T. Keleş, "Low-dose oral contraceptive-induced acute myocardial infarction," *The European Journal of Contraception & Reproductive Health Care*, vol. 21, no. 6, pp. 499–501, 2016.

[15] N. Braiteh, R. Chaudhry, I. Rehman, J. Breiteh, and A. Yarkoni, *Acute nonatherosclerotic coronary thromboembolism presenting with an inferior STEMI in a patient on oral contraception; A Case Report*, Authorea Preprints, 2020, https://www.authorea.com/doi/full/10.22541/au.160464799.92150144/v1.

50

Nonsurgical Management of a Papillary Fibroelastoma of the Aortic Valve

Antonino M. Grande,[1] Nicoletta Castiglione,[1] Adelaide Iervolino,[2] Francesco Nappi,[3] and Antonio Fiore[4]

[1]*Department of Cardiac Surgery IRCCS Fondazione Policlinico San Matteo, Pavia, Italy*
[2]*Department of Cardiovascular Sciences, Fondazione Policlinico Universitario A. Gemelli IRCSS, Italy*
[3]*Department of Cardiac Surgery, Centre Cardiologique du Nord de Saint-Denis, Paris, France*
[4]*Department of Cardiac Surgery, Henri Mondor University Hospital, Assistance Publique-Hôpitaux de Paris, Créteil, France*

Correspondence should be addressed to Francesco Nappi; francesconappi2@gmail.com

Academic Editor: Assad Movahed

We report the case of a 63-year-old woman who had an incidental echocardiographic diagnosis of papillary fibroelastoma (PFE) of the right coronary cusp of the aortic valve. The patient was informed about the embolic risk due to the pedunculated mass located on the aortic valve but she refused the proposed surgical removal. She was followed up yearly, and each follow-up included an echocardiographic evaluation of the mass. The lady is taking lysine acetylsalycilate 160 mg daily, and after more than 19 years later, she does not complain any symptoms or complications as a result of possible embolic episodes. If on one hand, our report is provocative for PFE nonsurgical management; on the other, we do believe that in symptomatic patients PFE located in the left heart chambers, the standard of care remains surgical excision after diagnosis. Anyway, our analysis shows that further data in this issue are needed in asymptomatic patients, and surgical indication should be proposed considering carefully the risk-benefit balance.

1. Introduction

Cardiac papillary fibroelastoma (PFE) represents 7.9% to 10% of all cardiac tumours and is the third most common primary benign cardiac tumour after myxoma (27%) and lipoma (10%) [1–4]. Before 1980, PFE was diagnosed as autoptic finding or incidentally at surgery [2, 3]. Echocardiography allows to diagnose most of these tumours antemortem with the possibility of curative surgical treatment. PFE mainly affects cardiac valves and as matter of fact represents more than 75% of valve tumours and occurs in almost all age groups, with a mean age of detection around 60 years, and its incidence is higher in men [5]. In addition, it is well known that PFE has the potential to determine embolic events that may jeopardize a patient's life. As a matter of fact, surgical removal of PFE is mandatory for all patients that have symptoms, but the treatment for those who are asymptomatic is still controversial.

2. Case Report

A 63-year-old woman was hospitalized in November 2001 in our department for surgical coronary revascularization. In 1998, she had an anterior acute myocardial infarction, and in January 1999, complaining exertion induced angina, she underwent coronary angiography and subsequently percutaneous transluminal coronary angioplasty of the left anterior descending (LAD) coronary artery. A year and a half later, she complained again exertional angina, and a repeated angiography showed a LAD occlusion and 90% stenosis of the first diagonal, while right and circumflex arteries showed a normal caliber; left ventricle ejection fraction measured by ventriculography was 50% and echocardiography showed only a mild mitral regurgitation. At that time, the lady underwent LAD grafting via a left anterior thoracotomy, with the left internal mammary artery (LIMA) as conduit. Two weeks later, she presented with recurrent exertional angina and coronary angiography showed occlusion of the LIMA graft. Reoperation was performed again via left anterior thoracotomy, and LAD bypass grafting was obtained using a tract of the saphenous vein. The cause of acute LIMA occlusion was due to technical issues at the level of the anastomosis. Postoperative course this time was uneventful, and the patient was transferred to rehabilitation department. Here, in January 2002, transthoracic echocardiography showed a small mobile mass on the right coronary cusp. The mass on the aortic valve was later confirmed by transesophageal echocardiography (TEE): a mobile, pedunculated, 0.8 cm round mass on the aortic side of the right coronary cusp of a trileaflet aortic valve, with an appearance most consistent with a PFE. She was afebrile and blood cultures were negative, ruling out endocarditis. Considering that we routinely use perioperative transesophageal echocardiography (TEE) during cardiac surgery, we may believe that PFE formed after the revascularization procedure.

Although the patient was adequately informed of the risk of stroke, systemic embolism, and the risk of myocardial infarct, she always refused surgery. Therefore, the patient was followed up at 12-month intervals, and each follow-up included an echocardiographic evaluation of PFE. She is under antiplatelet therapy with a daily 160 mg dose of lysine acetylsalycilate. In November 2011, a contrast computed tomography scan showed a mildly ill-defined, nonenhancing, hypodense nodular lesion, 11 mm in diameter, in the aortic root on the right coronary cusp of the aortic valve (Figure 1).

In 2015, she had a mastectomy for breast cancer followed by chemotherapy. The patient after more than 19 years later did not complain any symptoms or complications as a result of possible embolic episodes. Over the years, the echocardiographic size of the mass did not significantly increase: in October 2017, PFE diameter was 9 mm as indicated in Figure 2.

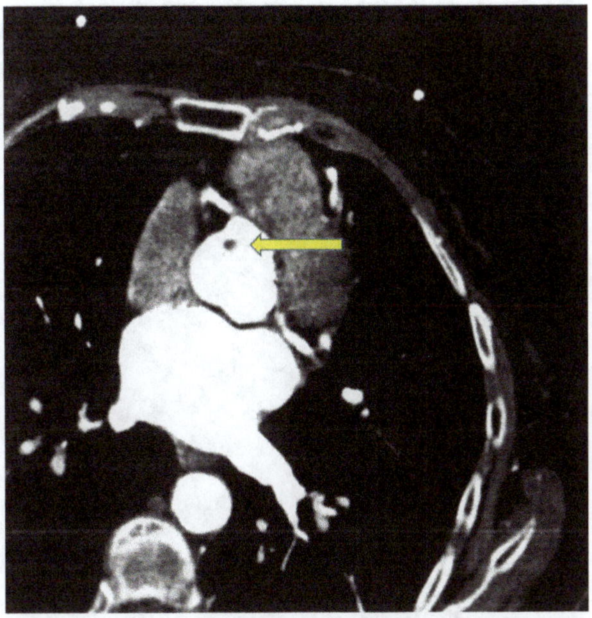

FIGURE 1: Computed tomography of the heart: the yellow arrow indicates the small round mass located on the right coronary cusp, 11 mm in diameter. Note the origin of the right and left coronary arteries.

3. Discussion

Erroneous diagnoses of a cardiac mass may lead to inappropriate treatment. There are several normal structures that may mimic a cardiac mass: the Eustachian valve, Chiari network, crista terminalis, pectinate muscles, moderator band, trabeculations, interatrial septal aneurysm, and lipomatous hypertrophy of the interatrial septum are some examples of normal structures that are frequently mistaken for pathologic entities [6, 7]. In the case of valvular mass, if valvular destruction or regurgitation is present, a vegetation rather than PFE should always be suspected.

Mutlu et al. [8] describe the case of a 63-year-old woman with an incidental echocardiographic 1 × 1 cm mass attached to the inferior wall of the left ventricle by a stalk, showing motion with cardiac cycle. The patient refused surgical removal, and she was kept on anticoagulation with warfarin and regularly followed up for 4 years without developing any symptoms or complications due to embolism. Küçükoglu et al. [9] reported a PFE located at the chorda of the anterior mitral leaflet in a 26-year-old woman complaining atypical chest pain: tumour diagnosis was made in 1988, and the patient was operated two years later but the attempt to remove the mass was unsuccessful. Therefore, the patient underwent conservative follow-up for the next 6 years, during which she complained palpitations and asthenia, until she went reoperation. At surgery, a 5 × 10 mm pedunculated polypoid mass attached to anterior mitral chorda was removed by simple excision, preserving mitral valve function.

Tamin et al. [10] evaluated the pathology and echocardiography database of Mayo Clinic (Rochester, MN, U.S.A.) for PFE and cardiac myxoma occurring between 1995 and 2010. This study showed that PFE is more common than cardiac myxoma, at a rate of approximately 2 : 1, for a rate of 1 PFE per every 1,100 echocardiograms; in more than 500 cases with a presumed PFE diagnosis, 185 patients had surgical tumour removal and 326 patients did not have surgical resection for different reasons. Furthermore, a significant association was found between clinically diagnosed PFE and neurologic events (NE); both mortality and risk of cerebrovascular accidents are greater in patients with PFE identified with echocardiography and not removed than with age- and sex-matched rates. In patients undergoing PFE surgical removal, median postoperative follow-up was 1.6 years showing a recurrent PFE in 3 cases (1.6%), at 1 year and 5 years, 95% and 86% of patients, respectively, were alive; overall risk of CVA was 2% at 1 year and 8% at 5 years; 10 CVA were found compared with 4.1 expected CVA on age- and sex-matched rates. In the conservative group, median follow-up was 1.7 years, and the CVA risk was 6% and 13% at 1 and 5 years, respectively, 29 CVA compared with 8

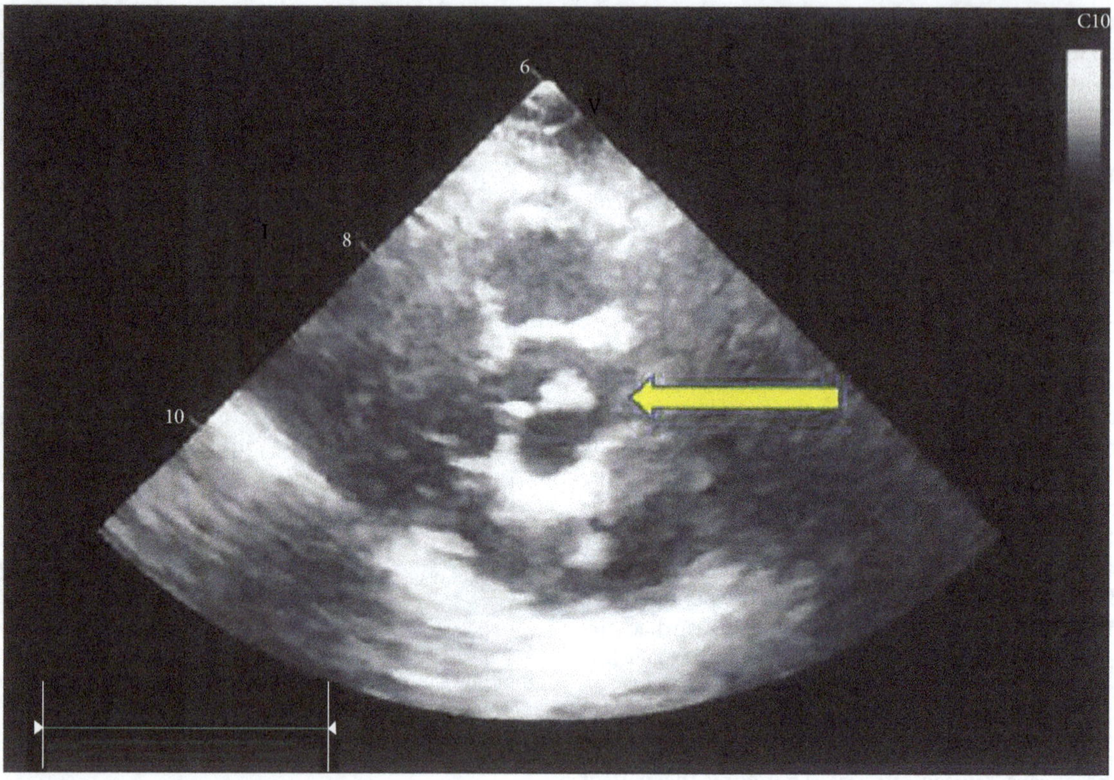

FIGURE 2: Transthoracic echocardiography: parasternal short axis shows a round mass, 9 mm in diameter (yellow arrow), on the aortic side of the right coronary cusp of the aortic valve.

expected in the matched control population; 1-year and 5-year survival were, respectively, 87% and 67%. Histological PFE study showed surface thrombi may occur, and for this reason, it suggested long-term antiplatelet agents. The study concludes that in patients with echocardiographically suspected PFE who do not undergo surgical removal, rates of cerebrovascular accident and mortality are increased.

In a comprehensive analysis of 725 cases found in the literature, Gowda et al. [3] found 25 cases not operated but with adverse outcomes: of these, 12 patients had PFE-related death.

Sang-Hoon et al. [11] reported a probable PFE with a stalk on the septal leaflet of the tricuspid valve in a 25-year-old woman that was followed at two months intervals for 3 years: she was asymptomatic and the tricuspid mass size decreased. PFE is located in the high flow and high pressure left heart, the risk of embolism is higher than the one located in the right cardiac system.

Our reported case presents a special interest because in the reviewed literature it is the longest follow-up, 19 years, in a patient with an echocardiographic PFE diagnosis who did not undergo surgical removal of the tumour. It is well known that most PFE reported are incidental findings in asymptomatic patients but embolic complications may be life-threatening. Our patient refused the proposed surgical treatment and was followed up yearly.

We do believe that in symptomatic patients, surgical PFE located in the left heart should be removed but our analysis shows that further data in this issue is needed in asymptomatic patients, and surgical indication should be proposed considering carefully the location of the mass, size of the mass, morphology and other clinical characteristics, and the risk-benefit balance.

References

[1] T. Flotte, H. Pinar, and H. Feiner, "Papillary elastofibroma of the left ventricular septum," *The American journal of surgical pathology*, vol. 4, no. 6, pp. 585–588, 1980.

[2] H. Frumin, L. O'Donnell, N. Z. Kerin, F. Levine, L. E. Nathan Jr., and S. P. Klein, "Two-dimensional echocardiographic detection and diagnostic features of tricuspid papillary fibroelastoma," *Journal of the American College of Cardiology*, vol. 2, no. 5, pp. 1016–1018, 1983.

[3] R. M. Gowda, I. A. Khan, C. K. Nair, N. J. Mehta, B. C. Vasavada, and T. J. Sacchi, "Cardiac papillary fibroelastoma: a comprehensive analysis of 725 cases," *American Heart Journal*, vol. 146, no. 3, pp. 404–410, 2003.

[4] F. H. Edwards, D. Hale, A. Cohen, L. Thompson, A. T. Pezzella, and R. Virmani, "Primary cardiac valve tumors," *The Annals of Thoracic Surgery*, vol. 52, no. 5, pp. 1127–1131, 1991.

[5] M. D. Cheitlin, M. A. HA, and C. M. de Castro, "Myocardial infarction without atherosclerosis," *JAMA*, vol. 231, no. 9, pp. 951–959, 1975.

[6] M. M. Ragland and T. Tak, "The role of echocardiography in diagnosing space-occupyng lesions of the heart," *Clinical medicine & research*, vol. 4, pp. 22–32, 2006.

[7] I. Nadra, D. Dawson, S. A. Schmitz, P. P. Punjabi, and P. Nihoyannopoulos, "Lipomatous hypertrophy of the interatrial septum: a commonly misdiagnosed mass often leading to unnecessary cardiac surgery," *Heart*, vol. 90, no. 12, article e66, 2004.

[8] H. Mutlu, I. E. Demir, J. Leppo, and W. K. Levy, "Nonsurgical Management of a Left Ventricular Pedunculated Papillary Fibroelastoma: A Case Report," *Journal of the American Society of Echocardiography*, vol. 21, no. 7, pp. 877.e4–877.e7, 2008.

[9] S. Küçükoglu, A. Arat, H. Mutlu et al., "A cardiac papillary fibroelastoma with chordal location," *Journal of the American Society of Echocardiography*, vol. 12, no. 11, pp. 1001–1004, 1999.

[10] S. S. Tamin, J. J. Maleszewski, C. G. Scott et al., "Prognostic and bioepidemiologic implications of papillary fibroelastomas," *Journal of the American College of Cardiology*, vol. 65, no. 22, pp. 2420–2429, 2015.

[11] S. Sang-Hoon, K. Dong-Soo, H. Yang-Chun et al., "Nonsurgical management of a tricuspid valvular pedunculated papillary fibroelastoma," *Cardiovascular Ultrasound*, vol. 7, no. 1, p. 44, 2009.

51

Long-Term Outcome of Thrombolytic Therapy for Massive Pulmonary Embolism in Pregnancy

Sy Van Hoang,[1] Anh Tuan Vo,[2] and Kha Minh Nguyen[1]

[1]*Department of Internal Medicine Faculty of Medicine, University of Medicine and Pharmacy at Ho Chi Minh City, Vietnam*
[2]*Department of Cardiovascular Surgery, University Medical Center, University of Medicine and Pharmacy at Ho Chi Minh City, Vietnam*

Correspondence should be addressed to Sy Van Hoang; hoangvansy@gmail.com

Academic Editor: Magnus Baumhäkel

A 25-year-old pregnant woman presented at 12 weeks of gestation with syncope and shortness of breath caused by massive pulmonary embolism. Due to persistent shock, fibrinolytic therapy with rtPA was administered. After fibrinolysis, clinical and hemodynamic response was excellent. No bleeding and fetal complications were recorded.

1. Introduction

Pulmonary embolism in pregnancy is still a leading cause of direct maternal mortality in the world [1]. During pregnancy, three pathophysiological mechanisms such as venous stasis, vascular injury, and hypercoagulability, known as Virchow's triad, that are together or in isolation may be responsible for the high incidence of pulmonary embolism in pregnancy [2]. Diagnosing of PE in pregnancy faces a number of difficulties due to clinical symptom overlaps due to hemodynamic changes during pregnancy period, as well as limitations of clinical indication (imaging) because it can affect the fetus [3].

In clinical trials, especially interventional trials, pregnant women are potentially vulnerable, and the fetus is faced with danger. Almost all clinical trials were done using methods regarding the diagnostic strategies and treatment of pulmonary embolism that exclude pregnant women due to moral and ethical standards by critics [4]. The recent guidelines for the management of cardiovascular diseases during pregnancy were developed by extrapolating the evidence for nonpregnant patients and had the weak-quality evidence [5]. A massive pulmonary embolism is an extremely life-threatening situation for the mother and fetus. The management of massive pulmonary embolism in nonpregnant patients is based on the acute removal of the thrombotic clot in the pulmonary arteries such as systemic thrombolysis, percutaneous catheter-based embolectomy, or surgical embolectomy. But clinicians face the challenge of treating pregnant patients with massive pulmonary embolism because of a lack of high-quality evidence to inform and guide their treatment decisions. Therefore, available data from case reports, case series, or retrospective observational studies are collected that is extremely helpful in treating massive pulmonary embolism in pregnant patients. In order to fill this important literature gap, we demonstrate a case report of massive pulmonary embolism in pregnancy treated by systemic thrombolysis (alteplase).

2. Case Report

A 25-year-old pregnant woman at 12 weeks of gestation was brought to the emergency department of our hospital by ambulance with worsening shortness of breath on exertion and onset of sudden syncope. The patient denied any cardiac disease and using any medication and had no relevant family history. She was having a swollen right leg from the ankle to the knee and dyspnea on exertion for the past week.

On admission, the patient was agitated and tired, and there is evidence of decompensation condition such as hypotension (70/40 mmHg), tachycardia (132 bbp), tachypnea (40 cpm), and low oxygen saturation in oxygen with a

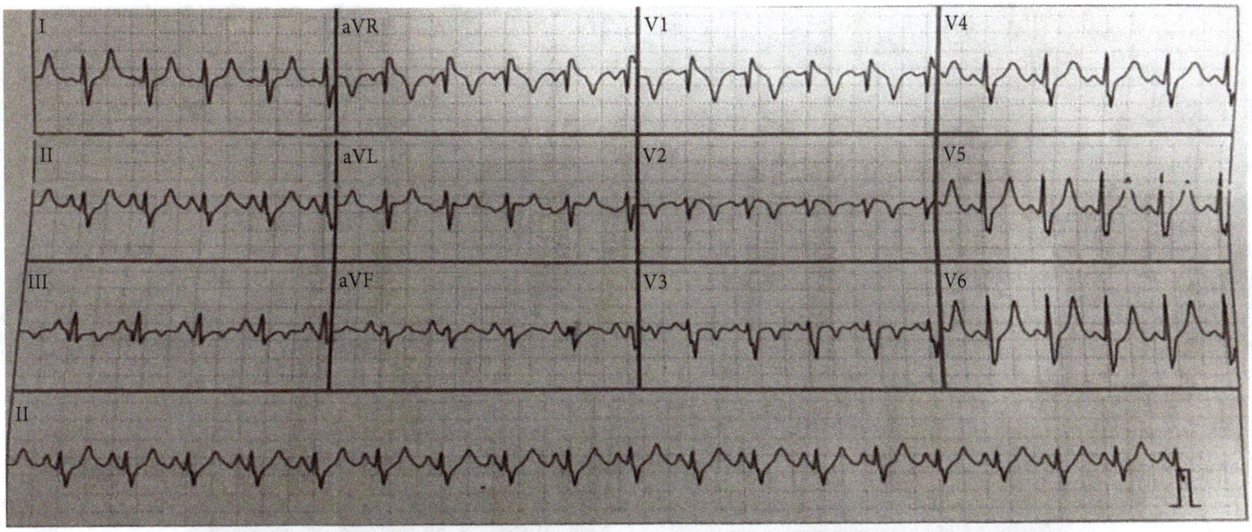

FIGURE 1: 12-lead ECG showing sinus tachycardia with a typical S1-Q3-T3 pattern.

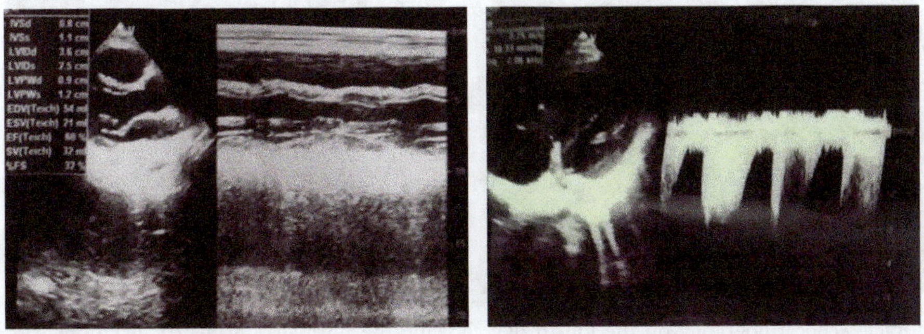

FIGURE 2: The transthoracic echocardiography on admission showing the right ventricular dilation, severity of tricuspid regurgitation, moderate pulmonary arterial hypertension with PAPs 50 mmHg, and normal left ventricular ejection fraction.

nonrebreather mask (8 L/min). She had signs of deep venous thrombosis in the unilateral leg. Jugular vein distention was visible, her lung fields were clear, and findings from cardiac examination were tachycardia, no gallop S3, S4, and existence of a 2/4 high-pitched systolic murmur heard along the upper left sternal border.

Laboratory tests revealed hemoglobin 132 g/L, WBC 12 G/L, PLT 155 G/L, D-Dimer >10,000 ng/mL, and Troponin I 1.482 ng/mL. The electrocardiogram showed sinus tachycardia and signs of right ventricular overload with a typical S1-Q3-T3 pattern (Figure 1). The transthoracic echocardiography performed on admission revealed signs of the right ventricular failure such as the right ventricular dilation, severity of tricuspid regurgitation, moderate pulmonary arterial hypertension with PAPs 50 mmHg, and normal left ventricular ejection fraction (Figure 2). Additional, deep venous thrombosis in the right leg was confirmed by duplex ultrasound, and obstetric ultrasound showed a fetus with cardiac pulsations inside the uterus at 12 weeks.

According to some evidence of clinical signs, laboratory tests, and initial imaging, a diagnosis of massive pulmonary embolism is suspected. In a patient with suspected massive pulmonary embolism who is in critical condition such as in an extremely life-threatening situation for the mother and the fetus, it was necessary to perform thoracic computed tomography (CT) with administration of intravenous contrast in the pulmonary arterial phase, with the fetus being protected from radiation by lead shielding. CT angiography revealed the right ventricular dilation (Figure 3(c)) and acute bilateral pulmonary thromboembolism (Figures 3(a) and 3(b)).

After first aid consisting of intravenous line placement, oxygen supplementation, subcutaneous enoxaparin 1 mg/kg, fluid infusion, and a vasoconstrictor agent (noradrenaline with dose of 0.5 mcg/kg/min), she was transferred to the CCU (coronary care unit) with a diagnosis of massive pulmonary embolism. Although there was a relative contraindication to thrombolysis, the condition of the mother and the fetus was extremely dangerous; systemic thrombolytic therapy was administered with alteplase (10 mg bolus, then 90 mg over 2 h) and according to partial thromboplastin time for the first 48 h, when enoxaparin 1 mg/kg twice daily was started. Within 2 hours, remarkable clinical and hemodynamic improvement was seen, with blood pressure 90/65 mmHg, heart rate 98 bpm, breathing rate 25 cpm, and decreasing need for oxygen supplementation, and dosage of noradrenaline was titrated based on the patient's response. After 6 hours of termination of fibrinolytic therapy, hemodynamic variables were stable, and she was weaned off noradrenaline infusion. She was discharged from the CCU on the third day.

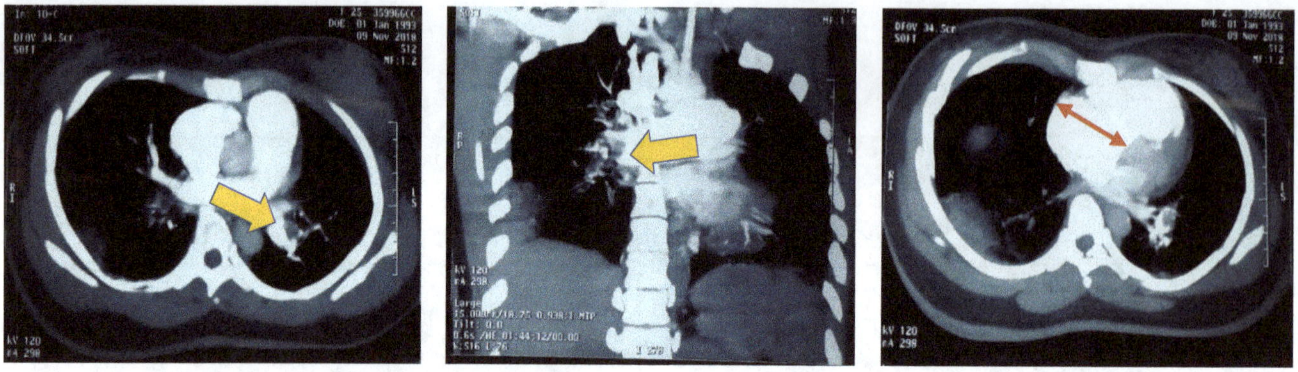

(a) (b) (c)

Figure 3: Thoracic computed tomography (CT) with intravenous contrast. Bilateral pulmonary thromboembolism (yellow arrow) in (a) coronal plane and (b) frontal plane; (c) shows the right ventricular dilation with the left ventricular compression (red 2-headed arrow).

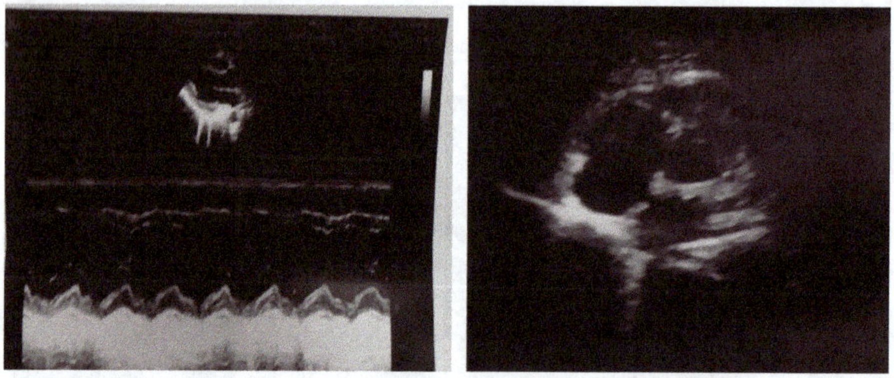

Figure 4: The transthoracic echocardiography on the fourth day showing the normal right ventricular dimension and the normal left ventricular ejection fraction.

On the fourth day, transthoracic echocardiogram (Figure 4) and obstetric ultrasound were performed, which revealed the normal right ventricular dimension, no signs of pulmonary hypertension, and no abnormal signs of pregnancy. She was discharged home on the 12th day at 14 weeks, medicated with acenocoumarol. Acenocoumarol was switched to subcutaneous enoxaparin from the 24th week of pregnancy to delivery. The patient was followed up regularly by experts in cardiology and obstetrics. On the 30th day after discharge, obstetric ultrasound revealed fetal growth in the same percentile curve and normal morphology with biparietal diameter 42 mm and the length of the femur 26 mm and amniotic fluid volume. At 36th week, the patient gave birth to a healthy 2.6-kilo baby boy. The anticoagulation was discontinued at 2 months postpartum.

3. Discussion

3.1. Diagnosis. It is usually difficult to evaluate the clinical signs of thromboembolism in pregnancy because most of them have bilateral leg edema, and there are 70% of pregnant women having dyspnea as well [6]. According to risk factor and clinical signs, it is reasonable to estimate the risk of pulmonary embolism in patients by using Wells score or Geneva score. These scores, however, are not used for pregnancy. In this case, the patient only had both leg edemas before presenting more severe symptoms and signs.

The clinical signs, laboratory tests, and initial imaging suggested the diagnosis of massive pulmonary embolism that could impair hemodynamics in this patient. The problem was that the fetus had to be exposed to radiation when performing thoracic CT with administration of intravenous contrast as a diagnostic test. The results would provide more information for the optimal and suitable treatment strategy to save the patient. Some studies showed that a fetus was exposed to the radiation of <0.01 mSv and 0.24–0.66 mSv with each chest X-ray and thoracic CT, respectively. However, the fetal vulnerability threshold is 50 mSv [7]. These necessary diagnostic imaging techniques have little effect on the fetus and conduct more benefits than risks for patients and fetuses [2]. In this situation, we requested a thoracic CT scan with pulmonary angiography at the recommendation level of IIA according to ESC 2014 guidelines [8].

3.2. Treatment. Regarding the treatment, this patient was diagnosed as having massive pulmonary embolism impairing hemodynamics at 12-week gestation. Pregnancy is a relative contraindication to thrombolysis [8]. The current treatment guidelines recommend that thrombolytic therapy is considered in pregnant patients whose life is at stake as this patient.

Up to now, no comparison of the efficacy between thrombolytic agents in pregnancy has been reported, but the current treatment guidelines recommend using rtPA or tenecteplase rather than urokinase/streptokinase because of their safety and efficiency [9]. If patients can be indicated to deliver (fetus can be alive), thrombolytic therapies should nốt be used except for the extremely life-threatening conditions or the case when thrombectomy and delivery cannot be carried out. The doctors have to consider the benefits and the risks when using thrombolytic therapies. The hemodynamic variables became gradually stable after usage of rtPA. In addition, the fetus was still alive and did not reveal any abnormalities according to obstetric ultrasound. Similarly, Ahearn et al. reported a case that a 12-week gestational 36-year-old woman who required massive pulmonary embolism with the shock condition was treated successfully with rtPA (dose of 100 mg IV in 2 hours) [9]. In 2019, a report about the outcome of thrombolytic therapies in 141 severe thromboembolic pregnant patients shows that there are 4 deaths (2.8%), 12 cases of severe hemorrhage (8.5%), 13 cases of mild/intermediate hemorrhage (9.2%), 9 cases of miscarriage (6.4%), 2 cases of stillbirth (1.4%), and 14 cases of premature delivery (9.9%) [10]. In our case, she gave birth to a healthy 2.6-kilo baby boy at 36th week. So this case was among the cases of premature delivery. At 36 weeks, this baby is considered late preterm then the risk of premature complications decreases significantly.

The method that thrombolytic agents are given locally via a catheter requires available instruments and experienced specialists, and there is no evidence that this method is more efficient than systemic thrombolytic therapy. Thrombectomy of pulmonary arterial embolism in impaired hemodynamic pregnancy has been reported in the world. However, the recommendation of surgery and criteria for patient inclusion are still controversial [11]. Many authors reported some cases of successful thrombectomy in pregnant women with massive pulmonary embolism. Blegvad et al. reported 10 cases of emergent thrombectomy for massive pulmonary embolism during pregnancy. Accordingly, there was no case of maternal death but 4 cases of miscarriage [12].

4. Conclusion

Pulmonary thromboembolism is common in pregnancy, and clinicians should keep a diagnosis of pulmonary embolism in mind, especially in the presence of suspicious clinical signs, laboratory tests, and initial imaging, including electrocardiogram and echocardiogram. Massive pulmonary embolism is associated with significant maternal and fetal mortality. Detecting early diagnosis and reasonable treatment strategies for massive pulmonary embolism improve the long-term outcome for the pregnant woman and fetus. Current evidence showed that the benefits of imaging tests outweigh the potential radiation risks when using radioactive sources such as thoracic computed tomography to diagnose pulmonary embolism. The thrombolytic therapy should be considered for life-threatening pulmonary embolism during pregnancy.

References

[1] J. S. Ginsberg, I. Greer, and J. Hirsh, "Use of antithrombotic agents during pregnancy," *Chest*, vol. 119, no. 1, pp. 122S–131S, 2001.

[2] M. Knight and UKOSS, "Antenatal pulmonary embolism: risk factors, management and outcomes," *BJOG: An International Journal of Obstetrics and Gynaecology*, vol. 115, no. 4, pp. 453–461, 2008.

[3] K. M. Moser, P. F. Fedullo, J. LitteJohn, and R. Crawford, "Frequent asymptomatic pulmonary embolism in patients with deep venous thrombosis," *JAMA*, vol. 271, no. 3, pp. 223–225, 1994.

[4] R. Meshaka, S. Jeffares, F. Sadrudin, N. Huisman, and P. Saravanan, "Why do pregnant women participate in research? A patient participation investigation using Q-methodology," *Health Expectations*, vol. 20, no. 2, pp. 188–197, 2017.

[5] V. Regitz-Zagrosek, J. W. Roos-Hesselink, J. Bauersachs et al., "2018 ESC guidelines for the management of cardiovascular diseases during pregnancy: the task force for the management of cardiovascular diseases during pregnancy of the European Society of Cardiology (ESC)," *European Heart Journal*, vol. 39, no. 34, pp. 3165–3241, 2018.

[6] S. E. Weinberger, S. T. Weiss, W. R. Cohen, J. W. Weiss, and T. S. Johnson, "Pregnancy and the lung," *American Review of Respiratory Disease*, vol. 121, no. 3, pp. 559–581, 1980.

[7] S. D. Chunilal and S. M. Bates, "Venous thromboembolism in pregnancy: diagnosis, management and prevention," *Thrombosis and Haemostasis*, vol. 101, no. 3, pp. 428–438, 2009.

[8] S. V. Konstantinides, A. Torbicki, G. Agnelli et al., "2014 ESC guidelines on the diagnosis and management of acute pulmonary embolism: the task force for the diagnosis and management of acute pulmonary embolism of the European Society of Cardiology (ESC)," *European Heart Journal*, vol. 35, no. 43, pp. 3033–3080, 2014.

[9] G. S. Ahearn, D. Hadjiliadis, J. A. Govert, and V. F. Tapson, "Massive pulmonary embolism during pregnancy successfully treated with recombinant tissue plasminogen activator: a case report and review of treatment options," *Archives of Internal Medicine*, vol. 162, no. 11, pp. 1221–1227, 2002.

[10] M. S. Gomes, M. Guimarães, and N. Montenegro, "Thrombolysis in pregnancy: a literature review," *The Journal of Maternal-Fetal & Neonatal Medicine*, vol. 32, no. 14, pp. 2418–2428, 2019.

[11] Z. Beckerman and G. Bolotin, "Surgical treatment of acute massive pulmonary embolism," in *Thrombosis and Embolism: from Research to Clinical Practice*, vol. 906 of Advances in Experimental Medicine and Biology, , pp. 75–88, Springer, 2016.

[12] S. Blegvad, O. Lund, T. T. Nielsen, and I. Guldholt, "Emergency embolectomy in a patient with massive pulmonary embolism during second trimester pregnancy," *Acta Obstetricia et Gynecologica Scandinavica*, vol. 68, no. 3, pp. 267–270, 1989.

Permissions

All chapters in this book were first published by Hindawi Publishing Corporation; hereby published with permission under the Creative Commons Attribution License or equivalent. Every chapter published in this book has been scrutinized by our experts. Their significance has been extensively debated. The topics covered herein carry significant findings which will fuel the growth of the discipline. They may even be implemented as practical applications or may be referred to as a beginning point for another development.

The contributors of this book come from diverse backgrounds, making this book a truly international effort. This book will bring forth new frontiers with its revolutionizing research information and detailed analysis of the nascent developments around the world.

We would like to thank all the contributing authors for lending their expertise to make the book truly unique. They have played a crucial role in the development of this book. Without their invaluable contributions this book wouldn't have been possible. They have made vital efforts to compile up to date information on the varied aspects of this subject to make this book a valuable addition to the collection of many professionals and students.

This book was conceptualized with the vision of imparting up-to-date information and advanced data in this field. To ensure the same, a matchless editorial board was set up. Every individual on the board went through rigorous rounds of assessment to prove their worth. After which they invested a large part of their time researching and compiling the most relevant data for our readers.

The editorial board has been involved in producing this book since its inception. They have spent rigorous hours researching and exploring the diverse topics which have resulted in the successful publishing of this book. They have passed on their knowledge of decades through this book. To expedite this challenging task, the publisher supported the team at every step. A small team of assistant editors was also appointed to further simplify the editing procedure and attain best results for the readers.

Apart from the editorial board, the designing team has also invested a significant amount of their time in understanding the subject and creating the most relevant covers. They scrutinized every image to scout for the most suitable representation of the subject and create an appropriate cover for the book.

The publishing team has been an ardent support to the editorial, designing and production team. Their endless efforts to recruit the best for this project, has resulted in the accomplishment of this book. They are a veteran in the field of academics and their pool of knowledge is as vast as their experience in printing. Their expertise and guidance has proved useful at every step. Their uncompromising quality standards have made this book an exceptional effort. Their encouragement from time to time has been an inspiration for everyone.

The publisher and the editorial board hope that this book will prove to be a valuable piece of knowledge for researchers, students, practitioners and scholars across the globe.

List of Contributors

Amit Alam
Division of Cardiology, Baylor University Medical Center, Dallas, TX, USA

Linle Hou and Deepa Iyer
Division of Cardiology, Rutgers-Robert Wood Johnson University Hospital, New Brunswick, NJ, USA

Dreamy James and Jesus Almendral
Division of Cardiology, Jersey Shore University Medical Center, Neptune, NJ, USA

Kanika Mody
Division of Cardiology, Hackensack University Medical Center, Hackensack, NJ, USA

Aziz Ghaly
Department of Cardiothoracic Surgery, Rutgers-Robert Wood Johnson University Hospital, New Brunswick, NJ, USA

Vanessa-Rose G. Turpin
Department of Kinesiology, College of Health and Human Sciences, Kansas State University, USA

Kyle Goerl
Lafene Health Center, Kansas State University, USA

Chen Hoe Chow
Cotton O'Neil Heart Center, Stormont Vail Health, USA

Carl J. Ade
Department of Kinesiology, College of Health and Human Sciences, Kansas State University, USA
Physician Assistant Studies, College of Health and Human Sciences, Kansas State University, USA
Johnson Cancer Center, Kansas State University, USA

Ali Shafiq, Fatima Samad, Eric Roberts and A. Jamil Tajik
1Aurora Cardiovascular Services, Aurora Sinai/ Aurora St. Luke's Medical Centers, Milwaukee, WI, USA

Jonathan Levin
BayCare Clinic Radiology, BayCare Health System, Green Bay, WI, USA

Ubaid Nawaz
Department of Hematology and Oncology, Vince Lombardi Cancer Clinic, Aurora Bay Care Medical Center, Green Bay, WI, USA

Christopher Nnaoma, Gurdarshan Sandhu, Christoph Sossou, Jose Bustillo and Anshu Garg
Newark Beth Israel Medical Center, Newark, NJ, USA

Ilan Vavilin
St. George's University, Grenada

José D. Martins, Guilherme Lourenço and Fátima F. Pinto
Pediatric Cardiology Department, Hospital de Santa Marta, Centro Hospitalar de Lisboa Central EPE, Lisbon, Portugal

Lídia Sousa
Cardiology Department, Hospital de Santa Marta, Centro Hospitalar de Lisboa Central EPE, Lisbon, Portugal

Xavier Galloo
Department of Cardiology, ZNA Middelheim, Antwerp, Belgium

Jan Stroobants and Esmael El-Abdellati
Emergency Department, ZNA Middelheim, Antwerp, Belgium

David Yeo
Emergency Department, University Hospital Birmingham, Birmingham, UK

Kosuke Saku , Keisuke Yamamoto, Hironori Inoue, and Masahiro Ueno
Department of Cardiovascular Surgery, Tenyokai Central Hospital and Central Clinic, Kagoshima, Japan

Hussein Al-Mohamad and Ronald Walsh
Department of Cardiology, Largo Medical Center, Largo, FL, USA

Kara Stout and Taryn Bolling
Department of Internal Medicine, Largo Medical Center, Largo, FL, USA

John Pueringer
Philadelphia College of Osteopathic Medicine, Philadelphia, Pennsylvania, USA

Joseph Cinderella and M. Greg Treuth
TidalHealth, Salisbury, Maryland, USA

S. Kumar
St. George Hospital, Sydney, Australia

S. Mahmood
Hornsby Hospital, Sydney, Australia

A. Madras
North Manchester General Hospital, Manchester, UK

A. Iyer
Northern Beaches Hospital, Sydney, Australia

Kyriacos Papadopoulos and Panayiotis Avraamides
Cardiology Department, Nicosia General Hospital, Nicosia, Cyprus

Murielle Bertin and Mohamed Aboukofa
Department of Anaesthesia, Mediclinic City Hospital, Dubai Health Care City, Building 37, Dubai, UAE

Pierre Francois Laterre
Intensive Care Department, Saint Luc University Hospital, UCL, Avenue Hippocrate 10, 1200 Brussels, Belgium

Zuhair Yousif
Department of Cardiology, Mediclinic City Hospital, Dubai Health Care City, Building 37, Dubai, UAE

Jelena Z. Arnautovic and Randy Ip
Division of Cardiovascular Medicine, St. John Providence Ascension Health System, Warren, MI, USA

Randi Connor-Schuler
Department of Emergency Medicine, Henry Ford Health System, Detroit, MI, USA

Ricardo O. Escárcega and David Bailey
Florida Heart Associates and Heart and Vascular Institute, Lee Health System, Fort Myers, FL, USA

Michael P. DeFrain
Shipley Cardiothoracic Center, Lee Health System, Fort Myers, FL, USA

Ashraf Abugroun, Safwan Gaznabi and Hussein Daoud
Department of Internal Medicine, Advocate Illinois Masonic Medical Center, 836 W Wellington Avenue, Chicago, IL 60657, USA

Ahmed Subahi
Department of Internal Medicine, Wayne State University/Detroit Medical Center, Detroit, Michigan, USA

Prathap Kumar, Blessvin Jino, Stalin Roy and Manu Rajendran
Department of Cardiology, Meditrina Hospital, Kollam, Kerala, India

Ebubechukwu Ezeh, Esiemoghie Akhigbe and Mackenzie Hamilton
Internal Medicine Department, Marshall University, Huntington WV, USA

Mohammad Amro
Internal Medicine Residency, The Palestinian Ministry of Health and Higher Education, State of Palestine

Mehrette Maru
Department of Cardiology, St. Mary's Medical Center, Huntington WV, USA

John Khoo and Paul Nguyen
Department of Cardiology, Liverpool Hospital, NSW, 2170 Sydney, Australia

David Ferreira and Craig Juergens
Department of Cardiology, Liverpool Hospital, NSW, 2170 Sydney, Australia
Department of Medicine, University of New South Wales, NSW, 2052 Sydney, Australia

Anthony Le and Manish Jain
Department of Cardiothoracic Surgery, Liverpool Hospital, NSW, 2170 Sydney, Australia

Timothy Spicer
Department of Medicine, University of New South Wales, NSW, 2052 Sydney, Australia
Department of Nephrology, Liverpool Hospital, NSW, 2170 Sydney, Australia

Hamza Hamayel and Yousef Hamshari
Department of Internal Medicine, An-Najah National University Hospital, Nablus, State of Palestine

Yahya Ismail, Sajed Majadla and Yunis Daralammouri
Department of Cardiology, An-Najah National University Hospital, Nablus, State of Palestine
Department of Medicine, Faculty of Medicine and Health Sciences, An-Najah National University, Nablus, State of Palestine

Robin Yeong Hong Goh, Stefan Buchholz and Allison Morton
Heart Care, Western Australia, Suite 21, St. John of God Bunbury Hospital, 700 Robertson Dr, College Grove, Western Australia, Australia

Shreeja Mehrotra and Deepak Mehrotra
Department of Cardiothoracic Surgery, Heart and Lung Centre, Mount Hospital, 150 Mounts Bay Rd, Perth, Western Australia, Australia

Talha Ahmed
University of Maryland Medical Center Midtown Campus, USA

Diljon Chahal, Ronson J. Madathil, David Kaczorowski and Anuj Gupta
University of Maryland Medical Center, School of Medicine, USA

Álvaro Herrera-Escandón
Internal Medicine Department, Universidad del Valle, Cali, Colombia
Cardiology Department, DIME Clínica Neurocardiovascular, Cali, Colombia
Heart Failure and Cardiac Transplant Unit, DIME Clínica Neurocardiovascular, Cali, Colombia

Orlando Castaño-Cifuentes
Cardiology Department, DIME Clínica Neurocardiovascular, Cali, Colombia

Carlos A. Plata-Mosquera
Heart Failure and Cardiac Transplant Unit, DIME Clínica Neurocardiovascular, Cali, Colombia

Alicia Shim and Ronald Henry
Cardiology Unit, Advanced Cardiovascular Institute, Port of Spain, Trinidad and Tobago

Rajeev Seecheran, Valmiki Seecheran and Sangeeta Persad
Department of Medicine, North Central Regional Health Authority, Mt. Hope, Trinidad and Tobago

Shiva Sreenivasan
School of Medicine, Dentistry, and Biomedical Sciences, Queen's University, Belfast, UK

Naveen Anand Seecheran
Department of Clinical Medical Sciences, University of the West Indies, St. Augustine, Trinidad and Tobago

Majken van den Handel Vestergaard and Ann Bovin
Department of Cardiology, SLB Vejle, Denmark

Erik Lerkevang Grove
Department of Internal Medicine, Faculty of Health, Aarhus University, Aarhus, Denmark
Department of Cardiology, Aarhus University Hospital, Palle Juul-Jensens Boulevard 99, 8200 Aarhus, Denmark

Aswin Srinivasan, Tusharkumar Pansuriya and Branden Wilson
Department of Internal Medicine, HCA Houston Kingwood/University of Houston College of Medicine, USA

Siva T. Sarva, Salman Alim and Ramesh Kesavan
Department of Pulmonology/Critical Care, HCA Houston Kingwood/University of Houston College of Medicine, USA

Turuvekere Jayaram
Department of Internal Medicine, HCA Houston Kingwood/University of Houston College of Medicine, USA
Department of Pulmonology/Critical Care, HCA Houston Kingwood/University of Houston College of Medicine, USA

Syed Raza
Department of Cardiology, HCA Houston Kingwood/University of Houston College of Medicine, USA

Dre Eleonore Campiche and David Carballo
Cardiology Department, University Hospitals of Geneva, 1205 Geneva, Switzerland

Jean-Paul Vallée
Radiology Department, University Hospitals of Geneva, 1205 Geneva, Switzerland

Nicolas De Schryver
Department of Intensive Care, Clinique St-Pierre, 1340 Ottignies, Belgium

Philippe Hantson
Department of Intensive Care, Cliniques St-Luc, Université catholique de Louvain, 1200 Brussels, Belgium
Louvain Centre of Toxicology and Applied Pharmacology, Université catholique de Louvain, 1200 Brussels, Belgium

Vincent Haufroid
Louvain Centre of Toxicology and Applied Pharmacology, Université catholique de Louvain, 1200 Brussels, Belgium
Department of Clinical Chemistry, Cliniques St-Luc, Université catholique de Louvain, 1200 Brussels, Belgium

Mélanie Dechamps
Cardiovascular Intensive Care, Cliniques St-Luc, Université catholique de Louvain, 1200 Brussels, Belgium

Sri Harsha Patlolla, Saraschandra Vallabhajosyula and Malcolm R. Bell
Department of Cardiovascular Medicine, Mayo Clinic, Rochester, Minnesota, USA

Bo Zhang, Laxman Gyawali, Zengzhang Liu , Huaan Du , and Yuehui Yin
Department of Cardiology, The Second Affiliated Hospital of Chongqing Medical University, No. 288 Tian Wen Avenue, Nan'an District, Chongqing 401336, China

Wajeeh ur Rehman , Altif Muneeb and Usama Sakhawat
Department of Internal Medicine, United Health Services Hospitals, Wilson Regional Medical Center, Johnson City, NY, USA

Pranava Ganesh, Nabil Braiteh, Vince Skovira, Waseem Sajjad and Afzal ur Rehman
Department of Cardiology, United Health Services Hospitals, Heart and Vascular Institute, Wilson Regional Medical Center, Johnson City, NY, USA

Fakilahyel S. Mshelbwala
Cardiology Fellow PGY4, Henry Ford Hospital, K-14 Cardiology, 2799 W. Grand Blvd, Detroit, MI 48202, USA

Brittany Fuller, Khaldoon Alaswad and Mir B. Basir
Department of Cardiology, Henry Ford Hospital, Detroit, Michigan, USA

Saad Sikanderkhel and Harish Manyam
Department of Cardiovascular Medicine, University of Tennessee College of Medicine Chattanooga, USA

Jon-Austin Ash, Kimberly O'Dell and Jacob Mok
Department of Internal Medicine, University of Tennessee College of Medicine Chattanooga, USA

John Golding
Heart and Lung Institute, Erlanger Baroness Hospital, Chattanooga, Tennessee, USA

Rohit Mody
Department of Cardiology, MAX Super Specialty Hospital, Bathinda, Punjab, India

Debabrata Dash
Department of Cardiology, Zulekha Hospital, AL Zahra Street, Sharjah 457, UAE

Bhavya Mody
Department of Medicine, Kasturba Medical College, Manipal, Karnataka, India

Aditya Saholi
Department of Medicine, Irwin Hospital, Surja Ram Market, Malout, Punjab, India

Gao Hao-kao and Li Cheng-xiang
Department of Cardiology, The First Affiliated Hospital of Air Force Military Medical University, Xi'an 710032, China

Mark I. Davis, Brian K. Courtney, Stephanie Poon and Mina Madan
Division of Cardiology, Department of Medicine, Sunnybrook Health Sciences Centre, University of Toronto, Toronto, Canada

Gideon Cohen
Division of Cardiac Surgery, Department of Surgery, Sunnybrook Health Sciences Centre, University of Toronto, Toronto, Canada

Evan Harmon, Yoo Jin Lee, Sula Mazimba, Kanwar Singh, Aditya Sharma and Younghoon Kwon
University of Virginia Health System, Charlottesville, VA, USA

Amanda Fernandes and Crystal Lihong Yan
1Division of Internal Medicine, University of Miami/ Jackson Memorial Hospital, Miami, FL, USA

Phillip Ruiz
Departments of Surgery and Pathology, University of Miami/Jackson Memorial Hospital, Miami, FL, USA

Nina Thakkar Rivera
Division of Cardiology, Miami Transplant Institute, University of Miami/Jackson Memorial Hospital, Miami, FL, USA

Haris Ahmed, Jonathan Brown, Brooke Walterscheid, Phebe Abraham, Junaid Alam and Nabeel Ahmad
Department of Internal Medicine, HCA Houston Kingwood/University of Houston College of Medicine, USA

Syed Arman Raza
Department of Cardiology, HCA Houston Kingwood/ University of Houston College of Medicine, USA

Fernando Montenegro Sá, Sara I. L. Fernandes, Rita J. R. Carvalho, Luís M. G. Santos, José A. S. Antunes, Joana M. Guardado, and João C. A. Morais
Cardiology Department, Leiria Hospital Center, Portugal

Khalil Kanjwal , Michael Soos, Daniel Gonzalez-Morales, Ibrahim Shah, Mohan Madala, Majid Mughal, and Muhammad Awais Kang
McLaren Greater Lansing Hospital, Lansing, MI, USA

Diana C. Ramírez-Mesías
Hospital Universitario San Ignacio, Bogotá 110231, Colombia
Pontificia Universidad Javeriana, Bogotá 110231, Colombia

Juan F. Contreras-Valero, Gabriel D. Pinilla - Monsalve and Carlos E. Vesga-Reyes
Fundaci6n Valle del Lili, Cali 760032, Colombia
Universidad Icesi, Cali 760031, Colombia

Claire Chakkalakal, Rezo Jorbenadze and Meinrad Gawaz
University Hospital, Department of Cardiology and Cardiovascular Medicine, University of Tübingen, 72076 Tübingen, Germany

Diego H. González-Bravo, Melanie Quintana-Serrano, Sergio Alegre-Boschetti and Juan Vázquez-Fuster
Cardiovascular Division, Department of Medicine, VA Caribbean Healthcare System, San Juan, Puerto Rico, USA

Pedro Colón-Hernández
Cardiovascular Center, Menonita Medical Center, Cayey, Puerto Rico, USA

José J. Acevedo-Valles
Cardiovascular Division, Department of Medicine, VA Caribbean Healthcare System, San Juan, Puerto Rico, USA
Internal Medicine Division, Department of Medicine, VA Caribbean Healthcare System, San Juan, Puerto Rico, USA

Eric Avilés-Rivera
Cardiovascular Division, Department of Medicine, VA Caribbean Healthcare System, San Juan, Puerto Rico, USA
Cardiovascular Center, Menonita Medical Center, Cayey, Puerto Rico, USA

Hideki Wada, Soshi Moriya, Manabu Ogita, Satoru Suwa and Hiroka Sasahara
Department of Cardiovascular Medicine, Juntendo University Shizuoka Hospital, Izunokuni-shi, Japan

Shoichiro Yatsu
Department of Metabolism and Endocrinology, Juntendo University Graduate School of Medicine, Tokyo, Japan

Eiryu Sai
Department of Cardiovascular Biology and Medicine, Juntendo University Graduate School of Medicine, Tokyo, Japan

Suguru Miyazaki and Kan Kajimoto
Cardiovascular Surgery, Juntendo University Shizuoka Hospital, Izunokuni-shi, Japan

Ehsan Aghaei Moghadam
Department of Pediatrics, Tehran University of Medical Science, Tehran, Iran
Children's Medical Center, Pediatrics Center of Excellence, Tehran, Iran

Helia Mojtabavi and Farnoosh Larti
Children's Medical Center, Pediatrics Center of Excellence, Tehran, Iran

Nahid Aslani
Department of Pediatrics, Isfahan University of Medical Science, Isfahan, Iran

Azin Ghamari
Growth and Development Research Center, Tehran University of Medical Science, Tehran, Iran

Vahid Ziaee
Department of Pediatrics, Tehran University of Medical Science, Tehran, Iran
Children's Medical Center, Pediatrics Center of Excellence, Tehran, Iran
Pediatric Rheumatology Research Group, Rheumatology Research Center, Tehran University of Medical Sciences, Tehran, Iran

Sangam Shah and Rukesh Yadav
1Maharajgunj Medical Campus, Institute of Medicine, Tribhuvan University, Maharajgunj 44600, Nepal

Rajan Chamlagain, Yagya Raj Adhikari, Sanjit Kumar Sah, Bipin Kandel and Subash Basnet
Tribhuvan University Teaching Hospital, Maharajgunj 44600, Nepal

Sutap Yadav
Department of Cardiology, Institute of Medicine, Tribhuvan University, Maharajgunj 44600, Nepal
Department of Cardiology, Manmohan Cardiothoracic Vascular and Transplant Center, Maharajgunj 44600, Nepal

Arash Hashemi and Arsis Ahmadieh
Erfan General Hospital, Tehran, Iran

Ashkan Hashemi
Weill Cornell Medicine, New York, New York, USA

Azin Alizadehasl
Rajaie Cardiovascular, Medical and Research Center, Iran University of Medical Sciences, Tehran, Iran

Mohammad Mostafa Ansari Ramandi
Cardiovascular Diseases Research Center, Birjand University of Medical Sciences, Birjand, Iran
Network of Immunity in Infection, Malignancy and Autoimmunity (NIIMA), Universal Scientific Education and Research Network (USERN), Tehran, Iran

Abdullah Rathur, Hussein Al-Mohamad and Jeffrey Steinhoff
Department of Cardiology, HCA Healthcare/USF Morsani College of Medicine GME Programs/Largo Medical Center, Largo, FL, USA

João Ferreira Reis
Department of Cardiology, Hospital de Santa Marta, Centro Hospitalar Universitário de Lisboa Central, Lisbon, Portugal

Petra Loureiro and José Diogo Martins
Department of Pediatric Cardiology, Hospital de Santa Marta, Centro Hospitalar Universitário de Lisboa Central, Lisbon, Portugal

Rita Lopes Silva
Pediatric Neurology Unit, Pediatric Department, Hospital de Dona Estefânia, Centro Hospitalar Universitário de Lisboa Central, Lisbon, Portugal

Nabil Braiteh and Alon Yarkoni
Department of Cardiology, United Health Services Hospitals, Wilson Regional Medical Center, NY, USA

Raheel Chaudhry
Department of Internal Medicine, United Health Services Hospitals, Wilson Regional Medical Center, NY, USA

braheem Rehman
Emory University School of Medicine, Atlanta, Georgia, USA

Jowana Breiteh
Department of Nutrition and Food Sciences, American University of Beirut, Beirut, Lebanon

Antonino M. Grande and Nicoletta Castiglione
Department of Cardiac Surgery IRCCS Fondazione Policlinico San Matteo, Pavia, Italy

Adelaide Iervolino
Department of Cardiovascular Sciences, Fondazione Policlinico Universitario A. Gemelli IRCSS, Italy

Francesco Nappi
Department of Cardiac Surgery, Centre Cardiologique du Nord de Saint-Denis, Paris, France

Antonio Fiore
Department of Cardiac Surgery, Henri Mondor University Hospital, Assistance Publique-Hôpitaux de Paris, Créteil, France

Sy Van Hoang and Kha Minh Nguyen
Department of Internal Medicine Faculty of Medicine, University of Medicine and Pharmacy at Ho Chi Minh City, Vietnam

Anh Tuan Vo
Department of Cardiovascular Surgery, University Medical Center, University of Medicine and Pharmacy at Ho Chi Minh City, Vietnam

Index

N

O

P

R

S

T

U

V

www.ingramcontent.com/pod-product-compliance
Lightning Source LLC
LaVergne TN
LVHW082152200926
848484LV00008B/2148